The Clinical Practice of Nephrology

☐ VOLUME III, Nephrology Today Series

The Clinical Practice of Nephrology

☐ VOLUME III, Nephrology Today Series

Edited by:

Harry G. Preuss, M.D.

Professor of Medicine and Pathology
Director of Research, Renal Division
Georgetown University Medical Center
Washington, DC

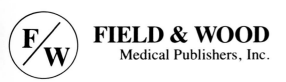

FIELD & WOOD
Medical Publishers, Inc.

Distributed by W. W. Norton & Company, Inc.

500 Fifth Avenue, New York, NY 10110

Distributed by:

W.W. Norton & Company, Inc.
500 Fifth Avenue
New York, New York 10110

Library of Congress Catalog Card Number: 89-080832

ISBN 0-938607-26-X

Printed in the United States of America

Printing: 1 2 3 4 5 6 7 8 9 10

NEPHROLOGY TODAY SERIES
VOLUME I —GERIATRIC NEPHROLOGY
VOLUME II —MANAGEMENT OF COMMON PROBLEMS IN RENAL DISEASE
VOLUME III—THE CLINICAL PRACTICE OF NEPHROLOGY
VOLUME IV—TUBULOINTERSTITIAL DISEASES (In preparation).

Volume 3
The Clinical Practice
of Nephrology
Harry G. Preuss, MD

Preface		vii
Contributors		ix
Advisory Board		xi
1.	**Laboratory Evaluation of Renal Patients** Harry G. Preuss, Gregory A. Threatte and Kamal Sethi	1
2.	**Renal Biopsy** Thomas A. Rakowski and Harry G. Preuss	20
3.	**Evaluation of Kidneys by Imaging Techniques** Erica A. George and Carroll R. Markivee	23
4.	**Acute Nephritic Syndrome** William P. Argy and Robert C. Mackow	34
5.	**Acute Renal Failure** Jack Moore, Jr. and John P. Johnson	40
6.	**Chronic Renal Failure** Harry G. Preuss and Steven J. Zelman	46
7.	**Nephrotic Syndrome** Kamal Sethi and Guido Perez	52
8.	**Urologic-Related Renal Diseases** Yutaka Saito and Atsushi Kondo	59
9.	**Pregnancy-Related Nephrology** Alexander C. Chester and Jeffrey P. Harris	69
10.	**Pediatric Nephrology** Pedro Jose, Antonia C. Novello and Jean Robillard	76
11.	**Geriatric Nephrology** Bernard B. Davis, Terry V. Zenser and Robert D. Lindeman	86
12.	**Primary Glomerular Diseases** John P. Johnson and Jack Moore, Jr.	90
13.	**Systemic Glomerulopathies** James E. Balow and Howard A. Austin	102
14.	**Tubulointerstitial Diseases** Jack Moore, Jr. and Harry G. Preuss	121
15.	**Renal Vascular Diseases** Rishpal Singh and Harry G. Preuss	129
16.	**Clinical Management of End-Stage Renal Disease (ESRD)** James F. Winchester and Michael C. Gelfand	133
17.	**Renal Transplantation and Rejection** Michael C. Gelfand, James F. Winchester and Antonia C. Novello	147

18. Total Parenteral Nutrition in Renal Failure   **159**
      Vinod K. Bansal and Leonard L. Vertuno
19. Poisoning   **165**
      James F. Winchester and Lester M. Haddad
Index   **175**

PREFACE

This volume was written as a companion to Volume 2 of the Nephrology Today Series. Together Volumes 2 and 3 comprise an overview of the practice of Nephrology. The two volumes were designed to appeal to a wide variety of medical professionals. The primary audience is intended to be practicing physicians, regardless of the area of expertise. The book should also aid third and fourth year medical students and house officers who require basic information about kidney diseases. Since the emphasis is clinical, the text will prove useful to trainees in Nephrology and finally, may serve as a guide for nephrologists to develop lectures for medical students. The book was not intended to replace the standard textbooks on renal diseases which are necessary to obtain an all-encompassing description of specific disorders.

While Volume 2 is problem oriented, many fundamentals of Nephrology are assessed in Volume 3. The 19 chapters are divided into 5 sections. The initial 3 chapters in section I discuss the tools used to diagnose and follow nephrological problems. This basic background is necessary to comprehend the overall assessment of renal problems. In section II, the 4 common syndromes of nephrology are presented and discussed. The last 3 sections contain a general overview of nephrological subjects which could not be assessed fully in the problem-oriented Volume 2. Problems and disorders occurring in unique situations that cross the boundaries between other specialties and Nephrology are discussed. These include urological and pregnancy-related problems and disorders. Also included are 2 chapters concerned with pediatric and geriatric patients. The fourth section deals with renal diseases. Only major entities are described. It is not intended that the chapters of section IV contain a comprehensive classification and description of every renal disease, for this is best left to the standard textbooks of Nephrology. The final section summarizes the management of nephrological disorders by conservative means, parenteral nutrition, dialysis and transplantation. Poisoning is included here since these patients are often managed by nephrologists. Some chapters are innovative. For example, Chapter 11 on Geriatric Nephrology and Chapter 18 on Total Parenteral Nutrition in Renal Failure discuss important clinical topics which are rarely detailed in other texts.

The same acknowledgements given in Volume 2 pertain to the present volume as well. This volume would not have been possible without the encouragement and cooperation of the other 30 contributors. To them I am most grateful. In addition, I would like to acknowledge the assistance of my wife, Bonnie Preuss, RN, MSN in helping with the editing of some chapters and the excellent secretarial work of Mrs. Elizabeth Lightfoot-Ergueta and Mrs. Betty Mendelson.

Harry G. Preuss, MD
McLean, Virginia, 1989

DEDICATION

To my parents, the late Mr. Harry G. Preuss, Jr., and Mrs. Mary Kumpon Preuss, and to my wife, Bonnie Coleman Preuss and my children Mary Beth, Jeffrey, Christopher and Michael.

Vol 3 NEPHROLOGY TODAY
THE CLINICAL PRACTICE
OF NEPHROLOGY

CONTRIBUTORS

William P. Argy, M.D.
Professor of Medicine
Georgetown University Medical Center
Washington, DC

Howard A. Austin, III, M.D.
Kidney Disease Section, NIDDK
National Institutes of Health
Bethesda, MD

James E. Balow, M.D.
Chief, Kidney Disease Section,
NIDDK and Senior Investigator
National Institutes of Health
Bethesda, MD

Vinod K. Bansal, M.D.
Professor of Medicine
Loyola University School of Medicine
Maywood, IL

Alexander C. Chester, M.D.
Clinical Associate Professor of Medicine
Georgetown University Medical Center
Washington, DC

Bernard B. Davis, M.D.
Professor of Medicine
St. Louis University Medical Center
Chief of Medicine
St. Louis, Veterans Administration
   Medical Center
St. Louis, MO

Michael C. Gelfand, M.D.
Clinical Associate Professor of Medicine
Georgetown University Medical Center
Washington, DC

Erica A. George, M.D.
Associate Professor of Medicine & Radiology
St. Louis University School of Medicine
Staff Physician, Nuclear Medicine
Veterans Administration Medical Center
St. Louis, MO

Lester M. Haddad, M.D.
Chief of Emergency Medicine
Beaufort Memorial Hospital
Beaufort, SC

Jeffrey P. Harris, M.D.
Winchester Medical Center
Winchester, VA

John P. Johnson, M.D.
Chief, Department of Nephrology
Walter Reed Army Institute of Research
Washington, DC

Pedro Jose, M.D., Ph.D.
Professor of Pediatrics
Head, Pediatric Nephrology
Georgetown University Medical Center
Washington, DC

Atsushi Kondo, M.D.
Emeritus Professor of Urology
Department of Urology
Nagasaki University School of Medicine
Nagasaki, Japan

Robert D. Lindeman, M.D.
Chief of Staff
Washington Veterans Administration Hospital
Professor of Medicine
George Washington Medical Center
Washington, DC

Robert C. Mackow, M.D.
Assistant Professor of Medicine
Georgetown University Medical Center
Washington, DC

Carroll R. Markivee, M.D.
Associate Professor of Radiology
St. Louis University School of Medicine
Chief of Radiology
Veterans Administration Medical Center
St. Louis, MO

Jack Moore, Jr., M.D.
Chief, Nephrology Service
Walter Reed Army Medical Center
Washington, DC

Antonia C. Novello, M.D., M.P.H.
Deputy Director
National Institutes of Child Health and Human
    Development
Clinical Associate Professor of Pediatrics
Georgetown University Medical Center
Washington, DC

Guido Perez, M.D.
Professor of Medicine
Chief, Dialysis Unit, Veterans
    Administration Hospital
University of Miami School of Medicine
Miami, FL

Harry G. Preuss, M.D.
Professor of Medicine and Pathology
Director of Research: Renal Division
Georgetown University Medical Center
Washington, DC

Thomas A. Rakowski, M.D.
Associate Professor of Medicine
Georgetown University Medical Center
Washington, DC

Jean Robillard, M.D.
Professor of Pediatrics
University of Iowa Medical Center
Iowa City, IA

Yutaka Saito, M.D.
Professor of Urology
Head, Department of Urology
Nagasaki University School of Medicine
Nagasaki, Japan

Kamal Sethi, M.D.
Associate Professor of Medicine
Georgetown University Medical Center,
Head, Georgetown Nephrology Division
D.C. General Hospital
Washington, DC

Rishpal Singh, M.D.
Head, Renal Division
Prince George's Hospital
Cheverly, MD

Gregory A. Threatte, M.D.
Associate Professor of Pathology
Director, Clinical Chemistry
SUNY, Health Science Center
Syracuse, NY

Leonard L. Vertuno, M.D.
Professor of Medicine and
Chief of Staff
Loyola University Medical Center
Maywood, IL

James F. Winchester, M.D.
Professor of Medicine
Georgetown University Medical Center
Washington, DC

Steven J. Zelman, M.D.
416 North 12th St.
Mt. Vernon, IL

Terry V. Zenser, Ph.D.
Geriatric Research Education & Clinical Center
Professor of Medicine & Biochemistry
Veterans Administration Medical Center
St. Louis University
St. Louis, MO

ACKNOWLEDGEMENTS

Chapter 1   *Figs 3E, 2F, 3D* Schreiner GE: Urinary Sediment, Med Com Inc. New York, NY.

Chapter 9   *Figs 1 & 2* Sims EAH, Hermit E: Social Studies of Renal Function During Pregnancy and in the Puerperium in the Normal Women. J Clin Invest 37:1764, 1958.
Fig 3 Harris JP, Chester AC, Schreiner GE: Kidney and Pregnancy. Am Family Phys 18:99–102, 1978.
Fig 4 MacGillivrary I, Rose GA, Rowe B: Blood Pressure Survey in Pregnancy. Clin Sci 37:395, 1969.
Fig 5 McFarlane C: An Evaluation of Serum Uric Acid Level in Pregnancy. J Obstet & Gynecol of Br Commonwealth 70:63, 1963.
Fig 6 Chesley LC, Annitto JE, Cosgrove RA: The Remote Prognosis of Eclamptic Women. Am J Obstet Gynecol. 124:446, 1976.

Chapter 10   *Fig 1* De Swiet M, Fayers P, Shinebourne EA: Pediatrics. 56:1028, 1980
Table 2 Moore ES, Galvey MB: J Pediatr 80:867, 1972.
Table 3 Goellner MH, Zeigler EE, Formon SJ: Nephron 28:174, 1981.
Table 4 Jose PA, Tina LU, Papadopoulou ZL, Calcagno PC: Neonatology, Pathophysiology and Management of the Newborn. Avery (ed). JB Lippincott Co., Boston, 1981, pp 677.

Chapter 14   *Fig 3* Lombardo J, Terlinsky A, Preuss HG: Tubulointerstitial Diseases. Am Family Phys, 21:128, 1980.

Chapter 19   *Fig 1 - Tables 2–5* Clinical Management of Poisoning and Drug Overdose. Ed. Haddad and Winchester, WB Saunders Co., Publishers Philadelphia PA 1983.

Harry G. Preuss
Gregory A. Threatte
Kamal Sethi

1

Laboratory Evaluation of Renal Patients

Besides eliminating waste products of metabolism, the kidneys maintain the tonicity, volume, acid-base balance, and chemical composition of the extracellular fluid through the formation of urine. In addition, kidneys have many known endocrine functions, such as the formation of 1,25 Vitamin D_3 and erythropoietin. Accordingly, assessment of the different functions often contributes to an understanding of a renal disorder and its ultimate diagnosis. Evaluation and management of patients with any degree of renal malfunction is achieved through carefully thought out use of urinalysis, serum urea, creatinine and electrolyte concentrations, clearance procedures, special renal function measurements, various imaging techniques (chapter 3); and renal biopsy (chapter 2). Many of these procedures are discussed in other chapters in relationship to specific renal problems. A chart of normal values is given at the end of this chapter.

ROUTINE EXAMINATION OF THE URINE

Collection and Handling of Sample

The first morning urine is the preferred specimen, as it represents several hours of collection not influenced by a recent meal, and generally should reflect an ability or inability to concentrate. The best specimen for examination is a clean-catch, midstream sample. In young children, females and incontinent patients, suprapubic aspiration of the bladder may be necessary to obtain an adequate urine specimen. Catheterization is rarely necessary for this reason alone and should be avoided, unless a good urine specimen cannot be obtained by the usual collection techniques.

The urine specimen should be taken to the laboratory as soon as possible for examination. If the assessment cannot be carried out quickly on the fresh urine, the sample should be refrigerated; since urine tends to become alkaline on standing. The latter causes destruction of casts. For best results, urinalysis should be performed by the physician as part of the physical exam.

The "three-glass test" is used in men to evaluate the location of urinary tract infection (Table 1). The patient voids 30 ml to 90 ml of urine into the first glass. This represents urethral washings. A similar volume is passed into a second glass and contains material coming from the bladder and upper urinary tract. The third glass is collected after gentle prostatic massage and contains material from the prostate. By determining whether pus is present in a given sample, the site of infection may be approximated. Pus only in the first glass suggests urethritis; in the third glass only, prostatic infection; and in all glasses, generalized urinary tract infection. Consistent findings of pyuria with few or no or-

Table 1-1   Diagnostic Implications of the Three Glass Test

	Glass I (Initial)	Glass II (Midstream)	Glass III (Prostatic Massage)
urethritis	+	0	0
prostatitis	0	0	+
bladder and/or renal infection	+	+	+

+ = cloudy urine containing pus
0 = relatively clear urine
See text for details

ganisms detected with routine culture suggests tuberculosis or nonbacterial infection.

Volume. Healthy individuals pass one to two liters of urine per day depending on their fluid intake. Abnormal diminution of urine output is a common sign of pre- and post-renal failure (chapter 5). Increased fluid intake and exposure to cold increases urine volume. Under normal circumstances, more urine is excreted during daytime than during the night. Overnight, normal individuals usually pass less than 500 ml with a specific gravity of 1.022 or greater. Nocturnal frequency of urination is called nocturia. This may be the first symptom of renal disease, because diminished concentrating power is an early sign of renal dysfunction. Polyuria is a characteristic feature of both diabetes insipidus and diabetes mellitus. A pathological increase in urine output can also result from the loss of concentrating ability.

Color and transparency of the urine. Normal urine has the color of amber or pale sherry from urochromes; acid urine or a concentrated urine is usually darker than an alkaline or dilute one. While small quantities of red blood cells in the urine can give it a smoky appearance, larger quantities color the urine brown or red. Free hemoglobin, myoglobin and porphyrins impart a dark red color to the urine or turn it brownish-black. Riboflavin and carotene turn urine dark yellow. Urine containing bile pigments produces a yellowish foam on shaking. Bile also turns urine brownish-black or black. Rarely, urine appears normal when passed, but upon exposure to air gradually darkens to take on a dark brown or black appearance, as in alkaptonuria. Green urine may be noted if bilirubin is converted to biliverdin by bacteria.

Drugs, dyes, and various foods impart colors to urine.

The urine is normally pale when it is very dilute. Usually, urine is clear but may be opalescent when various particles are in suspension. Turbidity may appear because of the presence of cells and/or debris. Urine allowed to cool may become cloudy from the presence of urate crystals, and after a heavy meal a similar appearance may be attributed to phosphate crystals in an alkaline urine. Urates are more soluble in an alkaline urine, while phosphates are more soluble in an acid urine. The addition of acid or alkali to the urine with subsequent clearing suggests that these crystals are causing the clouding.

Specific gravity. The specific gravity of the urine is measured usually by a urinometer. Normally, urine specific gravity varies from 1.005 to 1.030 depending on fluid ingestion. Since specific gravity is increased by cooling, we prefer to measure the urine when it has cooled to room temperature in order to obtain consistency. In normal urines, specific gravity relates closely to the amount of urea and chlorides present. A urine of high specific gravity despite great volume often denotes diabetes mellitus. Because glucose is a relatively heavy particle, the urine specific gravity may reach 1.040 to 1.050. After an IVP, the specific gravity may also be elevated due to contrast media. In diabetes insipidus, on the other hand, the specific gravity is low. Consistently low specific gravity in early morning urine samples can be a sign of a loss in concentrating ability.

The refractometer is an instrument used to measure the refractive index of the urine. Although less accurate than the urinometer, it requires only a drop of specimen. The refractive index correlates very closely with specific gravity in the normal range. Large molecules such as sugar and contrast media give a high specific gravity relative to osmolality; and substances such as urea measure lower relative to osmolality (Fig. 1). When precise accuracy is necessary, an osmometer should be used to determine true osmolality by freezing point depression or vapor pressure elevation.

Dipstick Examination. The dipstick can be used to estimate pH and to detect the presence of protein, glucose, ketones, blood, bilirubin, nitrite, leukocyte esterase and urobilinogen.

pH. Urine pH depends on [H^+] and is influenced by various buffers in the urine. Total H^+ excreted in one day, be it free, or bound as titratable acid or ammonium, averages approximately 1mEq/Kg body weight. The normal urinary pH range is between 4.4 and 7.8. Usually urine is acid, influenced considerably by the normal diet. Vegetarians tend to have alkaline urines, while heavy meat eaters usually pass markedly acidic urines. During the day urine pH varies, being alkaline following a heavy meal, the "alkaline tide." A urine pH above the high normal level of 7.8 usually signifies contamination with urea splitting organisms. The dip-

stick incorporates various combinations of dyes which show different colors at various pH. The hydrogen sensitive electrode is used when exactness is desired such as in a workup of RTA.

Proteins. The presence of protein in the urine is an important observation. Proteinuria, along with concentrating defects and an abnormal sediment, are signs of renal disease. The protein strip on the dipstick, tetrabromphenol blue, is specific for albumin. In rare cases, when only L-chains (Bence Jones Protein) or globulins are in the urine, one can miss proteinuria by this test. A more accurate evaluation of Bence Jones proteinuria can be made by immunoelectrophoresis. Fortunately for diagnostic purposes, albumin is usually present no matter what the major urinary protein.

In the qualitative dipstick test, a reading of trace or even 1+ (30 mg/dl) in a highly concentrated urine may not be significant; whereas it could be highly significant in a dilute urine. Therefore, one must evaluate dipstick readings in light of the urine concentration and the overall findings in the patient. A reading of 2+ (100 mg/dl), 3+ (300–800 mg/dl) or 4+ (> 1g/dl) is almost always pathological. Other tests for proteinuria include boiling supernate or the dropwise addition of sulfosalicylic acid to the urine (Table 2). To quantitate proteinuria, a 24h urine collection should be made, and the protein excretion over a fixed time measured. In most laboratories, upper limits of normal individuals are 150 mg/24h. Normal individuals excrete a small amount of protein, usually under 100 mg in a 24h period; and a good portion is a mucoprotein from the genitourinary tract called "Tamm-Horsfall Proteins." We have found that the procedure in Tables 3 and 4 works quite well for 24h protein determination.

Glucose. The Dipstick method to estimate glucose depends on the ability of glucose oxidase to convert glucose to gluconic acid and H_2O_2. This method is farily specific for glucose, while the presence of other sugars like lactose can be missed. Glucosuria occurs due to either renal overload or tubular malabsorption.

Ketone bodies. Ketone bodies may be elevated during uncontrolled diabetes, starvation, fasting, and during alcohol intoxication. In the Rothera test, acetone and aceto-acetate react with

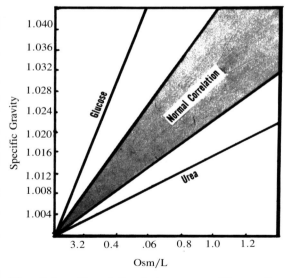

Fig. 1-1. Correlation between specific gravity and osmolality. When particles are mainly composed of glucose or urea, the correlation falls out of the expected range.

Table 1-2 Common Tests for Detecting the Presence of Protein in Urine

Boiling Test: Urine should be clear before testing, filtration may be required. A small test tube is filled with 7–8 ml of urine. This test is best carried out in acid urine, so that a few drops of 10% acetic acid may be necessary if the urine is alkaline. Boil the top half of the fluid over a flame. Cloudiness indicates protein or phosphates. Add 10% acetic acid dropwise and continue to boil. The cloud disappears if it is phosphates, but remains if due to albumin.

Sulfosalicylic Acid Test: To 7–8 ml of clear urine (filter if necessary), add 6 drops of 20% sulfosalicylic acid. A cloudy turbidity suggests the presence of albumin.

Test for Bence Jones Proteins (L-Chains): To 4 ml of clear urine, add 1 ml of 2M acetate buffer of pH 4.9. Heat specimen in water bath to 56° C for 5–10 min. If a precipitate appears, the presence of BJ protein is possible. Centrifuge the specimen and discard the supernate. Suspend the sediment in 2 ml of 3% sulfosalicylic acid. If the precipitate is BJ protein, it will disappear during boiling and reappear on cooling.

sodium nitroprusside to produce a purple color. The other ketone body, β-hydroxybutyrate may be missed. Addition of a few drops of H_2O_2 will convert the non-reactive β-hydroxybutyrate to the reactive aceto-acetate, thus allowing a better estimation of the amount of ketonuria.

Blood. The dipstick reaction for blood is positive in the presence of free hemoglobin and myoglobin. In hematuria, the urine always contains red cells on microscopic examination, whereas red cells are conspicuously absent or rare in myoglobulinuria or hemoglobinuria secondary to intravascular hemolysis.

Microscopic examination. Once the above assessments are made on the sample, the urine should be centrifuged at 450 × g for 5 minutes. When the supernate is poured from the centrifuge tube, a drop or two of urine is left behind. The sediment is mixed with the remaining drops by tapping the tube gently or mixing with a long glass rod. A drop of this mixture is placed on the slide and flattened with a cover slip. We prefer to put two drops of urine on the slide. To one, we add Sternheimer-Malbin Stain. Under high power, both preparations are studied. The sediment includes many findings and should be examined systematically (Table 5). A descrip-

Table 1-3 24 H Urinary Protein Determination

1. Spin urine aliquot in urine tube for 10 minutes at 2,000 rpm. Then use supernate for protein testing.

2. Test supernate initially with protein Dipstick to determine whether to use 4 ml or 1 ml urine for test.

3. If proteinuria is moderate to severe, use 1 ml urine, placed in Shevky-Stafford tube. Then add distilled water to 4 ml mark. Lastly, add Tsuchiya's Reagent* to 6.5 ml mark. Invert and mix thoroughly.

4. If proteinuria is slight, use 4 ml urine, add to S. S. tube. Add Tsuchiya's Reagent to 6.5 ml mark. Invert and mix thoroughly.

5. Spin S. S. tube for 5 minutes at 2,000 rpm.

6. Convert reading of precipitate (see Table 4) to mg/ml at 23 degrees C and multiply by 24 hour urine volume. If 4 ml of urine were used, the derived figure (mg/ml) must be divided by four prior to multiplying by urine volume.

* —Tsuchiya's Reagent is made by dissolving 1.5 g phosphotungstic acid in 5.0 ml concentrated hydrochloric acid and adding 95% ethyl alcohol to make a total volume of 100 ml.

Table 1-4 Milligrams of Protein Present in the Actual Amount of Urine Used

Ppt. Reading ml.	20° C.	21° C.	22° C.	23° C.	24° C.	25° C	26° C	27° C	28° C.
0.00	0.13	0.14	0.14	0.15	0.16	0.16	0.17	0.18	0.19
0.01	0.26	0.27	0.28	0.30	0.31	0.33	0.34	0.36	0.37
0.02	0.52	0.54	0.57	0.60	0.62	0.65	0.68	0.71	0.74
0.03	0.78	0.82	0.86	0.90	0.94	0.98	1.03	1.08	1.13
0.04	1.04	1.09	1.14	1.19	1.25	1.31	1.37	1.44	1.50
0.05	1.30	1.36	1.42	1.49	1.56	1.63	1.71	1.79	1.88
0.06	1.56	1.63	1.71	1.79	1.87	1.96	2.05	2.15	2.25
0.07	1.82	1.91	2.00	2.09	2.19	2.29	2.40	2.51	2.63
0.08	2.08	2.18	2.28	2.39	2.50	2.62	2.74	2.87	3.00
0.09	2.34	2.45	2.56	2.69	2.81	2.94	3.08	3.22	3.38
0.10	2.60	2.72	2.85	2.98	3.12	3.27	3.42	3.59	3.76
0.11	2.86	3.00	3.14	3.28	3.44	3.60	3.77	3.94	4.13
0.12	3.12	3.27	3.42	3.58	3.75	3.93	4.11	4.31	4.50
0.13	3.38	3.54	3.70	3.88	4.06	4.25	4.45	4.66	4.88
0.14	3.64	3.81	3.99	4.17	4.37	4.57	4.79	5.01	5.25
0.15	3.90	4.08	4.28	4.48	4.69	4.91	5.14	5.38	5.63
0.16	4.16	4.36	4.56	4.78	5.00	5.23	5.48	5.74	6.01
0.17	4.42	4.63	4.85	5.07	5.31	5.56	5.82	6.10	6.38
0.18	4.68	4.90	5.13	5.37	5.62	5.89	6.16	6.45	6.76
0.19	4.94	5.17	5.42	5.67	5.94	6.21	6.51	6.81	7.13
0.20	5.20	5.44	5.70	5.97	6.25	6.54	6.85	7.17	7.51
0.21	5.46	5.72	5.99	6.27	6.56	6.87	7.19	7.53	7.88
0.22	5.72	5.99	6.27	6.56	6.87	7.20	7.54	7.89	8.26
0.23	5.98	6.26	6.56	6.86	7.19	7.52	7.88	8.25	8.64
0.24	6.24	6.53	6.84	7.16	7.50	7.85	8.22	8.60	9.01
0.25	6.50	6.81	7.13	7.46	7.81	8.18	8.56	8.97	9.39
0.26	6.76	7.08	7.41	7.76	8.12	8.50	8.90	9.32	9.76
0.27	7.02	7.35	7.70	8.06	8.44	8.83	9.25	9.68	10.14
0.28	7.28	7.62	7.98	8.36	8.75	9.16	9.59	10.04	10.51
0.29	7.54	7.89	8.26	8.65	9.07	9.49	9.94	10.41	10.90
0.30	7.80	8.17	8.55	8.95	9.37	9.81	10.28	10.76	11.26
0.31	8.06	8.44	8.84	9.25	9.69	10.14	10.63	11.13	11.65
0.32	8.32	8.71	9.12	9.55	10.00	10.47	10.96	11.48	12.01
0.33	8.58	8.98	9.40	9.85	10.31	10.80	11.30	11.83	12.39
0.34	8.84	9.26	9.69	10.14	10.62	11.12	11.64	12.19	12.76
0.35	9.10	9.53	9.98	10.44	10.94	11.45	11.99	12.55	13.14
0.36	9.36	9.80	10.26	10.74	11.25	11.78	12.33	12.91	13.52
0.37	9.62	10.07	10.55	11.04	11.56	12.10	12.67	13.27	13.87
0.38	9.88	10.34	10.83	11.34	11.87	12.43	13.01	13.63	14.27
0.39	10.14	10.62	11.12	11.64	12.19	12.76	13.36	13.99	14.65
0.40	10.40	10.89	11.40	11.94	12.50	13.08	13.70	14.34	15.02

Table 1-5 Systematic Examination of urinary Sediment

1.	Cells—	RBC, WBC
		— renal tubular epithelial cells (RTE)
		— transitional, squamous epithelial cells
2.	Casts—	hyaline
		— granular
		— cellular — RBC, WBC, RTE cells
		— other — fatty, blood
3.	Crystals	— oxalate, uric acid, etc.
4.	Bacteria	
5.	Other—	lipids
		— parasites

tion of all these findings is beyond the scope of this chapter. (See Figures 2 and 3 for pictures of some of these elements). Suffice it to say, the presence of red and white cells, casts, red cells in clumps or included in casts, and/or white cells in clumps or included in casts, may be signs of renal parenchymal disease. Inclusion of cellular elements in casts localizes the origin to the kidney.

Casts are classified as hyaline casts, epithelial cell casts, white blood cell casts, red blood cell casts, and fatty casts. Hyaline casts are produced chiefly from Tamm-Horsfall mucoprotein and dissolve readily in alkaline urine. They are homogeneous, lucent and usually devoid of cells. Tubular epithelial cell casts are composed of desquamated cells from the tubular lining and they are seen in tubular disorders such as tubular necrosis and allergic interstitial nephritis. As the cells degenerate, they decompose into coarse or fine granules. White blood cell casts indicate pyelonephritis, while orange-red casts containing red blood cells are commonly seen in certain glomerulonephritides.

The presence of fat in the urine (cholesterol esters, oval fat bodies, and fatty casts) is the result of fatty metamorphosis of renal tubules and associated with the nephrotic syndrome. These can be detected by using polarized light and/or using stains specific for fats. Trichomonas vaginalis, schistosoma hematobium and/or sperm may be seen in urine. Bacteria are often seen. In addition, various crystals may suggest the etiology behind a renal problem.

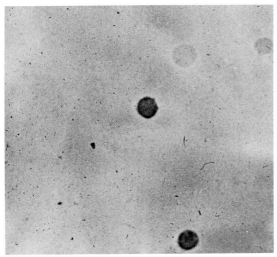

A

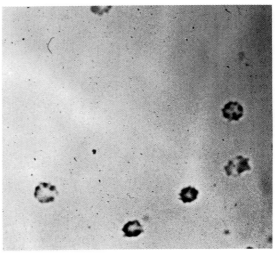

B

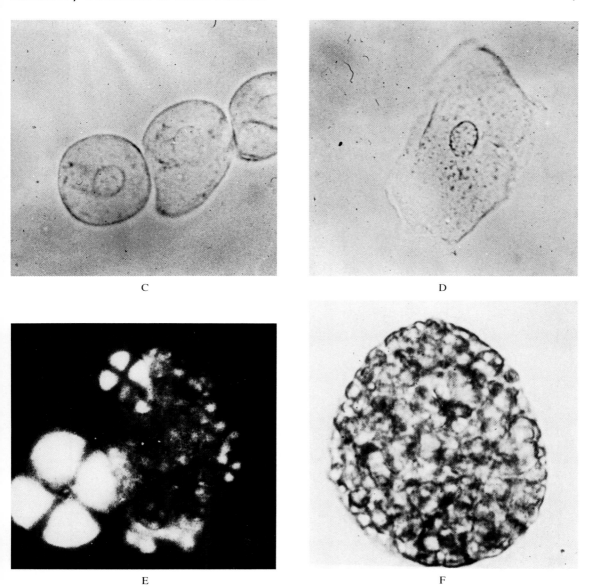

Fig. 1-2. (a) Red Blood Cells; (b) White Blood Cells; (c) squamous Epithelial Cells; (d) transitional Cells; (e) cholesterol esters show Maltese Crosses when polarized; (f) oval fat body
Panel E, F with permission. Schreiner, G.E.: Urinary sediment. Medcom Inc., New York, N.Y.

DETECTION OF BACTERIURIA

The detection of significant bacteriuria is sometimes difficult. Perhaps one half of patients with proven bacteriuria have no pyuria, and many with significant pyuria have no bacteriuria. Definitive culture procedures are often too expensive for routine use, and may introduce artifac-

tual bacterial growth when specimens are delayed in transit. Accordingly, it is helpful to utilize screening procedures.

Dipstick methodology has been adapted for bacterial screening. A firm plastic strip contains three separate reagent areas. One reagent pad is a chemical test for nitrite in the urine. This detects the conversion of nitrate to nitrite in the

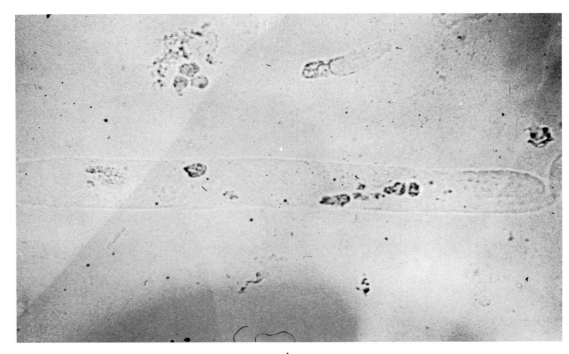

A

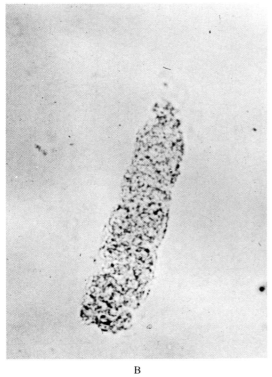

B

C

8

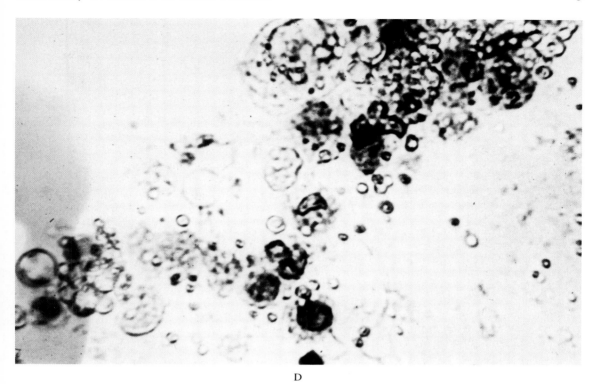

D

Fig. 1-3. (a) Hyaline Cast; (b) fine Granular Cast; (c) red Blood Cell Casts; (d) telescoped urine containing RBC, WBC, Fat Bodies, Red, White and Granular Casts, and Broad "Failure" Casts. Panel D with permission. Schreiner, G.E.: Urinary sediment. Medcom Inc., New York, N.Y.

urine by certain species of bacteria. At the acid pH of the strip, the nitrite from the urine reacts with other agents to form a pink color. The color conversion suggests the possibility of bacteriuria. A second area on the strip contains nutrients to support both gram-positive and gram-negative bacterial growth. The last area contains an inhibitor that prevents growth of gram-positive organisms but selectively allows gram-negative organisms to grow. Thus, if growth is present on both culture areas after 24h, a gram-negative organism is present. If there is growth on only one area, a gram-positive organism is suspected.

If this screening procedure is positive, the organisms must be identified. Another urine specimen should be obtained and plated within 30 minutes after collection or refrigerated promptly. Clean-voided midstream samples from healthy individuals characteristically contain fewer than 10,000 organisms per milliliter. The finding of 100,000 or more organisms per mil-

liliter in a urine sample is usually considered to be 95% positive for clinical infection. If a culture is found to contain between 10,000 and 100,000 organisms per milliliter, the physician must repeat the culture and make sure that the urine is obtained and transported correctly. Routine bacteriological culturing of the urine is still the main tool for definitive diagnosis of symptomatic patients and positive screens and often is carried out in the physician's office.

SPECIFIC RENAL FUNCTION TESTS

Renal blood flow (RBF) comprises approximately 20% of the cardiac output. From the RBF, the kidney filters approximately 180 liters of plasma each day and usually excretes less than one percent of the filtered solute. Some constituents of the ultrafiltrate, such as glucose and bicarbonate, are usually completely reabsorbed;

and only small amounts of amino acids are passed. Compounds such as penicillins, uric acid, and certain organic anions (PAH) and cations (tetraethylammonium) are secreted into the tubular lumen for excretion. The excretion of water, sodium, potassium, and hydrogen ion varies for the most part with the daily ingestion of these. Inability of kidneys to properly regulate the composition of the extra-cellular fluid (ECF) can lead to many undesirable effects. Almost all tests for evaluating specific functions can be performed at the bedside. Each measurement (GFR, RBF and tubular functions) affords an estimation of some aspect of renal function.

Glomerular filtration rate. Substances that are freely filterable and are neither reabsorbed nor secreted by renal tubules are used to assess glomerular filtration rate (GFR). Inulin is a polysaccharide with a molecular weight of 5100 daltons, and is the most commonly used substance to determine a true GFR. The average GFR is 125 ml/min/1.73 m^2 in men and 110 ml/min/1.73 m^2 in women. GFR is lower in children up to two years of age, even when corrected for surface area and may decrease progressively as the individual passes middle life. Since the GFR varies little from day to day, it is probably the best measure of functioning nephron mass. Once established, GFR offers a baseline for estimating changes in renal function of any individual patient.

Inulin has to be given as a constant infusion to maintain the level at around 0.25 mg/ml after a priming dose of 50 mg/kg. To maintain the plasma level at 0.25 mg/ml, one must replace the amount excreted. For example, if the GFR is estimated to be 120 ml/min, then 0.25mg/ml × 120 ml/min (30 mg/min) would be the infusion rate. Because inulin and other substances require a constant infusion to obtain a steady state, in practice, it is often necessary to use an easily measured substance that is endogenous to the body. Clinicians routinely use the creatinine clearance to estimate GFR, although it does not follow all the criteria necessary to obtain a true GFR. Because of tubular secretion, creatinine clearance can exceed the true GFR by as much as 40% especially in individuals with decreased renal function. Another problem with the creatinine clearance is that the chromagens present in plasma may give a falsely high reading of creatinine. An alternative in patients with

markedly decreased renal function is to measure both creatinine and urea clearance and average the values,

$$\frac{Cl_{urea} + Cl_{cr}}{2}$$

however, the inulin clearance is recommended when knowledge of the precise GFR is sought in patients with a GFR below 20 ml/min. All in all, the creatinine clearance offers a good clinical tool to estimate GFR and can be used to monitor changes in renal function if one is aware of its shortcomings. Normal values for Cl_{cr} in males are 85–125 ml/min/1.73 m^2 and 75–115 ml/min/1.73 m^2 for females. Our protocol for a two-hour hydrated creatinine clearance determination is shown in Table 6.

The major sources of error in the creatinine clearance occur if urine flow rates are variable or if the urine sample is not the entire urine volume produced during the timed collection. The 24 hour specimen averages the differences in GFR due to normal diurinal variations. In diseases where there are rapid changes in muscle metabolism, such as with muscle diseases, the creatinine levels change rapidly and create erroneous results. Drugs such as cimetidine and trimethoprim interfere with creatinine secretion and can influence the calculated GFR.

The clearance of any substance can be measured by the following equation:

$$Cl = \frac{U \times V}{S}$$

Cl = clearance (ml/min)

U = urine concentration (mg/dl)

V = volume (ml/min)

S = serum concentration (mg/dl)

For example, a patient passes 20 ml of urine over 20 minutes. The urinary concentration of creatinine is 120 mg/dl and the serum has 1 mg/dl. Substituting in the above equation:

$$Cl = \frac{120 \text{ mg/dl} \times 1 \text{ ml/min}}{1 \text{ mg/dl}}$$

Cl = 120 ml/min

Table 1-6 Creatinine Clearance Test

GENERAL INSTRUCTIONS:
1. Obtain height and weight.
2. No food or fluid other than water during the test period.
3. Water at room temperature is better tolerated than iced water,
4. Bedrest is observed except at the time of specimen collection.
5. Patients are to void directly into the containers provided. It is absolutely essential that the entire specimen be obtained.
6. The exact time of the voiding to the minute of completion must be recorded. Collection time extends from the end of one voiding to the end of the next voiding.
7. Symptoms of water intoxication should be reported to the physician in charge immediately (headaches, nausea, dizziness, chills).

PROCEDURES:
1. Withhold breakfast.
2. Patient is hydrated from 7:00 AM to 9:00 AM.

The amount of water to be given is calculated by multiplying the patient's weight in kilograms by 20 ml.

3. Collect U_0 and note the *exact time*—e.g., 9:00 AM, 9:05 AM.

Note the color and concentration. Urine should be dilute indicating that the patient is adequately hydrated.

4. 10 ml of blood is taken after U_0 has been collected.
5. Hydration should be continued throughout the test. One to two glasses of water every forty minutes.
6. Forty minutes after U_0 is collected, a voided specimen is obtained and labelled U_1. Note the exact time the voiding is completed, e.g., 39, 40, 41 minutes.
7. Repeat this procedure until U_2 and U_3 are collected.

At the end of this test which takes two hours, patient may eat and ambulate.

It is necessary that concentration units for U and S be identical so that they cancel out. Because clearance is dependent on parenchymal mass, it is often necessary to correct for this, i.e., a larger person should have a greater clearance than a child. Surface area correlates closely with kidney mass, and clearance is related to an average surface area of 1.73 m^2. Therefore, the clearance can be standardized by multiplying it by 1.73 and dividing by the surface area of the individual, calculated from a normogram which takes into account height and weight (see Fig. 4). Creatinine clearance can also be estimated from the serum creatinine using the formula,

$$\frac{(140 - age)\ wt\ kg}{72 \times S_{cr}}$$

for males and by multiplying the same formula by 0.85 for females.

Renal blood flow. The integrity of the renal circulation is critical in most every aspect of renal function. In addition to supplying kidneys with oxygen and nutrients, the renal circulation plays a significant role in the reabsorption of solids and water via tubular structures. Measurements of effective renal blood flow (ERBF) can be accomplished by determining the renal clearance of p-aminohippurate (PAH) at low plasma concentrations. The terminology "effective" is used because only 85% to 95% of PAH is extracted in a single passage through the kidney. The clearance technique requires an intravenous infusion of PAH at a constant rate. The priming injection of PAH is calculated from the volume distribution of PAH, approximately 400 ml/kg body weight. The initial loading bolus of PAH is 8 mg/kg, and an attempt is made to arrive at a plasma concentration of 0.02 mg/ml. Plasma concentration is then maintained by an infusion of PAH equivalent to the amount excreted. To

NOMOGRAM FOR THE DETERMINATION OF BODY
SURFACE AREA OF CHILDREN AND ADULTS*

$$ERBF = \frac{ERPF}{1-Hct}$$

Since 85% to 95% of PAH is extracted in a single passage through the kidney under most circumstances, one may divide the ERBF by 0.9 to obtain a rough estimate of the total RBF.

The filtration fraction (FF) is the ratio of the GFR (Cl_{in}) to ERPF (Cl_{PAH}). The GFR and ERPF usually vary in the same direction proportionately as renal mass decreases chronically maintaining FF in the range of 0.16–0.20. A decrease in FF indicates that relatively less ultrafiltration takes place. The opposite occurs when the FF increases. In general, FF falls with afferent arterial constriction and/or efferent arterial dilation; events which have been hypothesized to occur during ATN (chapter 5). A decrease in FF is also associated with acute glomerulonephritis. An increase in FF is associated with efferent arterial constriction in hypertension or in response to lessened renal circulation.

Tubular excretory maxima. Since the ability of tubules to secrete or reabsorb certain substances is limited, the maximal secretion or reabsorption of a substance (T_m) is used to assess tubular integrity.

$$T_m PAH = U_{PAH} \times V - S_{PAH} \times GFR$$

The secretion of PAH is used most often to obtain a secretory T_m. The desired plasma concentration of PAH is 0.4 mg/ml, achieved by priming the patient with 160 mg/kg of PAH and maintaining the plasma levels with a constant infusion. The prime is given *slowly* to avoid vasomotor and autonomic disturbances. To estimate the infusion rate, one must estimate the T_m PAH and the PAH filtration rate. The PAH filtration rate for a person with a GFR of 120 ml/min would be: 0.4 mg/ml (desired circulating concentration) × 120 ml/min (GFR) × 0.80 (filtration coefficient). The latter coefficient also corrects for PAH protein binding. The calculated filtration load is thus 38.4 mg/min, which added to the expected T_m of 75 mg/min for this normal individual yields an infusion rate of 113 mg/min to maintain steady state after prime. The normal range of T_m PAH is approximately 70–80 mg/min. For a T_m of a compound that is reabsorbed, glucose is frequently used. The av-

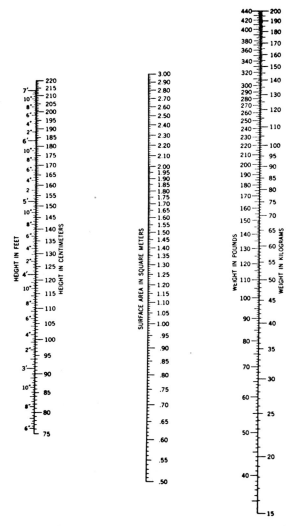

Fig. 1-4. Nomogram for the determination of body surface area of children and adults. (Brody WM, Sandiford RB: Boston Med Surg J 185:337, 1921.)

obtain this infusion rate, multiply 0.02 mg/ml by the estimated Cl_{PAH}. Effective renal plasma flow (ERPF) is about 600 ml/min for the average size adult. If Cl_{PAH} is 600 ml/min, then 600 × 0.02 yields an infusion rate of 12 mg/min. All clearances should be corrected to a standard body surface of 1.73 m². Effective renal blood flow (ERBF) can be calculated by erage for men is 375 mg/min/1.73 m^2; for women, 303 mg/min/1.73 m^2.

$$T_m \text{ Glucose} = S_{glucose} \times GFR - U_{glucose} \times V$$

Acidification of the urine. Although the acidification of the urine is a function of both proximal and distal tubules, the maximal acidifying capacity is used predominantly in the diagnosis of renal tubular acidosis (RTA) of the distal variety (dRTA). Patients with this disorder are unable to lower the urine pH normally (<5.3 in complete dRTA). The four tests described below, i.e., acid challenge, bicarbonate titration, (U − A)pCO$_2$, and sulfate or phosphate infusions are often used in various combinations for the complete workup of an RTA, distal, proximal, or due to an ammonia producing deficiency.

Acid challenge. NH$_4$Cl is administered orally (0.1 g/kg) as an acute acid challenge. If NH$_4$Cl is contraindicated (liver disease), CaCl$_2$ (0.1 g/kg) can be substituted. NH$_4$Cl forms H$^+$ through hepatic metabolism, and the CaCl$_2$ binds HCO$_3$ in the gut. Between 4 and 8 hours after acid challenge, urine pH should normally decrease to 5.3 or lower (see Table 7).

To challenge acid excretion maximally, NH$_4$Cl (0.1 g/kg) can be given for 4–5 consecutive days in divided doses. On the 5th day, the urinary pH should be 5.0 or lower and the total acid excretion should exceed 120 mEq/day. The total acid excreted is composed of the sum of excreted NH$_4^+$ plus titratable acid minus bicarbonate. The titratable acid is equal to the mEq of alkali required to titrate the urine to pH 7.4.

Bicarbonate titration. The T$_m$ for HCO$_3$ is decreased in pRTA but not dRTA. By infusing 7.5% NaHCO$_3$ (0.9M) at the rate of 2ml/min for 2 to 3 hours and producing a stepwise increment of serum HCO$_3^-$, one can determine the serum level of HCO$_3^-$ at which it first appears in the urine. Care must be taken to prevent an increase of serum HCO$_3^-$ of more than 2 meq/L in each 15 min period. In normal individuals, urinary HCO$_3^-$ does not appear until a serum concentration of 24 to 26 mEq/L is reached. Accordingly, excretion at a low serum HCO$_3^-$ concentration suggests pRTA. In practicality, urine HCO$_3^-$ does not necessarily have to be measured. It can be assumed that when urine pH exceeds 6.1, HCO$_3^-$ is being spilled.

(Urinary–Arterial)pCO$_2$. CO$_2$ may be present in the distal renal tubules, where carbonic anhydrase is lacking in the luminal borders. For valid measurements of urinary pCO$_2$ or HCO$_3^-$, urine must be collected anaerobically to prevent loss of CO$_2$ to the ambient air. This can usually be done by syringe aspiration directly from a catheter or immediately drawing the urine collected under oil into an air-free syringe. Hydrogen ion reacts with HCO$_3^-$ to form urine H$_2$CO$_3$, but CO$_2$ formation is delayed. NaHCO$_3$ is administered to raise the urinary pH above 7.4 and avoid the elevation of pCO$_2$ due to mixing of acid and alkaline urine (see method of giving bicarbonate under HCO$_3^-$ titration above). Normal alkaline urine contains some CO$_2$ because of this delay which prevents back diffusion across the tubules. In control subjects, the usual range of (U–A)pCO$_2$ is 40–70 mm Hg. The inability to excrete sufficient pCO$_2$ in a maximally alkalotic urine (pH 7.4–7.8) sug-

Table 1-7   Short Acid Load Procedure

1. Insure patient is well hydrated after breakfast. Draw blood for initial set of electrolytes.
2. From 8:00—10:00 AM, collect baseline urine for pH, NH$_4^+$ Titratable Acidity (TA) (rate and amount for NH$_4^+$ & TA).
3. At 10:00 AM, patient receives 100 mg/kg NH$_4$Cl orally over 1/2 hour (should be taken on a relatively full stomach). Volume is recorded for each specimen.
4. Urine then collected approximately every 2 hours for pH, TA and NH$_4^+$ as in step #2.
5. At 2:00 PM, draw blood for electrolytes (Na$^+$, K$^+$, Cl$^-$, HCO$_3^-$)
6. During the entire procedure, the patient should be encouraged to drink fluids.
7. Test terminates 6 hours after NH$_4$Cl at 4:00 PM.
8. To be normal, urine pH should be 5.3 or below, NH$_4^+$ excretion > 35 mEq/min, and TA > 25 mEq/min.

gests a distal tubular defect in hydrogen elimination. Factors known to influence the (Urinary–Arterial)pCO_2 are arterial pCO_2, serum K^+, and urine P and HCO_3^- concentrations. A low (U–A)pCO_2, however, does not distinguish a secretory (production defect) from a gradient (backleakage defect) cause. To determine whether low (U–A)pCO_2 concentrations are due to abnormalities in distal hydrogen production, or backleakage, a sodium sulfate or sodium phosphate infusion is used.

Sodium sulfate or phosphate infusion. Infusion of sulfate or phosphate increases distal sodium delivery, allowing for greater exchange with hydrogen. Because doubly charged anions are not readily absorbed, they capture hydrogen and prevent the backleakage into blood seen with gradient defects. Prior to a sulfate infusion, 1 mg of fludrocortisone can be given orally on the night preceding the test to enhance Na^+ avidity. After a baseline collection, 500 ml of 4% sodium sulfate solution is infused over 1 hour. Collections of blood and urine are made over the next 4 hours. With this sulfate infusion, titratable acidity will increase, and urine pH should decrease below 5.5 to be considered normal. In the case of neutral phosphate infusion, a solution of 0.2 M neutral phosphate (pH 7.4) is infused at a rate of 1–1.5 ml/min for 2 to 3 hours. The phosphate bound hydrogen is eventually released to react with urinary HCO_3^- and increase the pCO_2. pCO_2 measurements are made at 2, 3, and 4 hours after initiation of infusion. If the urine pH is close to 6.8, the (U–A)pCO_2 in normal subjects increases from 5–30 mm Hg. With a secretory defect, no significant increase in titratable acidity or pCO_2 will be noted after sulfate or phosphate infusion respectively, in contrast to gradient defects and normals.

Any pathological process that alters tubular function may limit the ability of the kidneys to excrete a maximal acid load. This is seen frequently with chronic renal disease and with diseases that cause chronic interstitial nephritis, e.g., pyelonephritis.

Renal concentrating and diluting. In central diabetes insipidus, the inadequate formation or release of ADH may be partial or complete. Partial central diabetes insipidus responds to chlorpropamide which stimulates ADH release and augments the renal tubular response to ADH.

Patients with psychogenic polydipsia do not respond normally at first to the administration of exogenous ADH as the renal medullary concentration gradient is not established completely until days after the abnormal water intake is halted. Nephrogenic diabetes insipidus is present when the renal tubular concentrating mechanism does not respond normally to ADH. Nephrogenic diabetes insipidus may be produced by drugs such as lithium or demeclocycline. Hypokalemia and hypercalcemia of sufficient degree can cause a similar problem. Other causes for nephrogenic diabetes are interstitial nephritis, arterionephrosclerosis, and chronic renal disease. Concentrating ability is one of the first functions to be impaired as a result of renal tubular damage.

Water deprivation test. The simplest test to assess concentrating ability is to withhold fluids overnight. In a normal individual, the specific gravity should exceed 1.025 after 16 hours. Urine osmolality must exceed 850 mOsm/kg water or the ratio of urine to serum osmolality (u/s) exceed 3.0 to also be considered normal. A specific gravity of 1.020 approximates 700 mOsm/kg. We test concentrating ability in the manner described in Table 8.

If the patient does not concentrate urine normally after Pitressin, nephrogenic diabetes insipidus is a possible cause. Patients with partial central diabetes can excrete a hypertonic urine after a maximal water deprivation and can concentrate their urine still further after administration of exogenous vasopressin.

The diluting ability of the kidneys is not routinely assessed. However, it can determine the renal effects of many drugs. Dilution of urine occurs when fluid ingestion decreases the plasma osmolality and/or increases ECF volume. Both inhibit ADH release.

To challenge the diluting mechanism, the following procedure is used. An oral water load of 20 ml/kg body weight is given, and the subsequent urine volume is replaced with an equal amount of water. With maximal water diuresis, urine osmolality decreases to 50–100 mOsm/kg. By excreting proportionately more water than osmotic particles (relative to serum), the plasma osmolality is returned toward normal. Water excreted in excess of osmolar clearance is called free water (Cl_{H_2O}). Cl_{H_2O} = urine flow rate (V) — the osmolar clearance (Cl_{osm}). The highest free water clearance is 10–15 ml/min. To maxi-

Table 1-8 Dehydration and Pitressin—Stimulation Procedure

1. Patient has evening meal.
2. After 6:00 PM, patient is deprived of all fluid intake, but allowed to consume solid food. He voids at 8:00 AM next day.
3. At 10:00 AM, serum(s) and urine(u) osmolality are determined. If u/s is greater than 3.0, or urine osmolality exceeds 850 mOsm, the test response is considered normal and no Pitressin is needed. Test is terminated.
4. If u/s is less than 3.0; or urine osmolality is below 850 mOsm, 5 units of Pitressin Tannate in oil is administered subcutaneously.
5. Urine and serum osmolality are then determined at 2:00 PM (20 hours) and 6:00 PM (24 hours).
6. If u/s osmolality ratio reaches or exceeds 3.0 or urine osmolality exceeds 850 mOsm at 2:00 PM, test is terminated and patient is allowed fluids.
7. If patient does not attain 850 mOsm/kg or a u/s osmolality ratio of 3.0 by 6:00 PM, test is terminated regardless.
8. Urine osmolality is determined on AM specimen the following day.

mally dilute urine, the ascending limb of Henle's Loop must function properly, and ADH release must be inhibited. A decrease in NaCl delivery to the distal diluting site due to diminished GFR (myxedema), excessive proximal tubular sodium reabsorption (congestive heart failure or liver disease) may decrease Cl_{H_2O}. Diuretics such as furosemide and ethacrynic acid interfere with renal diluting capacity while hypoglycemic agents such as tolazamide and glipizide enhance it.

Urinary sodium excretion. The renal tubule reabsorbs roughly 99% of the filtered sodium. In edematous states such as CHF, cirrhosis, nephrotic syndrome, etc., relatively more is reabsorbed. In some disease states, such as polycystic kidneys, medullary cystic disease, tubulo-interstitial diseases and chronic renal failure, urinary sodium wasting may become a severe complication.

Deficiency in the tubules' ability to regulate sodium excretion can be tested either by increasing or decreasing the intake of sodium and relating it to urinary excretion. The patient is initially placed on a normal diet containing a known quantity of sodium, e.g., 100 mEq/day and the daily urinary excretion is measured. Na^+ excretion should approximate 15 mEq/day less than the intake. This allows for loss of Na^+ in sweat and feces. After 3 days, the dietary intake of Na^+ is reduced to 10 mEq/day, which is the usual content of a hospital salt free diet. Within 7–10 days, urinary Na^+ excretion should be less than 10 mEq/day. Another measure of tubular ability to control Na^+ excretion is obtained by allowing the patient a normal diet and giving a

mineralocorticoid twice a day for two or three days. The urinary excretion of Na^+ should fall below 10 mEq/day. Daily decreases in body weight despite an adequate caloric intake suggests loss of Na^+ and water. Postural hypotension, signs of dehydration, or edema are indications to halt these tests.

As discussed in chapter 5 urinary Na^+ concentrations are used to differentiate pre-, post- and parenchymal acute renal failure. While a high urinary $[Na^+]$ suggests parenchymal damage, the fractional excretion of Na^+ is more reliable than simply measuring a spot urine $[Na^+]$.

$$Fe_{Na} = \frac{[Na^+]\ urine}{[Na^+]\ serum} \times \frac{[creatinine]\ serum}{[creatinine]\ urine} \times 100$$

A value below 1.0 is consistent with pre- and post- acute renal failure, while a number above 2.0 suggests parenchymal damage.

Urinary potassium excretion. About 90% of the normal intake, approximately 50–150 mEq/day, is excreted by kidneys. With low plasma $[K^+]$, the kidneys cannot completely conserve K^+ and urinary $[K^+]$ rarely drops below 5 to 10 mEq/L. In the hypokalemic patient, a spot urinary $[K^+] > 20$ mEq/L suggests that the kidney may be the source of K^+ loss or that the hypokalemia is acute, as the kidney takes 1–3 weeks to effectively conserve K^+. If under the same circumstances, the $[K^+]$ is < 20 mEq/L, then the kidney is usually not the source of K^+

Table 1-9   Nephrological Laboratory Values for Adults

Blood	Normal Range	SI Normal Range	
SUN	8–20 mg/dl	2.9–7.1 mmole/L	
Creatinine	0.6–1.6 mg/dl	53–141 μmole/L	
Uric Acid	3.0–8.0 mg/dl	0.18–0.48 mmole/L	
Sodium	135–143 mEq/L	135–143 mmole/L	
Potassium	3.7–4.7 mEq/L	3.7–4.7 mmole/L	
Chloride	95–105 mEq/L	95–105 mmole/L	
CO_2 Content (venous)	24–32 mmole/L	24–32 mmole/L	
Calcium, (Total)	9–10.5 mg/dl	2.2–2.7 mmole/L	
Magnesium	1.4–2.3 mEq/L	0.7–1.2 mmole/L	
pH (arterial)	7.36–7.44	36–44 mmole/L	
pCO_2 (arterial)	35–45 mmHg	—	
Phosphate	3.0–4.5 mg/dl	1.0–1.5 mmole/L	
Protein, (Total)	6.0–8.2 g/dl	—	
Albumin	3.5–5.0 g/dl	540–770 μmole/L	
Cholesterol	100–225 mg/dl	2.6–5.9 mmole/L	
Triglycerides	30–200 mg/dl	0.34–2.26 mmole/L	
Ammonia	—	40–70 μm/L	

RENAL FUNCTION TESTS: Based on 1.73 m² surface area

Cl Inulin (GFR)	110–150 ml/min	(male)
	105–132 ml/min	(female)
Cl Creatinine (GFR)	85–125 ml/min	(male)
	75–115 ml/min	(female)
Cl PAH (ERPF)	560–830 ml/min	(male)
	490–700 ml/min	(female)
Filtration Fraction (FF)	0.17–0.21	(male)
	0.17–0.23	(female)
Concentration and Dilution	1.025 (sp.g) or >850 mOsm/Kg	
	1.003 (sp.g) or <75 mOsm/Kg	
Maximal PAH Excretory Capacity (T_m PAH)	80–90 mg/min	
Maximal Glucose Reabsorptive Capacity (T_m Glucose)	300–450 mg/min	(male)
	250–350 mg/min	(female)

loss and the hypokalemia is of several weeks duration.

Urinary calcium excretion. Calcium reabsorption from the glomerular filtrate occurs mainly in the proximal tubule. Parathyroid hormone decreases calcium clearance and liberates calcium from bone. When excess urinary loss of calcium is due to a primary renal defect, the plasma ionizable calcium is always either normal or low. When the urinary loss is due to some other causes, the plasma calcium concentration is usually, but not always, raised.

With an ordinary diet, not containing excessive dairy products, the upper level of normal Ca^{++} excretion for men is 300 mg/24h; and for women, 250 mg/24h. The ability to conserve calcium in the face of restricted intake can be determined by placing the patient on a rigidly controlled diet containing 450 mg of calcium for five days. Twenty-four hour urinary excretion of calcium on the fourth and fifth day normally should not exceed 150 mg. A higher value indicates hypercalciuria.

Urinary magnesium excretion. About 1800 mg of Mg^{++} are filtered daily, and 3–5% is normally excreted by the kidney. Urinary excretion in excess of 100 mg/day in the presence of hypomagnesemia suggests urinary magnesium wasting. A T_m is present, and excretion depends a great deal on Na^+ excretion. Diuretics, like furosemide, enhance excretion and can lead to depletion.

Urinary phosphorus excretion. About 50%–60% of ingested phosphorus (P) is absorbed via the intestinal tract. Eighty to ninety percent of filtered P is reabsorbed primarily in the proximal tubule. Tubular reabsorption may vary depending on the concentration of PTH; but in advanced renal failure in spite of high levels of PTH, tubular regulation is insufficient to compensate completely.

One can calculate the percent P reabsorbed by measuring creatinine (Cr) and P concentrations in urine and serum.

$$\% \text{ P reabsorbed} = 1 - \frac{\text{P urine} \times \text{Cr serum}}{\text{P serum} \times \text{Cr urine}} \times 100$$

The urine is virtually free of P when serum [P] is below 2.0 mg/dl. A P reabsorption above 85% is considered normal and is lowered by PTH and in Fanconi Syndrome. Decreased tubular reabsorption of P is also found in familial hypophosphatemic rickets, when Na^+ intake is increased and extracellular fluid volume expanded, and during alkalosis.

Urinary uric acid excretion. Excretion of uric acid is often related to creatinine excretion (Cl uric acid/Cl creatinine). Values of 0.04–0.08 are normal, but the excretion varies with flow and serum uric acid concentration. Urinary uric acid excretion >1g/24h, especially with an acidic urine, is associated with a higher risk for the development of uric acid stones.

Urinary amino acid excretion. Amino acid excretion is characteristically elevated in Fanconi's Syndrome and in heavy metal toxicity. Specific amino acid excretory problems may be assessed by column chromatography.

Blood ammonia. Kidneys produce a significant proportion of circulating ammonia. In chronic renal failure, unaccompanied by CHF or liver disease, arterial ammonia concentrations are low. Blood ammonia can be determined enzymatically or by airation.

Miscellaneous urine tests. Serum amylase rises during renal insufficiency because of decreased amylase clearance. Urine activity increases with serum activity during pancreatitis. Excretory rates of over 1000 Somogyi units per hour indicate acute pancreatitis. For pancreatitis, the ratio of amylase clearance to creatinine clearance may be useful in the differential diagnosis.

$$\text{Clearance Ratio (\%)} = \frac{\text{U amylase}}{\text{S amylase}} \times \frac{\text{S creatinine}}{\text{U creatinine}} \times 100$$

The normal ratio of 2%–3% may be unchanged in 1/3 of the patients with pancreatitis and elevated in those with ketoacidosis, burns, duodenal perforations, and renal insufficiency.

Normal urine is free of fat. Cholesterol esters (Maltese Crosses) and epithelial cells filled with fat can be detected in the urine under polarized light. By specific histochemical techniques or chromotography, the characteristic glycolipid in Fabry's Disease can be found. Chyluria may also be associated with parasitic disease such as filariasis or retroperitoneal tumors such as lymphomas.

Enzyme Studies & β_2-Microglobulin

Increased urinary excretion of several proximal tubular enzymes has been used as a marker of tubular injury. The enzymes that can be measured include N-acetyl glucosaminidase, β-glucuronidase, alanine aminopeptidase, and lysozyme among others. Increased urinary enzyme excretion is non-specific and occurs in both acute and chronic tubulo-interstitial diseases with lesser increases seen in glomerular and vascular diseases. Urinary enzyme measurements are not useful as a screening test but may be helpful when measured sequentially. In patients receiving nephrotoxic drugs, such as aminoglycosides and cis-platinum, serial measurements may be helpful in predicting nephrotoxicity several days before the rise in serum creatinine occurs.

β_2-microglobulin (β_2M) is a low molecular weight protein that is filtered by the glomerulus and reabsorbed and catabolized by the proximal tubule. Increased urinary β_2M excretion is a very sensitive though non-specific marker of mild tubular injury. Unlike the urinary enzymes, it has been demonstrated to be a useful screening test for tubular dysfunction, as in cadmium nephrotoxicity. Serum β_2M levels are of value in transplant patients, rise with a fall in GFR, and have been shown to be a sensitive early indicator of acute rejection. The limitation of the serum and urinary β_2M is that the increases seen in renal insufficiency, can be the result of either glomerular or tubular damage, and levels may be difficult to interpret unless serial measurements are made.

A ratio of urinary β_2M and albumin excretion can also be used as a qualitative test for the assessment of the type of proteinuria. In tubular proteinurias, the β_2M:albumin ratios are high, commonly $\geq 2:1$; the reverse occurs in glomerular proteinurias, where albumin excretion is high and ratio of β_2M:albumin are usually $1:20$.

Serological tests. Serological testing is valuable in the diagnosis and management of glomerulonephritis. Several rheumatologic diseases are associated with glomerulonephritis; the one encountered most frequently is systemic lupus erythematous (SLE). The best screening laboratory test for SLE is the detection of antinuclear antibodies (ANA), positive in >95% of patients with SLE and often present in high titer. It may be positive in other diseases, as well, chiefly Sjorgren's ($\approx$75%) and scleroderma ($\approx$40%), although usually in low titer. Several ANA patterns are seen. The most common is a diffuse pattern which can be seen in a large number of rheumatic diseases. The peripheral and speckled pattern are common in SLE and the speckled pattern is also seen in scleroderma. Antibodies to the human glomerular basement membrane and pulmonary alveolar basement membrane are present in the serum of patients with Goodpasture's syndrome. High titers are associated with acute nephritis.

Serum complement measurements, both CH_{50} and C_3, are useful in monitoring acute glomerulonephritis. They are frequently low in SLE, shunt nephritis, bacterial endocarditis, cryoglobulinemias, post-streptococcal glomerulonephritis and membrano-proliferative glomerulonephritis (MPGN). Serial measurements in SLE can be used to assess the activity of disease and the response to therapy. In MPGN type I, the early components of complement, i.e., C_1, C_4 and C_2 may be markedly decreased. C_3 nephritic factor may be detectable in the serum of MPGN type II ($\approx$75%) and type I ($\approx$33%).

Cryoglobulinemia occurs in some patients with renal disease and is suggestive of the presence of immune complex disease. The cryoglobulins are monoclonal in multiple myeloma and lympho-proliferative disorders, and of the mixed type in bacterial, viral and parasitic infections, collagen disease like SLE, and essential mixed cryoglobulinemia. Symptoms associated with cryoglobulinemia include Raynaud's phenomenon, cutaneous ulcers, dependent purpura and cold-induced urticaria. In patients with high titers of cryoglobulin, especially essential mixed cryoglobulinemia, plasmapheresis may be beneficial.

The detection of circulating immune complexes provides an insight into the pathogenesis of some renal diseases. This is especially true in glomerulonephritis, about 75%–80% of which are immune-mediated. High titers are associated with active disease. Several methods are available for detection and quantitation, including the Cl_q binding, the Raji cell and the fluorescein labeled staphylococcal protein A tests.

The detection of specific antibodies to bacterial or viral antigens can assist in making an etiological diagnosis in glomerulonephritis. In post-streptococcal glomerulonephritis, specific antibodies are anti-streptolysin O (ASO), anti-hyaluronidase, anti-DNAse B and anti-DPNase. ASO titers are increased in >75% of patients with this disorder and almost all will have an elevated and or changing antibody titer to at least one streptococcal antigen. The FTA is used to make the diagnosis of syphilis which can cause several types of glomerulonephritis. In other infections, the specific antigen may be detectable in the serum, as in the acute glomerulonephritis associated with circulating hepatitis B surface antigen.

Other serological tests may be positive in renal disease, although they may not provide specific diagnostic information. One such test is the rheumatoid factor which is positive in several rheumatic, infectious and non-infectious diseases. Low titers may be present in patients with SLE, progressive systemic sclerosis, bacterial endocarditis and sarcoidosis.

SELECTED READINGS

1. McNeely, MDD: Routine Urinalysis. Drug Therapy Feb 1979 pp 37–40.

2. Murphey, JE: Preuss, HG; Henry JB: Evaluation of renal function and water, electrolyte, and acid-base balance in Clinical Diagnosis and Management by Laboratory Methods. Ed. Henry JB, WB Saunders Co., Philadelphia, PA 1984.

3. Reubi, FC: Clearance Tests in Clinical Medicine. Charles C Thomas, Springfield, Ill 1963.

4. Ware, F Renal Function Tests: A Guide to Interpretation. Hospital Medicine. June 1981, pp. 77–92.

Thomas A. Rakowski
Harry G. Preuss

2

Renal Biopsy

Renal biopsy can establish a histological diagnosis, suggest the prognosis of the renal disorder, and evaluate the course of therapy. Jungmann performed the first surgical renal biopsy in 1924. In 1944, Alwall began using a percutaneous technique. The modern biopsy era began in the early 50's after the successes of Iverson and Brun. Since then, examination of renal biopsy specimens has become a mainstay in the diagnosis and treatment of a wide variety of kidney disorders. The complication rate is low and diagnostic yield high when done by an experienced operator.

Examination of the specimen by light microscopy, immunoflourescent microscopy, and electron microscopy is mandatory for adequate pathological diagnosis. Pathologists experienced in viewing renal biopsies and familiar with immunomicroscopy must be involved. If adequate pathological support is not available, the patient or tissue should be referred to another center for evaluation. It is important that renal biopsy be performed by experienced hands and interpreted through trained eyes.

INDICATIONS AND CONTRAINDICATIONS

Indications for renal biopsy vary from center to center. In general renal biopsies are avoided where there is little chance of benefit, either therapeutically or prognostically. Some common reasons for attempting renal biopsy include: 1) Investigational studies into the natural histories of renal diseases or progression of treatment. 2) Histological diagnosis in patients with nephrotic syndrome or the nephritic syndrome (Chapters 4 & 7). 3) Histological diagnosis in states with pathological proteinuria and/or,a symptomatic hematuria. 4) Histological diagnosis in conditions of renal insufficiency of uncertain etiology. 5) Diagnosis in selected cases of acute renal failure and intra or post-partum renal failure. 6) Differentiating causes for decreased renal function after renal transplantation. 7) Evaluation of certain hereditary renal diseases.

All contraindications are relative. The presence of *only one* kidney is considered a general contraindication. However, if kidney tissue is vital to decisions regarding the patients course of therapy, an open biopsy may be obtained on a solitary kidney with meticulous care being taken with hemostasis. Biopsy should be delayed in patients with *coagulopathy* until correction is achieved. *Uremia* is not a contraindication to kidney biopsy *per se*; however, if possible, the uremic syndrome should be treated by dialysis prior to biopsy attempts to reverse the coagulopathy associated with uremia. Patients with *severe hypertension* are most likely to have a bleeding complication post biopsy, therefore, blood pressure should be controlled prior to biopsy. *Severe arteriosclerosis* or *amyloid* increase the possibility of hemorrhagic complications. Accordingly, patients with these disorders must be monitored more carefully. Known *renal malignancy* or *perirenal infection* often preclude renal biopsy. *Uncooperative patients* with *severe skeletal deformities* should forego percutaneous biopsy.

COMPLICATIONS

The most frequent complications are hemorrhagic; either gross hematuria or perirenal hematoma. Microscopic hematuria occurs in virtually 100% of cases and is not considered a complication. In fact, hematuria may be the first indication of a successful biopsy.

Strict bed rest for a period of 24 hours after biopsy minimizes complications. The patient should be cautioned to avoid straining or heavy lifting for a period of approximately two weeks after the procedure. If gross hematuria occurs, high fluid intake is maintained to facilitate the passage of small blood clots. All patients should have one or two units of typed blood ready prior to biopsy, as bleeding is sometimes brisk. Tissue from virtually every organ reachable has been inadvertently obtained with the biopsy needle. In general, these complications are not severe despite organ perforation. Other complications of the procedure include renal laceration necessitating nephrectomy or open surgical repair, and rarer still death (death rate is less than 0.1%).

RENAL BIOPSY TECHNIQUES

Closed biopsy is usually performed under local anesthesia with the patient lying prone. Two types of needles are in general use, one is a Franklin modification of a Vim-Silverman needle and the other is a modification of the Cope needle. The former is used more widely (Fig. 2-1). In both cases, an inner needle is introduced into the kidney. An outer cutting needle is advanced over this guide, trapping the specimen in the inner needle. One to three samples are usually taken. It is our policy not to exceed 3 "passes" with the needle at one sitting. We feel this conservative approach minimizes our complication rate.

Open biopsy is done in certain cases using a flank incision and a muscle splitting approach.

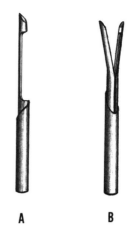

A   **B**

Fig. 2-1. A. Cutting head of Cope needle (A) and Franklin Modification of Vim-Silverman (B).

After kidney exposure, we prefer that needle biopsy be performed which obtains deep and superficial glomeruli rather than a shallow wedge biopsy.

LOCALIZATION OF THE KIDNEY

Initially closed biopsies were carried out using the intravenous pyelogram as a guide; transcribing measurements from the x-ray film onto the patient's back. More recently, other approaches to kidney localization have been widely used.

Kidney biopsy can be performed during an intravenous pyelogram using fluoroscopic guidance which affords direct visualization of needle and kidney. This approach has been very successful and decreases morbidity.

The use of ultrasound to outline the kidney for biopsy is becoming the most popular localization means. Its most obvious advantage is lessened radiation exposure, and the patient does not receive potentially nephrotoxic radiographic dyes. The location of the kidney can be marked on the patients back in the ultrasound laboratory and the patient then sent to his room for biopsy. As an alternative, the biopsy can be carried out under ultrasound guidance in the ultrasound room.

Importantly, the position and function of the kidneys should be assessed by intravenous pyelography or a combination of sonography and radionuclide scanning prior to biopsy, using any of the above localization techniques.

HANDLING OF SPECIMENS

Three samples of kidney tissue are taken, or preferably, one sample is divided into three portions. The individual portions are sent for routine light microscopy, immunofluorescent microscopy, and electronmicroscopy. Obviously, any non renal tissues removed with the needle should be sent for light microscopy as there are numerous case reports of diagnoses being made from non renal tissues obtained at renal biopsy, i.e., Hodgkins Disease being diagnosed by inadvertent aspiration of splenic tissue.

Light microscopy. The portion of tissue to be sent for routine microscopy is generally placed immediately in buffered formalin and sent to pathology. After fixation, 3 micron or less thick sections are stained with hematoxylin-eosin, PAS, methenamine silver stain and/or other special stains. Sections thicker than 3 microns are difficult to interpret.

If uric acid crystals are being sought, one portion of the specimen should be fixed in absolute alcohol prior to sectioning and staining. Formalin and other fixatives dissolve urate crystals.

Immunofluorescence. Tissue specimens sent for immunofluorescent microscopy must be frozen immediately or placed on gauze moistened with 0.9% saline solution and transported rapidly to the immunofluorescence laboratory.

In general, IgG antibodies to immunoprotein and albumin are layered on the slide sections and then stained with fluorescein labelled anti-IgG antibody (sandwich technique) prior to viewing under the fluorescence microscope. Routinely, antibodies to IgG, IgA, IgM, complement components, fibrin and albumin are used.

In certain cases, antibodies against hepatitis B surface antigen, Treponema pallidum, carcinoembyronic antigen, other tumor antigens, and a host of other specialized antigens can be used if necessary.

Electronmicroscopy. Specimens for electronmicroscopy are commonly fixed in glutaraldehyde or Zamboni solution and sent to the electron microscopy laboratory for embedding, sectioning, and staining. Ultrathin sections are then examined and photographed while under the electronmicroscope. Fine ultrastructural detail of the glomerulus can be examined: deposits and amyloid can be identified and localized. Good electronmicroscopy has made the use of special staining in light microscopy less necessary for evalution of renal biopsy specimens.

SELECTED READINGS

1. Curtis JJ, Rakowski TA, Argy WJ, and Schreiner GE. Evaluation of percutaneous kidney biopsy in advanced renal failure. Nephron 17:259–269, 1976.
2. Lindeman RA. Percutaneous renal biopsy. Kidney 7:1–6, 1974.

Erica George
Carroll Markivee

3

Evaluation of Kidneys by Imaging Techniques

The rapid growth of diagnostic imaging modalities and techniques has resulted in occasional indecision regarding the appropriate use of some of the newer imaging procedures. Preliminary consultation with imaging physicians can save time, increase the amount of information obtained, and improve cost effectiveness. In any given local setting, consideration of renal imaging modalities should be made in accordance with the availability of equipment, the experience and expertise of the physicians interpreting the various studies, and any potential hazard of a particular procedure.

RENAL IMAGING BY ULTRASONOGRAPHY

The relatively superficial posterior location of the native kidneys and the superficial anterior position of a transplant kidney in the iliac fossa allows ready examination by ultrasound.

Ultrasound does not involve the use of ionizing radiation or contrast material. The technique, however, is operator dependent. The sonographic transducer is moved by the operator over the patient's body surface and emits inaudible acoustic pulses and receives echoes of these pulses from the tissue interfaces. These are converted electronically into ultrasound images. Organ movement and vascular pulsation is easily identified by realtime equipment. The renal cortex contains relatively low amplitude homogeneous echoes. The kidneys are less echogenic than the liver. The renal pelvis and calyceal system are more echogenic than the renal cortex due to the presence of fibrous tissue and surrounding fat.

One of the most common indications for renal sonography is the evaluation of a space-occupying lesion seen on an intravenous pyelogram. Ultrasound can readily distinguish between solid and cystic masses in the kidney.

Ultrasound is the first examination of choice to rule out the possibility of obstruction in a patient with acute renal failure. Hydronephrosis is easily recognized by ultrasound. Polycystic kidney disease can be differentiated from hydronephrosis by the location of the sonolucent structures. In hydronephrosis the sonolucency is centrally located, whereas, in polycystic disease the sonolucencies are seen in the renal cortex. Renal cyst aspiration and renal biopsy are often performed under sonographic guidance.

Ultrasound is also performed for evaluation of kidney size. In a patient with chronic renal failure, the kidneys become more echogenic than the liver.

Renal transplant evaluation by real time sonography is particularly useful in the determination of hydronephrosis, hydroureter, and in size of renal graft and in the detection and differential diagnosis of perirenal fluid collections (Fig. 1). Doppler ultrasound assessing vascular impedance of the renal graft is useful for monitoring acute transplant rejection.

23

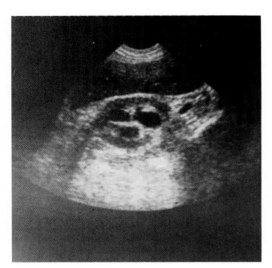

Fig. 3-1. Ultra-sonogram of renal allograft demonstrating hydronephrosis.

RENAL X-RAY EXAMINATION

Preliminary Films

PLAIN FILMS

The preliminary examination of the urinary tract should always begin with plain films made to include the adrenals above and the pubic bones below before any opaque medium is injected. If it seems that the patient is too large for these structures to fit on one film (14″ × 17″), then the plain film examination should consist of two films, a 14″ × 17″ made for the upper portion to include the upper poles of the kidneys and the adrenal gland areas, and a 10″ × 12″ placed transversely to include the bottom of the pubic bones.

One should determine if the plain film examination is complete so that renal and adrenal calcifications will not be missed at the upper end of the urinary tract and neither urethral calculi nor osteolytic metastasis from a tumor be missed at the lower end.

Renal parenchymal calcifications may be seen on the plain film. These may occur in tuberculosis, carcinoma, brucellosis and rarely in the wall of a benign cyst. Intrapelvic or intracalyceal calcifications are usually due to simple calculi, but rarely a calcification within the renal pelvis may be within an epidermoid carcinoma of the renal pelvis.

NEPHROTOMOGRAPHY

Nephrotomography is a radiographic technique (almost universally used) which requires tomography of the kidney during the nephrogram phase (Fig. 2A, B). This is defined as the first minute after the end of a rapid (15 seconds or less) IV bolus of urographic contrast medium. If more than 50 ml is injected as a bolus, the timing of the 1st exposure should begin no less than 45 seconds from the start of the injection, regardless of the amount of injectate. Usually at least three films are made at levels 1 cm apart such as 7, 8 and 9 cm above the table (the patient is supine and the kidneys are usually at these distances from the table top). At this time, all the films produced should be inspected by the physician for quality and to determine the size, shape, position and homogeneity of the renal parenchyma.

The size of the renal outline was measured in 165 healthy adults. The lengths was determined to be from 12.4 cm to 13.7 cm. The widths were 5.9 cm to 6.4 cm. The measurements refer to the size as seen as plain films made with the x-ray tube target at 100 cm above the film, and the patient no more than 3″ above the film (due to thickness of table top, Bucky, etc.). Table 1 lists causes of enlargement and Table 2 lists causes of decreased size of the kidneys.

The renal position is probably the most variable of the parameters discussed under this section, since the kidneys normally move 1 to 3 cm with respiration and may move up to 7 cm with change from supine to erect position.

As important as variation in size, shape or position of the kidney is alteration of the homogeneity of the renal parenchyma. During the nephrogram phase of capillary opacification, we may see a clearly outlined non-opacifying, filling defect or alternatively, a contrast enhanced irregular enlargement of the renal substance. These findings may indicate presence of a cyst or tumor, respectively. Table 3 lists causes of such changes.

Irregular enlargement should also be evaluated by ultrasound to exclude malignant tumor, even though the nephrotomogram film may be suggestive of renal cyst.

The thickness of the renal cortex and medulla from the edge of the calyces to subcapsular border can also be determined. Renal atrophic disease causes progressive decrease of cortical thickness, which is a reliable indicator from one

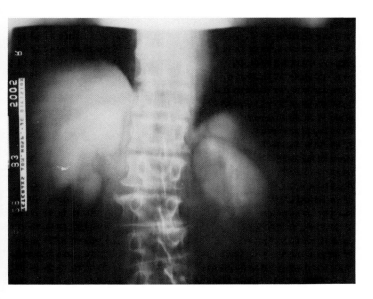

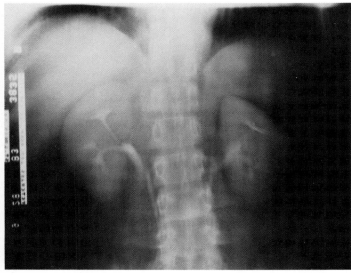

Fig. 3-2. Nephrotomography of normal kidneys; 2a. parenchymal cortical phase; 2b. medullary pelvic phase.

exam to another of further loss of renal substance. Chronic pyelonephritis, glomerulonephritis and nephrosclerosis will all show such changes indicating the progress of the disease.

Excretory Urography

Excretory urography demonstrates the pelvocalyceal system, ureters, urinary bladder and urethra. It may follow nephrotomography or be performed immediately after the plain film. Organic iodinated contrast medium is administered either by I.V. bolus injection of .5 to 1 ml/1b body weight of 60% to 76% solution or by I.V. drip infusion of 300 ml of 30% solution. In the presence of elevated SUN and serum creatinine levels greater than twice the maximal normal value and/or a urinary output of not less than 100 ml/day, the examination is contraindicated.

Contraindications to excretory urography are marked dehydration of the patient or the history of moderate or severe allergic reactions to the contrast medium. Types of reactions to contrast medium are listed in Table 4.

Glomerular filtration and tubular cell secretion both mediate the renal excretion of opaque

Table 3-1   Common Causes of Renal Enlargement

Diffuse generalized renal enlargement	1. Polycystic disease
	2. Multiple cysts in one or both kidneys
	3. Tumor of any type
	4. Renal vein thrombosis or thrombosis due to thrombocytopenic purpura
	5. Compensatory hypertrophy (due to absence of opposite kidney)
	6. Obstruction from any cause
	7. Acute glomerulonephritis
	8. Acromegaly
	9. Dysplastic renal disease (cystic)
	10. Goodpasture syndrome
	11. Hematoma
	12. Acute pyelonephritis
	13. Amyloidosis
	14. Parasitic infestation from schistosomiasis or echinococcus
Localized renal enlargement	1. Cyst or cysts
	2. Tumor
	3. Abscess
	4. Hematoma
	5. Hypertrophied columns of Bertin

contrast media. The rate of excretion is relative to the plasma concentration of the medium and glomerular filtration rate. Decreased renal blood flow and intraglomerular pressure may slow urinary flow which will cause a prolonged transit time of the contrast medium and produce a denser and/or persisting nephrogram.

The normal renal collecting system has great variations in shape and size. Subtle pathological changes may require sequential examinations for their detection. Oblique views are almost always necessary to complete any excretory urogram. If there is adequate glomerular filtration and/or tubular secretion of contrast medium, even a marked obstruction with dilatation of the collecting system, can be clearly defined, even if the obstruction is chronic.

Direct Opacification Urography

Direct injection of contrast material into the urinary collecting system allows greater opacification of the pelvocalyceal system and ureter on the side injected. It requires that each side be separately examined. Urine collection from the renal pelvis is possible from culture of cystological exam. There are two routes of injection, from below (retrograde pyelography) and from above (antegrade pyelography).

RETROGRADE PHELOGRAPHY

Injection of contrast medium may be made through the urethra and bladder into the ureteral orifices by means of a Braasch bulb inserted into the distal ureters or by insertion of radiopaque

Table 3-2   Common Causes of Decreased Renal Size

1. Congenitally small kidney
2. Renal atrophy from previous glomerulonephritis
3. Post operative (partial nephrectomy)
4. Scarring with local shrinkage after abscess, Tbc, or renal infarct.
5. Post traumatic (renal laceration)

Table 3-3 Causes of Other Abnormalities of the Renal Parenchyma on Nephrotomography

Types of Abnormalities	Comments
1. Radiolucent areas	
a. Cyst	May see 'beak' sign at junction of cyst wall and renal cortex.
b. Avascular tumor	Can mimic cyst
c. Dilated calyx or calyces	Negative filling defects seen where calyces should be. Indicates long term obstruction in a failed kidney.
d. Renal laceration	May see extravasation of contrast medium into perirenal space at point of laceration.
e. Renal parenchymal scar	Usually associated with irregular lobulation of renal outline. May be secondary to trauma, infection or radiation*
f. Amyloid deposit	
2. Radiodense areas	
a. Hypertrophied normal renal tissue ("columns of Bertin")	May mimic hypervascular tumor— differentiate by nuclear angiography.
b. Angiomyolipoma	Ultrasound and CT are both indicated; arteriography is also usually needed.
c. Arteriovenous malformation	Not usually well seen on nephrotomography due to intense arteriovenous shunting.
d. Other benign/malignant tumor	

*Radiation nephritis, secondary to radiation theraphy can produce scarring and irregularity of the renal outline if over 2300 rads are administered to the kidney in less than 5 weeks (B).

catheters into the ureters and injection of contrast material (Fig. 3). This procedure implies the ability of the surgeon to perform direct endoscopy of the bladder and thus to recognize primary or secondary changes related to upper tract disease. For example, a transitional cell carcinoma of the renal pelvis or ureter is often associated with similar changes in the bladder. Also, calculus disease of a kidney may be followed by presence of calculi in the bladder, or if recent passage of a stone has occurred, edema of the ureteral orifice may be seen at endoscopy. Retrograde pyelography is normally conducted with use of small amount of local anesthetic in the urethra. Rarely a greater degree of anesthesia is necessary. In the event of complete obstruction of the urinary tract, retrograde examination is the only means for examining the distal portion below the site of obstruction.

ANTEGRADE PYELOGRAPHY

As interventional radiological procedures increase in frequency and number, the use of fluoroscopically guided nephrostomy has become more wide spread. Radiologists can drain urine or pus collections from obstructed tracts, and outline the anatomy following the injection of contrast medium above. In addition, removal

Table 3-4   (Types of contrast medium reactions listed in order of significance)

A. Minimal Significance
   1. Sensation of body and head warmth
   2. Nausea
   3. Burning in the vein used for injection
   4. Sneezing and nasal mucosal congestion
   5. <10 mm Hg drop in systolic and/or diastolic blood pressure
   6. Hyperventilation

B. Moderate Significance
   1. Vomiting
   2. Headache
   3. <15 mm Hg drop in systolic and/or diastolic blood pressure
   4. Hyperventilation with transient productive cough
   5. Chest pain

C. Marked significance
   1. 15 mm or more drop in blood pressure
   2. Signs of edema of respiratory tract: "crowing," air hunger, cyanosis
   3. Shock
   4. Cardiac arrest*
   5. Respiratory arrest*
   6. Acute tubular necrosis

*frequency variously reported as 1 to 100,000 to 1 to 1,000,0000 injections

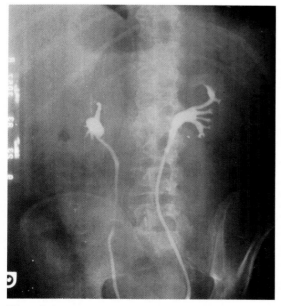

Fig. 3-3. Retrograde pyelography demonstrating normal pelvocalyceal system bilaterally.

of calculi from above through insertion of "basket" catheters can be accomplished by both retrograde and antegrade techniques, but is actually more easily carried out from above than below because of the ease of passage of the basket through the dilated region.

RENAL IMAGING BY COMPUTED TOMOGRAPHY

The technology and physics of image formation by computed tomography are complex and not an appropriate subject for this text, but certain fundamentals should be understood. The x-ray image is converted to electronic signals. Electronic signals are digitized, and transformed into image displays. Brightness of a structure seen on the video display unit corresponds to the degree of x-ray absorption in tissue. Spatial resolution is approximately 1 mm in both the plain and contrast enhanced images. CT can be useful in evaluating kidneys with poor function since only a small amount of excretion is needed to visualize the pelvis and ureters. Any low density calcifications in the parenchyma or calyces are seen with greater contrast than on plain radiography. A dilated pelvis is readily recognized and renal size and parenchymal cortical thickness can be determined by CT with intravenous injection of iodinated contrast medium. I.V. administration of contrast medium produces contrast enhancement in proportion to the vascularity of the tissue. It may detect hypervascular or ischemic areas in a normally perfused organ. Contrast enhancement allows better differentiation of solid masses from cystic lesions (Fig. 4). Hydronephrosis and perirenal fluid collection (urinomas, lymphocele) affecting renal allografts can be easily recognized on CT. In many respects, computed tomography of the kidney is complementary to sonography.

RENAL ANGIOGRAPHY

Transfemoral aortography, selective renal arteriography and digital subtraction angiography can opacify renal arteries and medullary, cortical and capsular arteries. The transfemoral aortogram is a screening study to demonstrate the number, size and condition of the main renal arteries and the evaluation of aortic disease.

Usually a selective renal angiogram is nec-

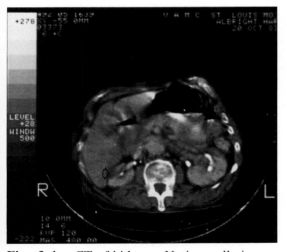

Fig. 3-4. CT of kidneys: Notice well circumscribed hypodense mass of right kidney which is a renal cyst (open arrow). There is a contrast enhancing mass lesion of the left kidney which is a renal cell carcinoma (black arrow).

essary for the evaluation of renal artery stenosis. Optimal visualization of the intrarenal vascular bed is also provided by selective renal arteriogram. Injection of a total of 12 ml of 60% to 76% opaque medium during a period of 1.5 seconds is the preferred method. When a renal cell carcinoma is suspected, a larger volume of contrast agent up to 25 ml may be injected and epinephrine used to constrict the normal vessels, leaving the tumor vessels filled for optimum visualization.

Reactions to the intravenous contrast medium are less common during angiography than with excretory urography. Local bleeding at the femoral insertion site of the catheter, arterial thrombosis, arterial dissection and dislodgement of plaques or thrombi in the aorta and renal artery, false renal artery aneurysm formation and arterio-venous fistula formation have all been reported in the past, but are seldom seen in modern practice.

The nephrographic phase of the selective renal arteriogram follows the arterial phase by 5 to 8 seconds, and shows a dense homogeneous band of renal cortex about 5-8 mm thick. A normal nephrogram indicates a normal renal vascular bed and displays the precise outline of the kidney. It shows any areas of absent vascularity due to small cysts, infarcts or scarring which may not be appreciated on an excretory urogram or any other imaging modality or on the arterial phase of the arteriogram. Seven to 12 seconds after injection of the contrast medium, major renal veins should become visible. Photographic subtraction should be performed routinely to optically enhance the images of the venous phase. The demonstration of multiple collateral veins is suggestive of renal vein obstruction.

Another indication for renal arteriography is the diagnosis of renal artery stenosis and/or renal artery aneurysm causing renal vascular hypertension. A stenotic lesion which reduces the vessel lumen by 80% appears to be directly related to the presence of clinically evident hypertension. The renal arteriogram is the diagnostic modality of choice for the demonstration of branch stenosis of the renal artery whether it is secondary to arteriosclerosis, dysplasia, thrombus, embolus or arteritis; it defines best the presence of tumor vessels associated with renal cell carcinoma and should be employed when other imaging modalities such as ultrasound and CT examinations are indeterminate.

NUCLIDE RENAL IMAGING AND COMPUTER ASSISTED FUNCTIONAL DATA ANALYSIS

The transitory or fixed deposition of renal radionuclide agents following intravenous administration relates to the interaction of extra- and intrarenal blood flow and renal extraction which depends on glomerular-capillary and tubular-cellular functional integrity. The nuclide renal scan adequately demonstrates in most instances anatomical alterations but is less sensitive and specific than other imaging modalities. Assisted by computer analysis, kidney function may be determined. Non-invasiveness and low radiation dose make radionuclide procedures useful when repeat examinations are anticipated. Increased specificity may be obtained by using multiple agents to define inflammatory conditions, abscess formation, and certain neoplastic lesions.

Presently, radiopharmaceuticals labeled with Technetium-99 in the form of Tc 99m-DTPA, glucoheptonate (GHA), DMSA and hippuran labeled with I-131 or I-123 are used primarily for renal imaging and function analysis. Glomerular filtration, effective renal plasma flow, renal perfusion and definition of cortical morphology may be determined by a single agent or combination of radioagents. With the availability of on-line computers, renal functional analysis may be performed (Fig. 5a,b,c,d). Many techniques appear to correlate well with creatinine clearance rates and are more sensitive and specific than the commonly used biochemical markers.

In certain clinical settings the nuclide renal scan and/or function analysis are the diagnostically preferred procedure.

a. Patients with acute pyelonephritis may present with a spectrum of clinical abnormalities, but only those with severe disease demonstrate compatible changes on an excretory contrast urogram. However, imaging with Tc-99m DMSA or Tc-99m GHA, demonstrates abnormal renal images. Radionuclide assessment of "single kidney" or split renal function may offer a sensitive marker of total and individual kidney injury. The additional use of gallium-67 citrate defines areas of inflammation or abscess formation.

b. In obstructive uropathy the excretory contrast urogram usually presents excellent anatomical information. However, a nuclear scan either prior to or with i.v. pyelography is recommended in this situation. Radionuclide agents, primarily excreted by glomerular filtration, Tc-99m-DTPA and -GHA or by tubular secretion, I-131 hippuran, demonstrate extrarenal obstructions. When parenchymal function and parenchynal excretion are poor, delayed imaging can demonstrate excretory activity proximal to the obstruction. In questionable cases where obstructive uropathy versus non-obstructive dilation is the differential, Lasix induced excretory Tc 99m-DTPA renography is a useful evaluation.

c. Renal artery stenosis is best established by arteriography. Radionuclide perfusion of the affected kidney is compared to the perfusion of the contralateral kidney to prognosticate the success of surgical reconstruction versus nephrectomy. Radionuclide perfusion and function analysis should be repeated following reconstruction of the stenotic artery.

d. Radionuclide renal function analysis and imaging is particularly well suited to pediatric renal problems due to dynamic processes requiring serial investigations. The absence of side effects and the low radiation have added to the popularity of radionuclide investigations in pediatrics. Their usefulness includes: to assess and distinguish between obstructive and non-obstructive hydronephrosis and to assess total renal perfusion and focal renal ischemia in children with hypertension or renal trauma. In addition, the nuclide renal image is probably the easiest and quickest assessment of congenital hydronephrosis, and polycystic disease and may be used as an emergency procedure in neonates.

e. Nuclide renal allograft imaging with perfusion and function analysis has been invaluable in the immediate post transplant period when medical and surgical complications are frequent. Serial nuclide examinations are important for optimal monitoring of renal graft rejection. Rejection is the most frequent post operative complications. In the early post transplant period, renal functional loss may be due to renal artery graft thrombosis, excretory obstruction at

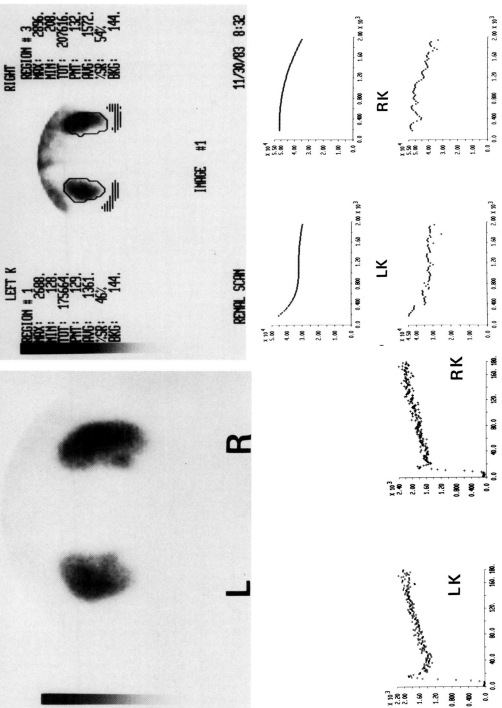

Fig. 3-5. Radionuclide renal scan. (5a.) Two hour delayed image with Tc-99m glucoheptonate; (5b.) Per cent ratios of perfusion and glomerular filtration of kidneys: 46% of total to the left kidney and 54% right; (5c.) Computer assisted time activity curves 0–3 minutes of renal perfusion and maximal glomerular filtration of glucoheptonate; upper row of curves are modified by computerized "curve-fitting"; (5d.) Time activity curves of excretory phase of kidneys demonstrating slower excretion on the right as compared to normal excretion slope on left.

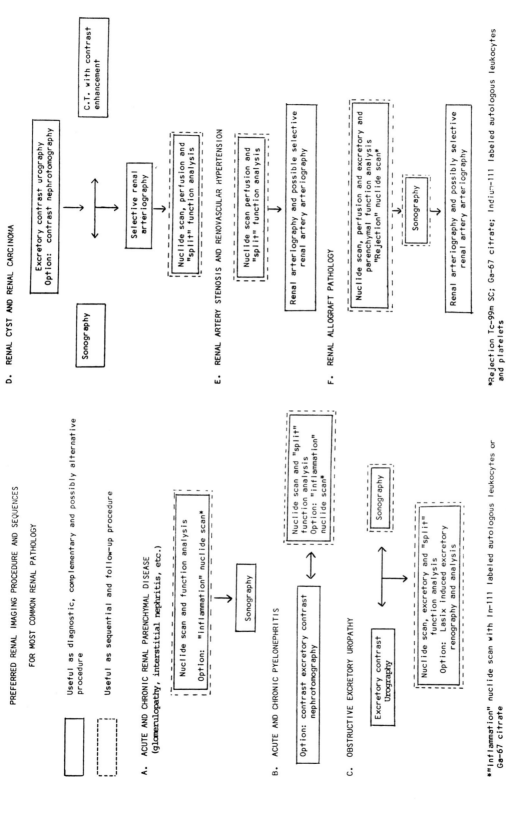

Fig. 3-6. Preferred renal imaging procedures and sequences for most common renal pathology.

PREFERRED RENAL IMAGING PROCEDURE AND SEQUENCES

FOR MOST COMMON RENAL PATHOLOGY

Useful as diagnostic, complementary and possibly alternative procedure

Useful as sequential and follow-up procedure

A. ACUTE AND CHRONIC RENAL PARENCHYMAL DISEASE
(glomerulopathy, interstitial nephritis, etc.)

Nuclide scan and function analysis

Option: "inflammation" nuclide scan*

Sonography

B. ACUTE AND CHRONIC PYELONEPHRITIS

Option: contrast excretory contrast nephrotomography

Nuclide scan and "split" function analysis

Option: "inflammation" nuclide scan*

Sonography

C. OBSTRUCTIVE EXCRETORY UROPATHY

Excretory contrast Urography

Sonography

Nuclide scan, excretory and "split" function analysis

Option: Lasix induced excretory renography and analysis

D. RENAL CYST AND RENAL CARCINOMA

Excretory contrast urography
Option: contrast nephrotomography

C.T. with contrast enhancement

Selective renal arteriography

Sonography

Nuclide scan, perfusion and "split" function analysis

E. RENAL ARTERY STENOSIS AND RENOVASCULAR HYPERTENSION

Nuclide scan perfusion and "split" function analysis

Renal arteriography and possible selective renal artery arteriography

F. RENAL ALLOGRAFT PATHOLOGY

Nuclide scan, perfusion and excretory and parenchymal function analysis

"Rejection" nuclide scan*

Sonography

Renal arteriography and possibly selective renal artery arteriography

*"Inflammation" nuclide scan with In-111 labeled autologous leukocytes or Ga-67 citrate

*Rejection Tc-99m SC; Ga-67 citrate; Indium-111 labeled autologous leukocytes and platelets

32

the vesico-ureteric junction, acute tubular necrosis, acute rejection and not infrequently some combination of the above. Tc 99m-DTPA and -GHA are useful in assessing overall renal function and excretory patency, urinary leaks, extravasation and are also helpful in defining photopenic areas in the vicinity of the allograft or urinary bladder. The latter may be due to hematomas, lymphoceles, and urinomas.

The most specific and sensitive evaluation of renal allograft rejection is via imaging with specific radioagents which interact with a specific aspect of renal allograft rejection such as thrombosis, vasculitis, interstitial cellular infiltrates, and alteration of allograft blood flow and distribution. Rejection radionuclides currently in use are gelatine stabilized, Tc 99m sulfur colloid, and autologous Indium-111 labeled leukocytes and platelets.

NUCLEAR MAGNETIC RESONANCE IMAGING

Nuclear magnetic resonance (NMR) imaging has already proven useful in early clinical trials of cerebral and spinal cord abnormalities. Spatial detail and resolution are similar to CT images and do not require contrast material. NMR imaging is dependent on hydrogen density, the motion of hydrogen and the relaxation time, T-1 and T-2, of hydrogen protons within tissue after being placed in a strong magnetic field. Hydrogen nuclei with an odd number of protons or neutrons act like small magnets in a strong magnetic field. A net magnetic vector or moment aligned with the magnetic field can be described for the population of nuclei affected. Application of radiofrequency pulse displaces the net magnetic vector by an amount determined by the amplitude and duration of the radiofrequency pulse. When the pulse is removed, protons emit the absorbed energy in form of radiofrequency signals and return to their original orientation. These signals are used to generate the NMR image. The type of surrounding tissue and the chemical state of the hydrogen atom dic-

tates the time it takes for the protons to regain their original orientation. Two basic forms of relaxation occur which are called T-1 and T-2. Each of them can be measured, and each reflects a distinct physical characteristic of the tissue imaged. Moving protons in blood flow return fewer signals because of the relatively poor hydrogen density. Preliminary NMR imaging of the kidneys shows great promise. It provides tomographic images of excellent spacial resolution; and the information demonstrated by NMR exceeds that of nonenhanced and in some instances, contrast enhanced X-ray CT. Compared with ultrasound, NMR has better spacial resolution and provides more specific tissue characterization. It is less operator dependent. In analyzing renal pathology, the main disadvantage of NMR is inability to recognize calcification. During forced diuresis, the distinction between cortex and medulla is most apparent. Pelvocaliectasis is easily detectable, and a dilated ureter can be followed to the level of obstruction. A distended ureter is easily differentiated from bowel, lymph nodes and blood vessel. This is not always possible with CT scanning if the kidneys do not excrete properly. NMR accurately distinguishes between solid tumor and renal cysts, sinus lipomatosis, and peripelvic cysts, and promises to have a major role in the assessment of renal medical disease.

The preferred renal imaging procedures and sequences for common renal pathology are outlined in Figure 6.

SELECTED READINGS

1. Campbell's Urology, W.P. Saunders and Company, Radiology of the Urinary Tract: 1:222-345, 1981
2. Fullerton GD: Basic concepts for Nuclear Magnetic Resonance Imaging 1:39-55, 1982
3. Hirocak H, Grooks L, Sheldon P, Kaufman L: Nuclear Magnetic Resonance Imaging of the Kidney. Radiology 146:423–432, 1983
4. Seminars in Nuclear Medicine, Grune & Stratton, Update on Radionuclide Assessment of the Kidney I XII:No. 3:246–279, 1982
5. Seminars in Nuclear Medicine, Grune & Stratton, Update on Radionuclide Assessment of the Kidney II XII:No. 4:308–386, 1982

William P Argy
Robert C Mackow

4

Acute Nephritic Syndrome

DEFINITION AND BACKGROUND

Acute nephritic syndrome is a constellation of signs and symptoms (Table 1) principally characterized by the presence of red blood cells, red blood cell casts and hemoglobin casts in the urinary sediment. Granular casts and other cellular elements may or may not be present. This describes a typical "nephritic" urine sediment. However, proteinuria is usually present and the patient is often oliguric. There is usually evidence of decreased glomerular filtration manifested by increased SUN and creatinine and frequently anemia, hypertension and at times pulmonary vascular congestion or frank pulmonary edema. The proteinuria is nonselective, i.e., less than 95% albumin and basically reflects high glomerular permeability to serum proteins. It is usually less than 2 g/24 hrs although on a given urine specimen it might be quite high. The patient is "protected" from high levels of protein loss by low output of urine.

Various etiologies of nephritic syndrome exist (Table 2). The prototype is post-streptococcal glomerulonephritis although other types of post-infectious glomerulonephritis occur, e.g., the nephritis associated with infectious endocarditis, shunt nephritis as seen with infected ventricular-atrial shunts constructed in the treatment of hydrocephalus, and staphylococcal osteomylitis. Other causes of nephritic syndrome include the idiopathic form of rapidly progressive glomerulonephritis and the antiglomerular basement membrane type of Goodpasture's Syndrome. Certain forms of collagen vascular diseases such as systemic lupus erythematosus and other types of systemic necrotizing vasculitis* may present as nephritic syndrome. Additionally Henoch Schöenlein purpura, a type of vasculitis, and acute hemolytic uremic syndrome often present in this manner.

Occasionally, other glomerulopathies associated with multi-system diseases such as mixed cryoglobulinemia or unassociated with multisystemic disease such as IgA nephropathy and membrano-proliferative glomerulonephritis manifest as the nephritic syndrome.

FEATURES

The features of nephritic syndrome will vary depending on the cause. Accordingly, the varying presentations will only be outlined here for purposes of differential diagnosis.

---

*Systemic necrotizing vasculitis (SNV) is subcategorized by various authors according to the size of the vessels that are pathologically involved. Types of SNV include polyarteritis nodosa of Churg & Strauss, SNV overlap, hypersensitivy angiitis, Wegener's granulomatosis and lymphomatoid granulomatosis.

Table 4-1 Nephritic Syndrome

—RBC, RBC casts, hemoglobin casts
—proteinuria
—increased creatinine and urea nitrogen
—oliguria
—anemia
—hypertension

Post-streptococcal   Glomerulonephritis.
The classical cause of nephritic syndrome is post-streptococcal glomerulonephritis. This presents 2–3 weeks after infection with a nephritogenic strain of streptococcus. It must be remembered that such an infection may be in the skin as well as the pharynx, particularly in warmer climates. Penetration of the disease is 20–50% after infection with a nephritogenic streptococcus. There is no convincing evidence that treatment of streptococcal infection prevents the occurrence of glomerulonephritis, however, screening and prophylatic antibiotic therapy for infected close-contacts should be considered. The patient usually comes to medical attention because of the presence of scanty amounts of smokey or tea colored urine. The sediment contains the "nephritic" elements mentioned above. These patients have salt and water retention due to decreased glomerular filtration and rather normal tubular function, hence, may present with edema in dependent areas and also in the periorbital region. Hypertension and/or pulmonary edema may also be present as a manifestation of volume overload. This does not necessarily imply intrinsic myocardial disease. Anemia in the acute stages is largely dilutional. Proteinuria generally occurs in amounts less than 2 g/day.

Oliguria usually persists for days to a few weeks followed by a diuretic phase. As the latter ensues, the other manifestations of nephritis tend to resolve. The urine sediment may continue to contain nephritic elements for a lengthy period of time, sometimes up to two years. Important to the prognosis of the disease is the res-

Table 4-2 Differential Diagnosis

Post-streptococcal glomerulonephritis
Rapidly progressive (crescentic) glomerulonephritis
Collagen vascular disease
Hemolytic uremic syndrome

olution of proteinuria. The persistence of proteinuria beyond two months after the acute phase is indicative of nonresolution of the acute nephritis. The prognosis for complete resolution in the younger patient is better than that of the older patient. Some few patients remain tightly oliguric with decreased glomerular filtration rate and will require renal replacement therapy, as will be discussed below.

The other forms of post-infectious glomerulonephritis may be diagnosed from their clinical setting. For a patient with a ventricular-atrial shunt in situ, who presents with a nephritic sediment in renal failure, the culprit is usually obvious. Improvement may occur with treatment of the bacterial infection.

Likewise, in the setting of valvular heart disease, positive blood cultures, increased Westergren Sedimentation rate, leucocytosis and echocardiography positive for valvular vegetations, the diagnosis of infective endocarditis is obvious. Thus, a nephritic sediment should make one think of the "post-infectious" type of glomerulonephritis associated with endocarditis. This may lead to fulminant glomerulonephritis with the presence of epithelial cresents in the kidney and tight oliguria. However, glomerulonephritis associated with endocarditis is probably very common and mild forms of "post-infectious" glomerulonephritis related to bacterial endocarditis may respond to appropriate antibiotic treatment.

RAPIDLY PROGRESSIVE GLOMERULONEPHRITIS (CRESCENTIC)

Rapidly progressive glomerulonephritis can be considered as a separate clinical entity characterized frequently by a "flu-like" prodrome followed by rapidly deteriorating renal function, oliguria, a nephritic urine sediment, volume overload and hypertension. Some cases presenting like this can be related to prior streptococcal infection. Most, however, are idiopathic. The hallmark on renal biopsy is the presence of epithelial crescents involving most glomeruli. The crescents arise from vascular leakage of fibrin and other serum proteins and a cellular proliferative reaction within the glomerular space. In a sizable series from our institution, rapidly progressive glomerulonephritis with oliguria secondary to streptococcal infection carries a better prognosis for return of kidney function than the idiopathic variety.

Treatment of both of these lesions is largely experimental at present. The efficacy of steroids and cytotoxic drugs as well as plasma exchange therapy is of unproven value.

The clinical presentation of rapidly progressive glomerulonephritis with concomitant pulmonary hemorrhage is called Goodpasture's Syndrome.* Circulating antibodies to glomerular basement membrane cause a variety of Goodpasture's Syndrome called, not surprisingly, "anti-glomerular basement membrane" (anti-GBM) disease. The renal presentation most frequently is the nephritic syndrome. Treatment remains controversial although steroids, cytotoxic agents, and plasma exchange therapy have been used with varying degrees of reported efficacy. The reader is referred to chapter 13 for details. Morbidity and mortality from the pulmonary complications are high even with careful management of renal insufficiency.

COLLAGEN VASCULAR DISEASE

Systemic lupus erythematosis (SLE) often presents as nephritis accompanied by other organ manifestations of lupus. The presentation varies but patients commonly show nephritic syndrome after several months of nonrenal manifestations of their disease. However, occasionally one presents predominantly with lupus nephritis as the sole manifestation of SLE. Although patients with SLE may have blood elements in their urine from time to time, a nephritic sediment in the setting of oliguria and decreased renal function is frequently a part of the more serious form of lupus nephropathology that may be amenable to therapy with corticosteroids and/or immunosuppressive drugs. Severe, difficult to control hypertension may be indicative of severe lupus glomerulonephritis, but the correlation of clinical presentation with pathology and prog-

nosis is not always clear. Accordingly, study of renal tissue by biopsy is indicated. For a patient presenting with nephritic syndrome and few systemic manifestations of SLE, the diagnosis can be made by serologic parameters including fluorescent antinuclear antibody titer, antibody titer against native double stranded DNA and decreased serum complement activity. On the other hand, in the patient with the history of positive serologies, arthralgias, alopecia, or other peripheral manifestations of SLE who presents with smokey colored urine and nephritic sediment, the diagnosis is more obvious.

The clinical syndromes associated with SNV (supra vide) may also have nephritic syndrome as part of their presentations. Vasculitis is an inflammatory lesion of small or medium size blood vessels in different organs and as such can manifest with systemic symptoms depending on organ and size of vessel involvement. Clinical manifestations vary, e.g., hypertension is more common with classical polyarteritis than with hypersensitivity angiitis. Hypertension when present is of the high renin variety and pathophysiologically is quite different from the volume overload and low renin state which occurs with the forementioned post-streptococcal glomerulonephritis. Since vasculitis is basically a necrotizing vasculopathy of the glomerular or preglomerular architecture, very frequently the findings on renal biopsy are nonspecific with necrotic changes seen in renal tissue. Findings must be taken in the context of the systemic symptom complex to "pigeon hole" the specific vasculitis syndrome. This becomes more important in terms of specific tailored therapy with immunosuppressive drugs.

HEMOLYTIC UREMIC SYNDROME

Hemolytic uremic syndrome may present with the characteristics of nephritic syndrome. The adult form is seen in four settings: a) idiopathic which may occur following a viral gastroenteritis-like prodrome, b) associated with parturition, c) a few weeks after parturition and d) associated with certain adenocarcinomas. The post-parturition variety carries a particularly ominous prognosis for long term renal dysfunction whereas that associated with parturition may resolve completely. At our institution, the he-

---

*We prefer to call Goodpasture's Syndrome any type of Glomerulonephritis associated with pulmonary hemorrhage. This would include anti-glomerular basement membrane disease, systemic lupus erythematosus with nephritis, Wegener's granulomatosis, etc.

molytic uremic syndrome associated with adenocarcinoma seems to occur most commonly with gastric or colonic adenocarcinoma after treatment with mitomycin C.

The hemolytic uremic syndrome is characterized by an acute course and by evidence of microangiopathy, intravascular coagulation, oliguria and frequently hypertension. There is also evidence of multiple organ system involvement. Intravascular coagulation is seen on renal biopsy in the small arteries and even glomerular arterioles and is accompanied by arterial intimal hyperplasia. Treatment with steroids, in some cases, has been beneficial. The value of anticoagulation is questionable. In some cases prostacyclin infusion, plasma infusion, or plasma exchange therapy, is beneficial.

LABORATORY

Laboratory values of concern are outlined in Table 3. In the nephritic syndrome, glomerular filtration rate is decreased as evidenced by a rise in serum creatinine and SUN. It must be remembered that creatinine clearance measured by a timed urine collection is not a valid estimate of renal function when the serum creatinine is rapidly rising. Creatinine clearances are best performed when the concentrations of serum creatinine are constant—not when they are rising rapidly from changes in production and/or excretion. In the case of glomerular injury from immunological processes, the level of total hemolytic complement may be depressed as is C_3*. Changes in complement activity are transient in post-infectious glomerulonephritis. Measurement of changing antibody titers to components of the streptococcus bacterium such as anti-streptolysin O, anti-hyaluronidase or anti-DNA'ase can be helpful, although these markers can be altered by antibiotic therapy.

The urinalysis is obviously important. The spun urine sediment may contain granular, hyaline or waxy casts, but the nephritic elements are the hallmark: red blood cells, red blood cell

---

*The hypocomplementemic nephritities include those associated with post-streptococcal glomerulonephritis, infective endocarditis, shunt nephritis, SLE, membranoproliferative glomerulonephritis, and cryoglobulinemia.

Table 4-3 Laboratory Values of Concern

Creatinine
Serum urea nitrogen
Complement
ASLO Titer
Antihyaluronidase titer
Urinalysis

casts or hemoglobin casts. The diagnostic import of the nephritic elements are great enough that the sediment should always be examined by the physician. The usual method of performing a urinalysis may be changed in an attempt to collect more cellular cast elements. To accomplish this, one may: a) centrifuge 10 ml of urine in the usual fashion, b) carefully decant the supernate until the pellet of sediment is nearly dry, c) carefully aspirate the pellet and d) place on a glass slide with a cover slip. It is of importance to use a freshly voided urine, i.e., less than two hours old. Proteinuria is usually present in a nephritic syndrome but is less than 2 g/24 h. In a given voided specimen it may be up to 4+; but because of oliguria, net excretion is not great.

In most cases of rapidly progressive glomerulonephritis, complement, including C_3, is normal. However, C_3 is often depressed and may remain so for along periods of time in the glomerulonephritis associated with systemic lupus erythematosus, cryoglobulinemia or membranoproliferative glomerulonephritis. In systemic lupus erythematosus one finds depression not just in C_3 but of the earlier components such as Clq and C_4. See chapter 13 for greater details.

Serum complement is usually not depressed in the systemic necrotizing vasculitities, unless cryoglobulinemia is present. In all forms of vasculitis with nephritic syndrome, the urinalysis is similar to that of post-infections glomerulonephritis.

Complement depression is not a prominent feature of hemolytic uremic syndrome. Rather, evidence of microangiopathy including fragmented cells on peripheral blood smears, fibrin split products in the urine, frequently depressed levels of fibrinogen and varying degrees of prolongation of the protime and partial prothromboplastin time are seen. The urine shows the nephritic features mentioned above.

PATHOLOGY

The nephritic syndrome is a manifestation of decreased glomerular filtration and glomerular or vascular immune-mediated inflammatory disease. Specific or nonspecific histopathology may be found. One must combine the clinical picture with the various findings on light, immunofluorescent and electron-microscopy to arrive at the diagnosis.

In the case of post-infectious glomerulonephritis, large subepithelial immune complexes are seen in the glomerulus which stain for immune globulin, predominently IgG as well as complement. A proliferative cellular response of endothelial and mesangial cells occurs with evidence of infiltration of the glomerulus with white blood cells.

In the fulminant form of post-infectious glomerulonephritis and other forms of rapidly progressive glomerulonephritis, the predominant lesion is the proliferative epithelial cell crescent. Some have postulated that this cellular reaction occurs from release of fibrin into Bowman's space. The normal architecture of the glomerulus is distorted by the expanding crescent. In the form of rapidly progressive glomerulonephritis associated with antiglomerular basement membrane antibody, the basement membrane of the glomerulus shows a smooth linear pattern on immunofluorescent microscopy. Commonly, but not always, this lesion is associated with pulmonary hemorrhage.

In systemic lupus erythematosus, finer deposits are present in a mesangial distribution. They frequently are seen in the subendothelial area of the capillary wall. Immune globulins can be identified which are usually IgG and IgA along with complement. Glomerular proliferative response is variable. Usually with nephritic syndrome, proliferation of mesangial and endothelial cells predominates and at times epithelial cell crescents are present.

In hemolytic uremic syndrome, intra-arterial and arteriolar thrombi are present with necrosis of glomeruli. Proliferation of the intima of small arteries may be present.

TREATMENT

Specific treatment for the causes of nephritic syndrome are mentioned above and are

Table 4-4   Treatment

—Supportive
—Treat hypertension
—Limit protein and adjust sodium and potassium intake
—Dialysis when indicted

detailed in other chapters. General treatment should be supportive and directed at volume overload, hypertension, and uremia (Table 4).

The primary functional deficit in nephritic syndrome is a decreased glomerular filtration rate. Tubular function is generally intact. Some patients may have concentrated urine and low urine sodium. The uses of moderate doses of loop diuretics, e.g. furosemide, up to 300 mg* in a given dose, may be efficacious in the treatment of excess volume. The need to treat excessive volume acutely is a function of the cardiovascular status of the patient. Clearly, in a patient evidencing incipient pulmonary edema, one is more pressed to treat volume than with simple peripheral edema.

Hypertension may respond to volume contraction, but if not controlled well, antihypertensive agents are warranted.

Finally, the patient's renal failure should be appropriately treated. This includes restriction of fluid intake to net loss plus 5 ml/kg/day as insensible loss. In addition, there should be dietary restriction of sodium, potassium and protein. In a nondialyzed, oliguric patient whose renal function is deteriorating, a diet containing 25 mEq Na, 25 mEq K, and 25 g of protein may be appropriate. Such a diet can be given in parenteral fluid therapy if the patient cannot take feedings by mouth. Such a restrictive diet, however, is difficulty to maintain for long periods and could easily lead to protein-calorie malnutrition. In some types of nephritic syndrome, the period of oliguria is short. In contrast dialytic treatment of volume overload, electrolyte imbalance and uremia becomes necessary in many patients. Emergency dialysis is indicated for pulmonary edema, severe hyperkalemia and severe acidosis. Although not as pressed clinically, the uremic patient generally should be di-

---

*Large doses should be infused slowly to avoid ototoxicity.

alyzed at a serum creatinine of approximately 10 mg/dl or when symptomatic aspects of uremia such as nausea, vomiting and somnolence are evident.

SELECTED READINGS

1. Cameron JS. The national history of glomerulonephritis. In: Black DAK (ed) Renal Disease, 3rd Edition, Blackwell Scientific Publications, Ltd., Oxford pp. 295–337

2. Lien JWK, Mathew TH, Meadows R. Acute poststreptococcal glomerulonephritis in adults—a long term study. QJ Med 48:00, 1979

3. Newgarten J, Baldwin DS. Glomerulonephritis in bacterial endocarditis. Am J Med 77:297, 1984

4. Briggs WA, Johnson JP, Teichman S, Yeager HD, Wilson CB. Antiglomerular basement membrane antibody—mediated glomerulonephritis and Goodpasture's Syndrome. Medicine 58:348, 1979

5. Peters DK, Rees AJ, Lockwood CM, Pusey CD. Treatment and prognosis in antibasement membrane antibody mediated nephritis. Transplant Proc 14:(3):513, 1982

6. Glassock RJ, Cohen AH, Bennett CM, Martinez-Maldonado M. Primary Glomerular Diseases. In: Brenner BM, Rector FC, Jr. (eds), The Kidney, Philadelphia, WB Saunders, 1981, pp. 1351–1492

7. Glassock RJ, Cohen AH, Secondary Glomerular Diseases. In: Brenner BM, Rector FC, Jr., (eds), The Kidney, Philadelphia, WB Saunders, 1981, 1493–1570

8. Fauci AS, Haynes BF, Katz P. The spectrum of vasculitis: clinical, pathologic, immunologic, and therapeutic considerations. Ann Intern Med 89:660, 1978

9. Madaio MP, Harrington JT. Current concepts: The diagnosis of acute glomerulonephritis. N Engl J Med 309:1299, 1983

10. Felson DT, Anderson J. Evidence for the superiority of immuno-suppressive drugs and prednisone over prednisone alone in lupus nephritis. N Engl J Med, 311:1528, 1984

Jack Moore, Jr., M.D.
John P. Johnson, M.D.

5

Acute Renal Failure

INTRODUCTION

Acute renal failure (ARF) is a clinical syndrome of diverse etiologies. It is characterized by a sudden decline in renal function as assessed by glomerular filtration rate (GFR), is clinically manifested by rising concentrations of blood urea nitrogen (BUN) and creatinine, and is frequently associated with decreased urinary output. The purpose of this chapter is to provide the reader with a stepwise approach to the differential diagnosis and management of clinical ARF. As do many others, we advocate an initial clinical evaluation aimed at distinguishing between prerenal, post-renal, and intrinsic renal causes of ARF. A list of the major causes of ARF based on such a mechanistic approach is given in Table 1.

It is apparent that the differential diagnosis of this syndrome involves consideration of a wide variety of possible etiologies. It is the clinician's task to orchestrate the findings of history and physical examination, in conjunction with laboratory and imaging data, so as to strive at a reasonable diagnosis. Surprisingly, in view of the breadth of the differential diagnosis and the acute nature of the problem, this can usually be accomplished. Accurate diagnosis is important, as accurate therapy is dependent upon it. Although the majority of hospital-acquired ARF

may require only supportive care, most forms of pre-renal and post-renal failure require specific interventions which may result in dramatic resolution of the clinical syndrome. Moreover, some forms of intrinsic ARF may benefit from specific therapy directed at the underlying disease, as in rapidly progressive glomerulonephritis, or an alteration in current therapy, as in allergic interstitial nephritis. It is beyond the scope of this chapter to discuss all the entities in Table 1 in any detail, thus we will focus primarily upon the process of differential diagnosis and the general principles of the management of the patient with hospital-acquired ARF.

Scope of ARF

The incidence of ARF in the general population is not well described. In hospitalized patients the incidence ranges between 1–5%. This indicates ARF is a relatively common disorder in these patients, and highlights the fact that in many cases, ARF occurs as a complication of other serious medical disorders. As such, it is an ominous prognostic factor, and is associated with excessive morbidity and a high mortality. Mortality from ARF varies significantly depending upon etiology, thus accurate diagnosis has prognostic as well as therapeutic implications.

The mortality of ischemic ARF, often called acute tubular necrosis (ATN), in trauma patients or patients with medical or surgical illness—associated shock, is around 60%. There has been no substantial reduction in this mortality in re-

---

The opinions of the authors are not official, and are not to be construed as representing the official views of the Department of the Army or the Department of Defense.

cent years, even with the evolution of more effective forms of dialytic therapy. In post-partum
ARF or ARF due to nephrotoxic injury, as with
radiocontrast or antibiotics, the mortality is much
lower, ranging from 2–15%. Those forms of ARF
associated with substantial urine output (non-
oliguria) are associated with a more favorable
survival rate than oliguric forms. The explanation for this is uncertain, but may reflect less
severe injury conferred by toxins compared to
ischemia, or that non-oliguric patients' fluid
balance and nutrition is easier to manage.

Pathogenesis

The pathogenesis of ATN, referring to
ischemic or nephrotoxic forms of intrinsic ARF,
is not well understood, but is the subject of considerable experimental study. In most all experimental models, both renal blood flow and
GFR decline early after the initial insult. This
period, lasting from hours to days, is termed the
initiation phase. Gradually, renal blood flow returns towards normal, while GFR remains depressed. This is called the maintenance phase.
The degree of renal failure which results is variable, and depends upon the nature and severity
of the insult. Over days to weeks, renal function
returns towards normal as the kidney repairs or
regenerates. In clinical ARF, recovery occurs
after two to three weeks unless the patient suc-
cumbs to uremia or other complications. The
reason for the persistent high mortality of ARF,
despite seemingly adequate dialytic support, is
not clear. To some degree this reflects the se-
riousness of comorbid medical conditions, but
the presence of ARF itself seems to be a poor
prognostic factor.

Some experimentalists feel that the course
of ATN may be modified during the initiation
phase by using vasodilators to improve renal
blood flow or diuretics to establish a solute diuresis. Results of such maneuvers have been
variable and inconsistent, as have such maneuvers when attempted in the clinical setting, possibly because it is difficult to distinguish between the initiation and maintenance phases of
ATN clinically, thus salutary efforts may have
been made too late. It is generally agreed that
there is no currently available method of re-
versing established ATN, although efforts directed towards improving renal cellular metabolism or minimizing oxidative damage to

Table 5–1   Causes of Acute Renal Failure

I. Pre-renal Failure
  A. Hypovolemia
  B. Cardiovascular failure
    1. myocardial failure
    2. vascular pooling
  C. Inadequate plasma oncotic pressure
    1. nephrotic syndrome
    2. cirrhosis and hepatorenal syndrome

II. Vascular Obstruction
  A. Arterial obstruction
    1. renal artery emboli
    2. atheroembolic renal disease
  B. Venous obstruction

III. Intrinsic Renal Disease
  A. Glomerulonephritis
  B. Tubulointerstitial nephritis
  C. Acute presentation of chronic renal failure
  D. Intrinsic acute renal failure
    1. Ischemic
      a. hemorrhagic hypotension
      b. severe volume depletion
      c. surgical aortic cross-clamping
      d. cardiac and biliary surgery
      e. defective cardiac output
      f. crush syndrome and other trauma
      g. septic shock
      i. pregnancy
      j. pancreatitis
    2. Nephrotoxic
      a. antibiotics
      b. heavy metals
      c. endogenous pigments: hemoglobin,
        myoglobin
      d. radiographic contrast agents
      e. drugs
      f. organic solvents
      h. fungicides and pesticides
      i. uric acid
      j. ethylene glycol and methanol

IV. Post-renal Failure
  A. Urinary bladder obstruction
  B. Extrinsic obstruction of the ureters
  C. Intraluminal obstruction of the ureters
  D. Retroperitoneal fibrosis

reperfused kidneys show some promise in the laboratory. In contrast, it is widely accepted that establishing a solute diuresis prior to renal insult may abort or attenuate the severity of resultant ATN. This knowledge is reflected by the use of mannitol in vascular surgery and volume repletion prior to radiocontrast studies.

Differential Diagnosis

The differential diagnosis of ARF is quite broad, as diverse conditions can result in the abrupt cessation of renal function. Structural disorders of blood vessels subserving the kidneys, inflammation of the glomeruli or tubulointerstitium, and obstruction of the kidneys may each present as ARF. Nearly all of these disorders can be rapidly excluded by a careful history, physical examination, simple renal imaging procedures, and a carefully examined urinary sediment.

The aorta or renal arteries can be occluded by dissection, thrombosis, or emboli. The two former conditions are seen often in patients with obvious evidence of atherosclerotic disease. The latter results either from dislodgement or a mural cardiac thrombus or disruption of atheromatous plaques in the aorta or renal arteries. A nuclear medicine renal blood flow study is the initial diagnostic imaging test, however, it may be non-diagnostic, and arteriography may be required. Whether to proceed to thrombolytic therapy or revascularization requires careful thought, and the patient's medical condition may dictate a conservative approach.

Acute glomerulonephritis (GN) and acute tubulointerstitial nephritis (TIN) are uncommon but important causes of ARF. If acute GN results in ARF, the presumption must be that the patient has rapidly progressive (crescentic) GN, and renal biopsy is indicated as soon as medically feasible. The urinary sediment examination is crucial to the accurate and rapid diagnosis of these disorders, as it will commonly demonstrate cellular casts, including red cell and/or white cell casts. Acute TIN often results from drug injury, in which case, eosinophiluria is an important clue.

ARF can occasionally be the mode of presentation of long-standing chronic renal disease, particularly when the patient has had little medical care. In this condition, the urinary sediment may reveal proteinuria and cylinduria, particularly broad, waxy casts. Renal ultrasound demonstrates small, shrunken kidneys, and other tests, including biopsy, are seldom helpful.

Notwithstanding the diagnostic considerations above, operationally, the major diagnostic decision is to determine whether the patient has intrinsic renal failure, usually from an ischemic or nephrotoxic insult, or whether renal function has been affected by inadequate delivery of blood to the kidney or obstruction of the urinary tract. When renal function can resume if blood flow were restored, the patient is said to have "prerenal azotemia." Similarly, if renal function can resume if the urinary tract were unobstructed, the patient is said to have "post-renal" azotemia. If either of these processes is allowed to continue untreated, the kidneys may be subject to ischemic injury of sufficient severity that renal function remains depressed even when the insult is removed. These patients have established ARF.

Pre-renal azotemia results from an absolute or relative deficiency of blood volume, so that renal blood flow is substantially reduced. An absolute reduction in blood volume is often seen as a consequence of renal salt loss from excessive diuretic therapy, from vomiting, overt blood loss, or sequestration of extracellular volume as in hemorrhagic pancreatitis. A relative reduction in blood volume may occur when there is inadequate plasma oncotic pressure to maintain effective blood volume, as in nephrosis or cirrhosis, or when cardiac function is insufficient to provide for effective renal perfusion.

Post-renal azotemia results from obstruction, at any level, of the urinary tract. Bladder outlet obstruction from prostatic hypertrophy is the most common cause of this condition in men, while pelvic cancer accounts for most cases in females. The kidneys may be intrinsically obstructed by infilterative processes, or may be obstructed along the course of the ureters by tumor or retroperitoneal fibrosis from drugs or as a result of a leaking aortic aneurysm. Finally, renal calculi can be bilateral and cause obstruction or the patient may only have a single kidney. It is important to recognize that ARF rarely results from an insult to a single kidney if another kidney is present and normal. In the vast majority of cases, renal ultrasound is both highly sensitive and specific for obstruction. With retroperitoneal fibrosis and intrarenal obstruction from infiltrative disorders, the ultrasound may be non-diagnostic, thus computerized tomography or retrograde ureterography may be required.

Diagnostic Assessment

The history, physical examination, basic laboratory information, and the microscopic and biochemical analysis of the urine are the mainstays of the evaluation of the patient with ARF. Review of the complete medical record, including flow sheets and nurses' notes is essential, particularly in hospital-acquired ARF.

The history may suggest recent hypotension, either profound or subtle, but sufficient to cause decreased renal profusion. Such hypotension may be associated with overt or covert volume losses, as with bleeding, or from excessive diuretic therapy or decompensated cardiac function, respectively. A history of drug therapy is also important, as many drugs, particularly antibiotics and non-steroidal anti-inflammatory agents, may cause nephrotoxic injury alone, or commonly in concert with decreased renal perfusion.

Patients with ARF have few symptoms and signs which contribute to establishing the diagnosis except those related to the causative disorder. Symptoms are related to the rapidity of onset and severity of dysfunction, and the patient's underlying condition. Azotemia, hyperkalemia, and acidemia are often asymptomatic unless the patient is very catabolic. Many patients quickly have symptoms of volume overload, which may reflect aggressive fluid therapy. Urine volume is an important sign, as anuria (≤ 100 ml/d) is common in vascular catastrophes or complete obstruction, while polyuria (≥ 1 liter/d) is characteristic of nephrotoxic injury. Since ischemic injury is operative in most patients with ARF, oliguria (≤ 400 ml/d) is usual.

The physical examination should primarily focus on the questions of whether the patient is in a state of volume depletion or volume overload, or obstructed. Crucial elements of the examination include skin turgor, the cardiac and pulmonary exam, edema, and genitourinary examination as keys to these important questions. Accurate weights, blood pressure assessment for orthostatic hypotension, and proof of a properly draining urinary tract are essential.

The concentrations of blood urea nitrogen (BUN) and creatinine increase steadily during the course of ARF as production remains relatively constant while excretion is profoundly diminished. Daily increments of BUN and creatinine average 20–30 mg/dl and 1.3–1.5 mg/dl, respectively. More rapid incremental changes in the BUN may reflect excessive catabolism or gastrointestinal hemorrhage, while excessive increments in the serum creatinine often reflect muscle necrosis (rhabdomyolysis). Metabolic acidosis results from retention of endogenously produced acid, thus the serum bicarbonate concentration averages 17–18 meq/L in uncomplicated cases. Hyperkalemia (5.0–6.0 meq/L) may result from limited excretion and acidemia. Hyperphosphatemia occurs since phosphate excretion is negligible. This, in conjunction with inhibition of the gastrointestinal effects of Vitamin D, leads to hypocalcemia. The hematocrit falls over 5–7 days to a level of 23–27%, and may reflect volume overload, blood loss, and bone marrow supression.

Examination of the urine is extremely important in patients with ARF, since it may provide evidence of pre-renal or post-renal azotemia, or support the diagnosis of established ARF. The information gleaned from the urine is so critical that the physician should examine it personally.

The patient with pre-renal azotemia should have a concentrated urine with high urine to plasma ratios of urea, creatinine, and osmolality, and a low urinary sodium concentration. Similar values are found in patients with acute urinary obstruction. The patient with established ARF usually loses concentrating ability and the ability to conserve urinary sodium, with low urinary to plasma ratios of solute and high urinary sodium concentrations. Similar values are found in patients with ARF from chronic obstruction of the urinary tract. Indices of renal function such as the fractional excretion of sodium and the renal failure index are manipulations of these basic data, which should be interpreted cautiously if the patient has received diuretics in the 12–18 hours prior to their measurement. Nonetheless, biochemical analyses of urine accurately distinguish between pre- and post-renal failure in nearly 90% of cases.

The urine sediment is unremarkable in pre- and post-renal azotemia, and contains hyaline, and rarely, granular casts. Hematuria may be present if a catheter is in place. Conversely, the sediment in ARF demonstrates many granular casts, and most importantly, renal tubular epithelial cells and other cellular debris, giving rise to a very "dirty" sediment. Experienced observers distinguish between pre- or post-renal failure and established ARF on the basis of the sediment in 85–90% of cases.

Imaging of the kidneys in patients with ARF should be limited to those studies which demonstrate whether there are two kidneys, whether there are calculi, and whether the urinary tract is obstructed. In our view the imaging test of choice is a technically well-done renal ultrasound. Plain films of the abdomen are often not helpful, and contrast procedures can be quite harmful. The nuclear scan should be reserved for anuric patients in whom arterial catastrophe is suspected.

Collectively, the history, physical examination, biochemical analysis of serum and urine, urinalysis, and renal ultrasound provide the necessary information needed by the clinician to determine whether the patient truly has established ARF or whether there is a readily reversible cause of acute renal dysfunction. At times the volume status of the patient is difficult to assess, and measurement of central venous pressure or pulmonary capillary wedge pressure is necessary. In our judgment these procedures are both over-utilized and time-consuming, and may often delay fluid resuscitation with perpetuation of renal ischemia.

Repetitive small challenges of isotonic saline, with close clinical assessment of effect, are often simultaneously diagnostic and therapeutic. In the pre-renal azotemia patient who is clinically volume depleted, fluid therapy with saline or blood may restore renal function. Similarly, improvement in cardiac function if heart failure is present may achieve the same result. Drainage of the urinary tract must be adequate in obstructed patients.

The use of diuretics and vasoactive hormones is widespread, but efficacy is lacking. The use of diuretics such as furosemide can be harmful if the patient is volume depleted. However, we believe that furosemide, if administered to euvolemic patients early in the course of ARF, may make oliguric patients non-oliguric and assist in their subsequent management. We administer graded doses of 1, 5, and 10 mg/kg of furosemide at hourly intervals over three-four hours to clearly euvolemic patients; restoration of urine output at any dose obviates further doses. Low-dose dopamine (1–3 mcg/kg/min) will promote urine flow in some patients, even without affecting systemic arterial pressure.

The use of mannitol prior to procedures associated with the development of ARF is widespread, and is probably efficacious in vascular surgical procedures. We advocate the use of isotonic bicarbonate and 100 ml of 20% mannitol in the fluid resuscitation of patients in whom ARF is due to rhabdomyolysis. There are no data of which we are aware which demonstrate that furosemide or dopamine have attenuated the mortality of established ARF.

TREATMENT OF ESTABLISHED ACUTE RENAL FAILURE

The fundamental assumption made in the treatment of ARF is that injured kidneys can recover. The major goal of therapy is to support the patient until this occurs. A secondary goal is to provide the proper metabolic milieu in which the patient can maintain adequate nutrition and resistance to infection, which is by far the major cause of death in ARF. To these ends, the assistance of experts in nutritional care and infectious diseases is critical in the management of these patients.

Some patients with ARF, particularly those who remain nonoliguric and in whom catabolism is not excessive, can be treated with fluid and protein restriction, in conjunction with adequate caloric support. Hyperkalemia can be controlled with exchange resins, glucose and insulin, and bicarbonate. The patient must be closely managed, however, and attention to routine details of patient care requires considerable effort. Moreover, the severity of renal dysfunction may limit the quantity and quality of nutritional support, with resultant catabolism of an unacceptable severity.

Dialytic support is required in many patients with ARF, and in our experience, is often required for a volume indication more so than for relief of symptoms of uremia. Generally accepted indications for dialysis include metabolic acidemia, hyperkalemia, hypercatabolic ARF, severe azotemia, volume overload, and uremia. Most nephrologists institute dialysis when the BUN and creatinine reach 110–130 mg/dl and 8–10 mg/dl, respectively.

Hemodialysis is widely available, and can be conducted with acceptable morbidity. Angioaccess is achieved with percutaneous catheters, and anticoagulation regimens are associated with minimal risk of bleeding. The procedure is usually performed on alternate days, although daily dialysis may be required if solute load is excessive or if required fluid volume administration results in volume overload.

Peritoneal dialysis, particularly if conducted with automatic cycling machines, offers similar efficacy without the risks of hypotension and bleeding which sometimes occur with hemodialysis. Additionally, peritoneal dialysis can be performed without the highly trained technical personnel needed for hemodialysis.

Recently artificial membranes have been made available which are sufficiently permeable to make fluid removal rates in excess of 1.5 L/hour possible. The membranes perform adequately at blood flow rates of 60 ml/min, and thus do not require flow augmentation with a blood pump. When connected to an artery and vein by means of special catheters, a functioning circuit is achieved with minimal cardiovascular stress. If the filter is used solely to remove fluid, the procedure is known as slow continuous ultrafiltration (SCUF). Pressure can be applied across the membrane to augment fluid removal, and the patient can receive sufficient quantities of electrolyte solution so that the con-

centrations of BUN and creatinine can be lowered. When conducted in this fashion, the procedure is known as hemofiltration. Operationally, the membrane is utilized continuously for several days. In our view its major use is in the patient who requires several liters of parenteral nutrition and antibiotic therapy each day. When used in this manner, volume overload is controlled. In many patients solute removal needs are sufficiently minimal, and the major personnel requirements of frequent hemodialysis are avoided.

SUMMARY

Properly managed, the mortality of ARF ranges from 2–65%, with higher mortalities being related to post-operative or traumatic ARF, underlying age and comorbidity, and infection. Patients rarely die of renal failure, but instead, die of their underlying disease or infection. The high mortality of ARF, persistent despite putatively adequate renal replacement therapy, suggests that future therapeutic success may depend upon advances in fighting infectious diseases, nutritional support, and in prophylactic measures effective in decreasing the incidence and/or severity of ARF.

Harry G. Preuss
Steven J. Zelman

6

Chronic Renal Failure

DEFINITION AND BACKGROUND

When the kidneys are no longer able to maintain a normal internal environment due to a persistent, gradual impairment of glomerular and tubular function, CHRONIC RENAL FAILURE, one of the major syndromes seen in Nephrology, ensues. Chronic renal failure may arise from any number of disorders which lead to severe renal parenchymal damage. Common etiologies are listed in Table 1. Since the onset of chronic renal failure is gradual, many clinicians divide the functional deterioration into four stages:

1. *Diminished Renal Reserve:* There is mild or modest reduction in function such that a normal or near normal internal environment is still maintained.
2. *Renal Insufficiency:* Some evidence of impaired capacity to maintain the internal environment appears, i.e., slight azotemia, impaired concentrating ability and perhaps mild anemia.
3. *Renal Failure:* A chronic and persistent perturbation of the internal environment is obvious.
4. *Uremia:* A number of different signs and symptoms appear that develop in the patient with renal insufficiency (see below).

DIAGNOSTIC EVALUATION

The physician responsible for the care of a patient with chronic renal failure should evalu-

ate, a) the nature of the renal disease, b) the extent of the disease, c) the existence of aggravating factors, and d) the type and magnitude of associated medical problems. Reversible factors that aggravate the chronic renal failure should always be sought. (Common reversible factors are listed in Table 2).

The diagnostic evaluation of the persistently azotemic patient is outlined in Table 3.

History. The history should include risk factors for renal disease, urinary tract symptoms, systemic diseases, and the patient's medications and analgesics. The family history may suggest a hereditary disorder and should include inquiries about renal disease, hypertension, gout, collagen diseases and deafness.

Physical examination. Of particular importance in the physical examination of the renal patient is the detection of cachexia, hypertension, extracellular fluid volume expansion, muscular atrophy, neuropathy, pruritis; an ammonia odor to the breath, and abnormalities of skin color or texture. The physician should always search for signs of an underlying renal or systemic disease.

Urinalysis. The physician may consider examining the urine for the presence of proteinuria, urinary sediment, abnormalities in renal acidification and concentrating ability. A urinary culture may be necessary.

Laboratory evaluation. In addition to the urinalysis, a measurement of renal function

Table 6-1 Common Etiologies of Chronic Renal Failure

I. Glomerular Diseases
  1. Focal glomerulosclerosis
  2. Membranous glomerulopathy
  3. Proliferative glomerulonephritis
    a. Acute post-streptococcal glomerulonephritis
    b. Membrano-proliferative glomerulonephritis
    c. Bergers Disease (IgA-IgG nephropathy)
  4. Anti-glomerular basement membrane disease
  5. Crescentic Glomerulonephritis
  6. Glomerulonephritis associated with systemic diseases
    a. Connective tissue disorder
      1) systemic lupus erythematosus
      2) polyarteritis nodosa
      3) Wegener's granulomatosis
      4) scleroderma
      5) Henoch-Schoenlein purpura
    b. Disorders of coagulation
      1) toxemia of pregnancy
      2) post-partum renal failure
      3) hemolytic-uremic syndrome
      4) thrombotic thrombocytopenic purpura
    c. Metabolic disorders
      1) diabetes
      2) amyloidosis
    d. Glomerulopathies associated with malignancies
  7. Glomerulopathies in hereditary-familial diseases
    a. Hereditary nephritis (Alport's Syndrome)
    b. Fabry's disease (Angio Keratoma Corporis Diffusa)

II. Tubulo-interstitial Diseases
  A. Chronic Interstitial Nephritis
  B. Obstructive Uropathy
  C. Reflux Nephropathy
  D. Radiation Nephritis
  E. Hypersensitivity Nephritis
  F. Disorders associated with metabolic derangements
    1. Hypercalcemic nephropathy
    2. Hyperuricemic nephropathy
    3. Hypokalemic nephropathy
  G. Analgesic Nephropathy
  H. Toxic Nephropathy
    1. Heavy metals
    2. Solvents and glycols
    3. Antibiotic and other drugs

III. Cystic Renal Diseases
  A. Polycystic Kidney Disease (adult form)
  B. Medullary sponge kidney
  C. Medullary cystic disease

IV. Vascular Disease of the Kidney
  A. Nephrosclerosis
  B. Renal arterial occlusion

V. Miscellaneous Disease
  A. Displacement of Renal Parenchyma by Tumors
    1) Renal cell carcinoma
    2) Metastatic tumors
    3) Lymphoma
  B. Congenital Anomalies
  C. Partial Nephrectomy

should be obtained. This might include the SUN or serum creatinine, and perhaps a creatinine clearance (Chapter 1). As the patient is followed, serial serum creatinines or the reciprocal of the serum creatinine versus time may be useful for evaluation. Electrolytes, Ca^{++}, P, uric acid, Mg^{++}, and glucose are part of a thorough laboratory profile. The patient's blood count and hemoglobin type should be determined. A 24 hr urine collection for protein and creatinine may be indicated. Other occasionally useful tests include anti DNA-antibody, hepatitis surface B antigen, and serum complement levels. A urine immunoelectrophoresis should be obtained if myeloma is suspected. (See Chapter 1 for more details.)

Secondary diagnostic procedures. Radiographical procedures valuable when assessing

Table 6-2 Reversible Problems in Chronic Renal Failure

Pre Renal
  a) Volume Depletion
  b) Renal Artery Obstruction
  c) Cardiac Failure
  d) Hypertension

Parenchymal
  a) Nephrotoxins
  b) Infections of the Kidney
  c) Potassium, Uric Acid, Calcium Imbalances
  d) Collagen Vascular Diseases (SLE, PAN)
  e) Amyloid?, Diabetes mellitus?

Post Renal
  a) Obstruction of ureters
  b) Obstruction of urethra
  c) Renal vein thrombosis

Table 6-3 Diagnostic Evaluation of the Azotemic Patient

A. History
  1. Systemic or chronic disease
  2. Medications (analgesics, Vit D, Ca^{++})
  3. Family history
  4. Occupational exposures (lead, mercury, gold, solvents, radiocontrast dyes).

B. Physical Examination (BP, abdominal mass or bruit, low set ears, evidence of uremia).

C. Urinalysis
  1. Proteinuria
  2. Sediment
  3. Specific gravity

D. Laboratory Evaluation
  1. SUN, creatinine, creatinine clearance, log or reciprocal of creatinine plot
  2. Chemistries: Na, K, Cl, CO_2, Phos, Uric Acid, Mg, glucose
  3. Hematologic: hemoglobin, hemoglobin electrophoresis
  4. 24-hour protein excretion, urine culture
  5. Immunologic: Anti-DNA, complement, HbsAG, urine immunoelectrophoresis

E. Secondary Diagnostic Procedures
  1. Abdominal plain film
  2. IVP (caution if serum creatinine >1.8 mg/dl)
  3. Renal sonogram
  4. Voiding cystourethrogram
  5. Renal biopsy
  6. Miscellaneous procedures—bone marrow biopsy, rectal biopsy, skin biopsy.

patients with renal problems include the abdominal plain film, IVP, renal sonogram, and voiding cystourethrogram (Chapter 3). Renal, bone marrow, rectal, and skin biopsies are occasionally necessary. An early diagnosis of a renal disorder allows for the best prognosis.

CLINICAL MANIFESTATIONS

The onset of chronic uremia is usually insidious. Characteristic features include weakness, fatigability, loss of appetite, and dyspnea. Patients may appear pale and have a uriniferous breath odor. Polyuria and nocturia are common. Patients in late stages of uremia may bleed into their skin and the mucous membranes of their gastrointestinal tract. Uremic patients are often somnolent. Fluid retention may precipitate congestive heart failure.

NEUROLOGICAL MANIFESTATIONS

Peripheral neuropathy. A mixed motor and sensory peripheral neuropathy is not uncommon in patients with end-stage renal disorders. Some patients experience the "restless leg syndrome," an unpleasant feeling of movement in the limbs associated with a burning sensation. Others complain of muscle weakness and cramps. The neuropathy is more common in males than females and symmetrically involves the lower extremities more than the upper. An early sign is a prolonged nerve conduction time. The disorder may progress rather rapidly. Eventually, impaired vibratory sense and diminished deep tendon reflexes develop. Vitamin supplementation is not helpful; however, intensive hemodialysis may slow the progression of the disease. Recovery is possible following successful renal transplantation.

Encephalopathy. The central nervous system abnormalities of uremia have been attributed to uremic toxins, hyponatremia, acidosis, water intoxication, hypertension and dehydration. Early manifestations of uremic encephalopathy are usually quite subtle and include insomnia, loss of concentrating ability, lethargy and slowing of cerebration. Eventually, memory loss, confusion, hallucinations, and delirium may occur. Tremulousness may appear, followed by asterixis. A sudden, gross twitching of the muscles is a late development. Tetany is not uncommon in severe uremia and rarely responds to calcium injections. Convulsions that occur in patients with terminal uremia respond occasionally to phenytoin or phenobarbital.

CARDIOVASCULAR MANIFESTATIONS

Hypertension. About 75% of the patients with end-stage renal failure have hypertension. This may be due to accumulation of a pressor substance such as angiotensin. The impaired kidney may also not synthesize vasodepressor substances, such as prostaglandins, or may be unable to regulate the extracellular fluid volume. Hypertension due to fluid overload, can usually be controlled by potent loop diuretics or when appropriate, ultrafiltration during dialysis. Persistent hypertension may cause additional renal damage. However, vigorous diuretic therapy may cause Na^+ depletion and hasten the onset of uremia.

Pericarditis. Uremic pericarditis may appear in up to half of undialyzed patients reaching end-stage renal failure. Hemorrhagic pericarditis is also not infrequent in patients receiving maintenance hemodialysis.

Cardiovascular complications. Almost 50% of chronic dialysis patients die from myocardial infarction and other cardiovascular complications. Arteriosclerosis may be accelerated in dialysis patients by such risk factors as hypertension, hyperuricemia, hyperlipidemia, carbohydrate (CHO) intolerance, altered lipoprotein metabolism, and vascular calcification from secondary hyperparathyroidism. Most dialysis patients develop atherosclerosis. Hyperkalemia occurring in end-stage renal disease patients may precipitate various arrhythmias. Fluid overload, anemia, and hypertension may precipitate congestive heart failure.

Gastrointestinal manifestations. Patients with uremia are often anorectic with persistent nausea and vomiting. Oral ulcers and parotitis may develop as a result of high concentrations of ammonia produced during urea metabolism, mouth breathing, acidosis, and dehydration. Hiccups are frequent. Peptic ulceration is common and may, in part, be due to hypergastrinemia. This along with the bleeding tendency of uremia may account for the frequency of gastrointestinal bleeding. Atrophic gastritis and pancreatitis are not uncommon. Diagnosis of pancreatitis is difficult since patients with renal insufficiency often have a reduced amylase clearance and hyperamylasemia. Persistent ascites in hemodialysis patients without liver disease has been a problem.

HEMATOLOGICAL MANIFESTATIONS

Anemia. The hematocrit usually ranges between 20% and 35%. A rough inverse correlation exists between the SUN and the hemoglobin level. Spontaneous nose bleeds, menorrhagia, and gastrointestinal bleeding are manifestations of a generalized bleeding ten-

dency and may contribute to the anemia. However, the classical anemia of uremia is normochromic and normocytic. The reticulocyte count in the peripheral blood is low and the bone marrow is hypoplastic. Suppression of erythropoiesis may be due to a direct toxic effect of urea or other uremic toxins on the bone marrow. In addition, inadequate renal production of erythropoietin may contribute to the anemia. Blood transfusions may further suppress erythropoiesis. Other possible causes for anemia in dialysis patients are iron deficiency, folic acid deficiency, and lost blood or hemolysis during the dialysis procedure. Red cell destruction is increased in uremia. Many renal patients have hypersplenism. A circulating factor may also be responsible for the reduced half life of red cells in the azotemic patients. However, uremic red cells themselves are probably normal since after washing they may have a normal half life when infused into normal recipients.

Bleeding tendencies. Approximately 20% of patients with chronic renal insufficiency have bleeding difficulties. Coagulation defects include a prolonged bleeding time, abnormal prothrombin consumption, thrombocytopenia, abnormal platelet adhesiveness, and decreased platelet factor III activity. Regular dialysis only partially corrects the platelet dysfunction. Guanidinosuccinic acid has been proposed to be the dialyzable factor that accumulates in uremia and inhibits platelet factor III release.

Use of transfusions. There has been much debate over transfusions in renal patients. Frequent transfusions can result in volume overload and congestive heart failure. Transfusions increase the risk of acquiring hepatitis, of sensitization to tissue antigens and of hemosiderosis. Transfusions may also inhibit erythropoietin production. Nevertheless, there are indications for transfusion. These include both acute blood loss and chronic anemia when it contributes to angina pectoris, intermittent claudication, or extreme weakness. In addition, frequent transfusions probably increase the success of subsequent renal transplantation.

Skin. The classic cutaneous appearance of uremic patients is that of a sallow, yellow-colored, pruritic individual. The coloring is due to both anemia and the deposition of carotene-like uremic pigments (urochromes). Severe itching has been attributed to deposition of Ca^{++} in the skin when the product of the $[Ca^{++}]$ and $[P]$ exceeds 55. This may be improved by parathyroidectomy, or by lowering the $[Ca^{++}]$ and $[P]$ product through the use of oral P binders. However, the itching can also be treated by daily baths, lubricating ointments, phototherapy, oral activated charcoal and antipruritic agents such as the antihistamines.

Immunological and infectious complications. Infections are a common cause of death in dialysis patients. These patients have several potential risk factors. Among these are depressed cellular immunity, leukopenia, lymphopenia, pulmonary congestion, coma, malnutrition, vascular insufficiency, chronic peritoneal catheters, or frequent vascular access. Uremia suppresses the lymphocyte response to phytohemagglutinins and impairs the chemotactic function of polymorphonuclear leukocytes. On the other hand, the immune suppression or uremia may improve the success of renal transplantation. However, this benefit is balanced by an increased incidence of malignancy. Antibiotic treatment of the uremic patient must be carefully considered. Many popular antibiotics are nephrotoxic. In addition, their dosage usually must be adjusted because of reduced renal excretion.

Nutrition and growth. Children requiring maintenance hemodialysis are threatened by growth retardation. In part, this can be attributed to dietary restrictions. Successful renal transplantation, if performed early, allows children to grow normally.

Renal osteodystrophy, altered calcium and phosphorus metabolism. Hypocalcemia, hyperphosphatemia, decreased synthesis of active renal metabolites of vitamin D $(1,25\text{-}(OH)_2 D_3)$ and increased parathyroid hormone secretion commonly accompany end-stage renal failure. Patients with renal osteodystrophy may have lesions of osteitis fibrosa cystica, osteomalacia, osteoporosis, osteosclerosis, osteopetrosis, or combinations of these. Patients with uremia can develop metastatic calcifications and intractable pruritus from Ca^{++} deposits in the skin.

Biochemical alterations. Mild CHO intolerance is present in more than half of chronically uremic patients. However, dialysis may improve the CHO intolerance. Fasting blood sugars are usually not greatly elevated, and ketosis is uncommon. The CHO intolerance is due predominately to resistance by skeletal muscle and other tissue to the glucose transport of insulin. Hypoglycemia also occurs in dialysis patients. An elevated growth hormone level and abnormalities in the glucose counterregulatory hormones may be responsible for the hypoglycemia. In severe renal insufficiency, impaired insulin degradation by kidneys reduces the overall rate of insulin clearance. This is seen in diabetic patients whose need for exogenous insulin diminishes as they become more uremic. Weight loss and a reduced caloric intake also contribute to the diminished insulin requirements. Many uremic patients have hypertriglyceridemia and type IV hyperlipoproteinemia. This has been associated with decreased activity of lipoprotein lipase and a reduced rate of triglyceride clearance from plasma. Furthermore, hepatic synthesis of low density lipoproteins is increased.

Endocrine alterations. End-stage renal failure disrupts both renal and nonrenal hormonal systems. Decreased renal erythropoietin production contributes to the anemia of uremia. Increased renin production elevates plasma angiotensin and contributes to hypertension in patients with end-stage renal disease. Severe renin dependent hypertension may necessitate removal of end-stage kidneys. Loss of functional renal tissue reduces production of 1,25 dihyroxy D_3, a regulator of Ca^{++} and P metabolism. Since the medullary areas of the kidney produce prostaglandins, the hypertension of end-stage renal disease may also be partially mediated by a deficiency of vasopressor prostaglandins.

As has been mentioned, PTH secretion is increased due to P retention in patients with reduced renal function. PTH may also be elevated due to failure of the kidneys to degrade PTH. High levels of PTH have been implicated in central nervous system dysfunction, pruritis, soft tissue calcification, renal osteodystrophy, and aseptic necrosis of bone.

Patients with chronic renal failure are usually euthyroid, but various alterations of thyroid hormones are found in end-stage renal disease. Plasma inorganic iodine levels are elevated. This may be the result of prior radiocontrast studies. Triiodothyronine concentrations are low because of reduced conversion of T4 and T3. Goiters are not uncommon in azotemic patients. Renal failure patients are also reported to have elevated plasma calcitonin, gastrin, glucagon, growth hormone, and insulin levels. During chronic renal failure, a compensatory hypersecretion of aldosterone increases K^+ excretion. Elevation of a proposed natriuretic hormone during chronic renal failure may help maintain the body's Na^+ balance.

Miscellaneous metabolic derangements. Hypothermia in azotemic patients is frequent and complicates the diagnosis of acute infections. A hyperchloremic metabolic acidosis develops during the early stages of chronic renal failure. With advanced renal failure, retention of organic and inorganic anions results in a metabolic acidosis with an increased anionic gap. Occasionally, salt wasting may occur in patients with end-stage renal failure.

TREATMENT

Whenever possible, a specific therapy should be prescribed for the primary renal disease. Further renal damage may be prevented by early treatment of the factors contributing to the renal disease. These may include urinary tract infections, hypertension, or drug nephrotoxicity. When the patient enters the final phase of renal failure, more aggressive therapies such as dialysis, transplantation, or symptomatic therapy for uremic manifestations may be undertaken. Therapies for chronic renal failure are discussed in Chapters 16–18.

SELECTED READINGS

1. Kurtzman, NA. Chronic Renal Failure: metabolic and clinical consequences. Hosp Prac 108–122, August, 1982
2. Naets, JP. Hematologic disorders in renal failure. Nephron 14:181–184, 1975
3. Platt, R. Structural and functional adaptation in renal failure. Br Med J I:1313–1317 and 1372–1372, 1952
4. Raskin, NH, Fishman, RA. Neurologic disorders in renal failure. N Engl J Med, 294:143–148, 204–210, 1976

Kamal Sethi
Guido Perez

7

Nephrotic Syndrome

DEFINITION

Nephrotic syndrome is defined as protein excretion greater than 3 g/day with a normal glomerular filtration rate, which is often accompanied by hypoalbuminemia, lipiduria, hyperlipidemia and edema. All the features may not be present in every patient, but heavy proteinuria is a consistent feature. When none of the associated features are present and isolated heavy proteinuria > 3 g/day occurs, it is called nephrotic proteinuria. No difference exists between the two from the etiological standpoint, and the diagnostic approach is similar in both.

PATHOPHYSIOLOGY

The concept of glomerular permselectivity has been reviewed in Chapter 2 Volume II of this series, along with the mechanisms of proteinuria. All the major manifestations of the nephrotic syndrome—proteinuria, lipiduria, hyperlipidemia, hypoalbuminemia and edema are secondary to an increased or altered glomerular permeability to plasma proteins. Their interrelationships are shown in figure 1.

ETIOLOGY AND DIFFERENTIAL DIAGNOSIS

Nephrotic syndrome occurs most commonly in glomerular diseases, which may be primary or secondary. Nephrotic range protein-

uria, on the other hand, occurs in both glomerular and non-glomerular diseases—an important example of the latter is the overflow proteinuria in multiple myeloma which may exceed 3 g/day. Nephrotic syndrome may be primary or secondary. The etiology and clinicopathological features of the idiopathic nephrotic syndrome are listed in table 1. The relative incidence in adults and children of the different morphological lesions in the idiopathic type is shown in table 2.

Fig. 7-1.   Pathophysiology of Nephrotic Syndrome

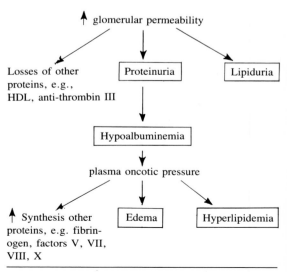

Major manifestations of the nephrotic syndrome are in rectangles

Table 7-1   Causes of the Idiopathic Nephrotic Syndrome or Proteinuria

CAUSE	CLINICAL CORRELATES	LAB FINDINGS INCLUDING HISTOLOGY	PROGNOSIS
1) Minimal change or nil disease	Peak incidence ages 2–4. Young adults, history of allergy, atopy, no systemic disease or hypertension	Nephrotic syndrome common, selective proteinuria; U/A-benign or occasional microscopic hematuria; normal renal function LM-normal EM-foot process fusion	Good. No CRF. Characterized by spontaneous remission and relapses
2) Membranous glomerulopathy	Commonest cause of adult nephrotic syndrome, males > females, hypertension occurs late	Maybe massive proteinuria with nephrotic syndrome, microscopic hematuria common, azotemia occurs late. Histology-spikes on silver stain with subepithelial deposits	Slowly progressive. 50% with renal failure at 10 yrs.
3) Focal & segmental sclerosis	Children or adults. Hypertension common.	As with membranous except histology which shows segmental sclerosis and immunoglobulin deposits.	As with membranous. Maybe better in children
4) Proliferative glomerulonephritis, Diffuse or focal			

a) Mesangiocapillary
  b) Endocapillary
  c) Endocapillary & extracapillary
	Hypertension, azotemia occurs early	Hematuria almost invariably present. Nephrotic-nephritic picture common but nephrotic syndrome may be present alone. ↓ C_3, C_3NEF	Not good. Progression to renal failure can be rapid.

The most common cause of the secondary nephrotic syndrome in adults in this country is diabetic glomerulosclerosis and in the world, malaria. The secondary causes, clinical features and histology are detailed in table 3. As is clear from a review of tables 1 and 3, the histological lesion can be identical in primary and secondary nephrotic syndrome. Very careful clinicopathological correlation and laboratory evaluation are

Table 7-2   Idiopathic Nephrotic Syndrome in Adults & Children

	Adults	Children
Minimal change	15–25%	70–90%
Membranous	30–50%	1–3%
Focal sclerosis	10–20%	10–20%
Proliferative	20–35%	15–20%

Table 7-3 Causes of Secondary Nephrotic Syndrome—1

Cause	Clinical Correlates	Common Histology
1. Metabolic		
—diabetes mellitus	History of diabetes for several years, retinopathy	Modular or diffuse glomerulosclerosis
—amyloidosis	Chronic suppurative disease, dysproteinemias, Mediterranean origin	Amyloid deposits with birefringence
2. Neoplasms		
—carcinoma	GI, lung, renal	Membranous
—lymphomas	Hodgkin & non-Hodgkin	Minimal change, in Hodgkin's disease
		Membranous or proliferative in Non-Hodgkins lymphomas
3. Collagen Vascular disease		
—SLE	Arthritis, skin rash, +ANA	Minimal, membranous, proliferative
—Polyarteritis	Arthritis, skin nodules	Proliferative
4. Drugs		
—heavy metals	Gold therapy, mercury	Membranous
—heroin	Drug abuse, track marks	Focal sclerosis & mesangiocapillary
—Captopril	Hypertension	Membranous
—non-steroidal, anti-inflammatory drugs	History of arthritis	Minimal change
5. Allergens		
Bee stings, pollen, immunizations, poison ivy	History of allergy, atopy, children	Minimal change
6. Infectious		
—bacterial		
post-streptococcal	recent impetigo, ↓ complement, sore throat, ↑ ASO titers	Subepithelial humps
bacterial endocarditis	rheumatic heart disease or drug abuse, ↓ complement, +blood cultures, ↑ rheumatoid factor	Proliferative
syphilis	secondary or congenital, +FTA	Membranous, focal proliferative
—viral		
hepatitis B	active hepatitis; carriers	Membranous, focal proliferative
—parasitic		
Malaria schistosomiasis	Usually in quartan malaria common in endemic areas	Membranous, focal proliferative

54

Table 7-3   (Cont.)

Cause	Clinical Correlates	Common Histology
7. Heredofamilial		
—Alport's disease	Family history, visual and auditory problems, hematuria	Proliferative, split basement membrane
8. Miscellaneous		
—Malignant hypertension	Severe hypertension, papilledema, renal failure, hematuria, microangiopathic hemolytic anemia	Fibrinoid necrosis
—Pre-eclampsia	Third trimester, hypertension, ↑ serum urate	Glomerular endothelial cell swelling
—Allograft rejection		

usually necessary to make an accurate diagnosis and develop an appropriate therapeutic plan.

COMPLICATIONS OF NEPHROTIC SYNDROME

The complications of the nephrotic syndrome are numerous and are depicted in figure 2. The most significant ones are thromboembolism, hypercoagulability, increased susceptibility to infection, refractory edema, hypovolemia, and hyperlipidema and accelerated atherosclerosis.

Thromboembolism. Renal vein thrombosis is the most common thrombotic event in the

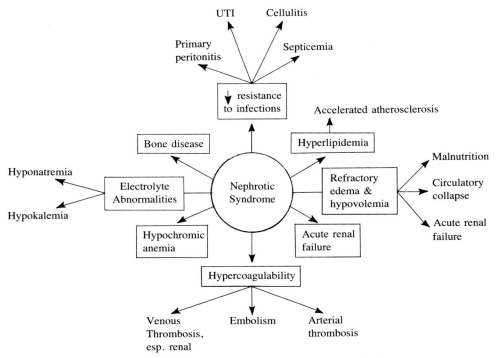

Fig. 7-2.   Complications of Nephrotic Syndrome

nephrotic syndrome. The highest incidence (~30%) is seen in membranous nephropathy, although it may occur uncommonly with other types of glomerulonephritis. Renal vein thrombosis may be associated with acute renal failure and increased proteinuria, especially if it is acute. Anticoagulation is indicated to prevent pulmonary embolism. Arterial thrombosis can occur too. However, its incidence is relatively low. Hypercoagulability is of multifactorial etiology and there is an increase in factors V, VII, VIII and X, fibrinogen and platelets along with increased platelet aggregation, all of which favor thrombosis. There may also be a decrease in inhibitors of coagulation such as anti-thrombin III. The hypercoagulable state may be aggravated by steroid therapy.

Infections. There is increased susceptibility to bacterial infections, the reasons for which are not totally understood. The severe malnutrition, acquired immunoglobulin deficiency and steroid therapy are undoubtedly important contributory factors.

Refractory edema & hypovolemia. Ongoing heavy proteinuria and hypoalbuminemia can lead to circulatory collapse and severe prerenal azotemia and rarely acute renal failure. Malnutrition because of massive urine losses is common and persists unless a remission in proteinuria occurs.

Accelerated atherosclerosis. In the hyperlipedemic nephrotic state, cholesterol, triglycerides and VLDL are increased and HDL often reduced because of urinary losses. Steroid therapy and primary diseases such as diabetes can only worsen the hyperlipidemia. Accelerated atherosclerosis with a high incidence of cardiovascular disease would then seem a logical consequence. The data are somewhat inconclusive however, and more prospective studies are necessary to elucidate the extent of this problem.

EVALUATION OF NEPHROTIC SYNDROME

Some routine studies merit special attention. A fasting glucose must be obtained to exclude diabetes mellitus, the most common cause of the secondary nephrotic syndrome. Serum and protein electrophoresis should be obtained in all adult patients with nephrotic syndrome because myeloma can be associated with amyloidosis, and thus heavy proteinuria.

The evaluation of the nephrotic syndrome requires some special studies, additionally (table 4), and those will be discussed here.

1. *Serology.* Serum complement levels, if low, suggest one of several diagnoses—infection-related glomerulonephritis, mesangiocapillary glomerulonephritis and lupus nephritis. ANA positivity suggests lupus, and elevated ASO and anti-DNAaseB titers suggest recent streptococcal throat or skin infection, respectively. Hepatitis B screen should be obtained in those with suspected drug abuse. VDRL, rheumatoid factor and cryoglobulins may also be indicated in some patients.

2. *Heavy metal screen.* Gold and mercury can produce membranous glomerulonephritis and can be readily detected in the urine. Gold therapy is used in rheumatoid arthritis and mercury is a common constituent of skin preparations.

3. *Hemoglobin electrophoresis.* Sickle cell anemia can be associated with the nephrotic syndrome. Hemoglobin electrophoresis

---

Table 7-4 Evaluation of Nephrotic Syndrome

Routine tests

- complete history & physical
- complete urinalysis
- 24 hr. urine protein × 3
- Renal function tests
- CBC, serum electrolytes
- Fasting glucose
- Protein studies: serum & urine protein electrophoresis
- Renal sonography

Special studies

- Serology: ASO, anti-DNAaseB, hepatitis B screen, ANA, complement, VDRL
- Heavy metal screen, if suspected toxicity
- Hemoglobin electrophoresis, in blacks
- Renal venography, if indicated
- Renal biopsy

should be performed in black patients with anemia and a positive family history.

4. *Renal venography.* It may be necessary in those with membranous glomerulonephritis, especially if there is sudden increase in proteinuria or pulmonary embolism or development of acute renal failure.

5. *Renal biopsy.* It is important for diagnostic, prognostic and often, therapeutic reasons in both idiopathic and secondary nephrotic syndrome. In secondary nephrotic syndrome, it may be necessary to assess the histologic activity of the renal disease, as in lupus nephritis. If the nephritis is active with few chronic changes, aggressive immunosuppressive therapy can be administered with the potential for recovery of renal function. It may not be necessary in those conditions where the clinical features strongly suggest a presumptive diagnosis, as in the long-standing diabetic with proliferative retinopathy, renal failure, normal sized kidneys and nephrotic syndrome. Renal biopsy for the most part, can only permit a morphological and not an etiological diagnosis. Occasionally, however, it may be possible to differentiate a primary and secondary lesion. This may have important therapeutic implications, because the management of the secondary disorders is directed at treatment of the primary problem. For example, patients with tumor-related membranous glomerulopathy may go into remission with treatment of the tumor and should not be considered to be candidates for even short-term steroid therapy.

MANAGEMENT OF THE NEPHROTIC SYNDROME

General Measures

Bed rest. This is important in initiating a diuretic response in the severely edematous patient.

Diet. A low salt, fluid-restricted diet is useful in minimizing edema formation. In the patient with relatively normal renal function, a high protein (1.5–2 g/kg/d) diet is usually prescribed to offset the urinary losses.

Diuretics. Great care should be exercised in the use of diuretics, especially in patients with contracted plasma volume because severe hypovolemia and circulatory collapse can occur. The loop diuretics, such as furosemide should be used only in the patient with severe edema and anasarca. The combination of furosemide and metolazone and sometimes aldosterone antagonists is useful in refractory edema. Albumin infusions may be used as a temporizing measure to maintain intravascular volume or to initiate a diuretic response. Hospitalization is recommended for the severely edematous patient who is to be given combination diuretics.

Specific Therapy

Treatment of the complications

1. Hyperlipidemia—clofibrate and cholestyramine have been used without much success. Gemfibrozil appears to be a promising new drug.

2. Thromboembolism—anticoagulation is indicated in renal vein thrombosis especially if associated thromboembolic complications occur. The value of surgical intervention has not been determined.

3. Infections—prophylactic antibiotics and vaccines are not indicated but pulmonary or peritoneal infections with encapsulated bacteria should be promptly investigated and treated.

4. Hypertension—if it persists after edema has disappeared, antihypertensives should be used.

5. Bone disease—Vitamin D metabolites may be required to treat hyperparathyroidism and/or osteomalacia.

Treatment of Idiopathic Nephrotic Syndrome

Corticosteroids. Steroids are the mainstay in the treatment of minimal change disease. Daily or alternate day steroids may be used. Responders can have a protein-free urine in 4–8 weeks and steroids should be tapered rapidly, after a 2 week protein-free period. The response rate is 70–75% in adults. Children have a better prognosis with 90% response rate, albeit with high incidence of relapses. The role of steroids in the management of other forms of the nephrotic syndrome is not clearly established. One study showed that alternate day steroid therapy for 8 weeks slowed the progression of renal failure in patients with GFR's > 50 ml/min. In membrano-proliferative glomerulonephritis one study describes an apparent benefit of continuous low-dose steroids on survival. These findings have not been confirmed by other investigations, however.

Immunosuppressive agents. Cyclophosphamide and chlorambucil can reduce remissions in relapsing, steroid-dependent minimal change disease. The effect of cytotoxics alone or in combination with other forms of therapy such as anticoagulants and plasmapheresis remains under active investigation. Corticosteroids and immunosuppressives are also used to treat secondary nephrotic syndrome associated with connective tissue diseases like SLE, polyarteritis and Wegener's granulomatosis.

SELECTED READING

1. Abuelo JG. Proteinuria: Diagnostic Principles & Procedures. Ann. Int. Med. 98:186–191, 1983
2. Brenner BM, Hostetter TM, and Humes DH. The Molecular Basis of Proteinuria of Glomerular Origin. N.E.J.M. 298:826–833, 1978
3. Eagen JW & Lewis EJ. Glomerulopathies of Neoplasia. Kidney Int. 11:297–306, 1977
4. Hricik DE and Kassirer JP. The Nephrotic Syndrome. Disease-A-Month Vol. 28, April 1982
5. Llach F, Paper S, Massry SG. The Clinical Spectrum of Renal Vein Thrombosis: Acute and Chronic. Am J Med 69:819–827, 1980
6. Peters DK. The Major Glomerulopathies. Hospital Practice 16:117–133, October 1981

Yutaka Saito
Atsushi Kondo

8

Urologic-Related Renal Diseases

TUMORS OF THE KIDNEY AND RENAL PELVIS

Abdominal or flank pain, gross or microscopic hematuria, and tumor mass are the classic triad for renal tumors (Table 8-1). However, it is rare to simultaneously find these clinical manifestations in the same patient. In fact, many patients show no specific symptoms in the early stages of their disorders. Fever, hypertension, weight loss, anorexia, nausea, vomiting, constipation, and lassitude are found occasionally, but it is only in the advanced stages that more specific signs and symptoms suggest renal tumor.

Renal Cell Carcinoma

Symptoms. Ten to 20% of cases with renal carcinoma show the complete symptomatic triad—hematuria, flank pain, and tumor mass. Incidental gross or microscopic hematuria is present in 30% to 60%, flank pain in 30% to 35%, and palpable mass is observed in 20% to 40%. Not infrequently, fever is the only clinical sign of disease. Persistent or intermittent fever is found in 20% of patients with renal tumors. Renal carcinoma is associated with a 10% to 25% incidence of hypertension. When hypertension is present, renal tumors are considered to be the direct cause, since blood pressure is normalized after nephrectomy. Other nonspecific complaints such as weight loss, anorexia and weakness are noted in 25% of effected patients.

Diagnosis. Renal cell carcinoma develops most commonly in patients between 50 years to 70 years of age, with a mean of 57 years. Only 1% of patients are under 20 years old, and the male to female ratio is 3:1.

Diagnosis of renal cell carcinoma is accomplished mainly by radiological techniques, combined with finding symptoms such as hematuria, proteinuria, and anemia. Elevated erythrocyte sedimentation rates are observed in many cases of renal cell carcinoma, and usually indicate an advanced tumor stage. Additional frequent associations are high erythropoitin concentration, polycythemia, and hypercalcemia.

The gold standard for diagnosis of any renal tumor is intravenous pyelography (IVP). (Fig. 1-A). Nephrotomography enhances the accuracy of the diagnosis. The most frequently observed deformities seen on pyelography are enlargement and/or irregularity of the renal outline, elongation of calyces, irregular filling defects of calyces and/or the pelvis, and calcification.

To determine whether the deformity of calyces found on pyelography is caused by a tumor or a cystic mass, ultrasonography is helpful. However, ultrasonography alone cannot distinguish renal cell carcinoma from benign lesions. To accomplish this, percutaneous needle puncture with ultrasonography is necessary. A diagnosis of cyst by ultrasonography may be incomplete. Even though cytological evidence of malignancy is lacking, percutaneous puncture of cysts revealing a bloody aspirate or high lipid,

Table 8-1   Classification of Renal Tumor

1. Tumors of the Renal Parenchyma	
i) Benign Tumors:	Adenoma, Fibroma, Lipoma, Leiomyoma, Hemangioma, Lymphangioma, Hamartoma.
ii) Malignant Tumors:	Renal Cell Carcinoma, Nephroblastoma, Sarcoma.
2. Tumors of the Renal Pelvis	
i) Benign Tumors:	Papilloma
ii) Malignant Tumors:	Transitional cell carcinoma, Squamous cell carcinoma, Adenocarcinoma.
3. Tumors of the Renal Capsule	
i) Benign Tumors:	Lipoma, Fibroma, Leiomyoma.
ii) Malignant Tumors:	Sarcoma
4. Secondary Malignant Tumors	

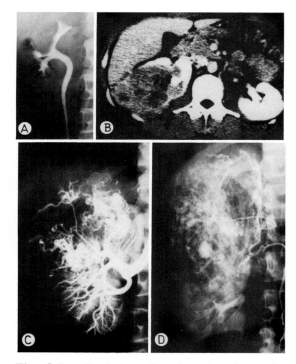

Fig. 8-1.   Depiction of various imaging techniques used for diagnostic purposes. (a) IVP; (b) Computerized tomography and (c/d) Angiography.

cholesterol, and LDH concentration are suspicious. After aspiration of the mass contents, further radiological examination is carried out by injecting a contrast medium into the cyst cavity. A smooth wall rules out malignancy; but if the wall is irregular, neoplasia may be present. Computerized tomography (CT) is useful for the primary diagnosis of renal tumors, recognizing perinephric extension, and determining enlargement of regional lymph nodes (Fig. 1-B).

Selective renal angiography plays an important role in the diagnosis of renal cell carcinoma. Even comparatively small tumors can be uncovered by angiography. Typical vascular patterns suggesting the diagnosis are neovascularity, pooling of contrast medium, arteriovenous fistula, intrarenal microaneurysms, and tumor blush. However, one must remember that avascular or minimally vascular patterns are observed in approximately 10% of renal cell carcinomas (Fig. 1-C,D).

Venacavography is employed to determine caval invasion of renal cell carcinoma. Caval invasion is a problem in approximately 5% of renal cell carcinomas.

Pathology.   According to cytoplasmic appearances, renal cell carcinoma is classified into a clear cell type, a granular cell type, a mixed type composed of both clear cells and granular cells, and an anaplastic cell type. Roughly, 25% of renal cell carcinoma is pure clear cell type, and about 15% consists of granular cells. The 5-year survival rate of pure clear cell tumors surpasses that of granular or mixed cell tumors.

Treatment. At present, radical nephrectomy is the only treatment which offers the possibility for a complete cure of renal cell carcinoma. Radical nephrectomy requires removal of the kidney with an intact Gerota's fascia. For patients with large renal tumors, preoperative renal artery occlusion is carried out. Tumor vascularity decreases, and the surgical procedure becomes easier, as blood loss and operating time are lessened. Preoperative and postoperative radiotherapy do not improve the survival rate of renal cell carcinoma. Accordingly, radiotherapy is used only for palliation of symptomatic metastases.

Chemotherapy of renal cell carcinoma has proven generally ineffective. Vinblastine, hydroxyurea, chloroethyl-cyclohexy-nitrosourea, and other combinations produce no more than a 20% response rate.

Hormonal therapy for disseminated renal cell carcinoma is not, as yet, established. A 10% to 20% objective response rate has been obtained by using androgens and progesterones. However, recurrence is possible even after 10 years or more of therapy.

Nephroblastoma (Wilms' Tumor)

Nephroblastoma is a renal tumor found in children. Ninety percent of nephroblastomas are found in children under 5 years of age with 70% of the victims under 3. Predilection for males or females and the right or left side has not been noted. Bilateral renal involvement occurs in 2% to 5%.

Symptoms. Nephroblastoma has no characteristic symptoms in initial stages. In 40% to 50% of cases, the mother or the physician finds the tumor mass accidentally. Pain is certainly not an early symptom. When colicky pain occurs, it does so because of distention of a renal capsule, ureteral obstruction from a clot, or partial intestinal obstruction.

Hematuria occurs in 20% of nephroblastoma cases, but once more is rare in its early stage. Associated hypertension has an incidence

of 70% to 90%. Fever is observed in 50% of cases, and patients frequently complain of irritability, fretfulness, loss of appetite, and weakness.

Diagnosis. The tumor surface is smooth and round, and its consistency ranges from hard to soft. Roentgenological examinations are essential for diagnosis. Calcification of the tumor is found in 10% to 15% of nephroblastomas. Excretory urography is important. Roentgenological changes include distortion of the pelvis—calyces, and displacement and compression of the ureter. Other possible findings are a renal mass showing a smooth radiographic contour and homogeneous density, obliteration of the psoas muscle outline, and displacement of the abdominal viscera. Ten% to 20% of nephroblastoma cases have severe renal dysfunction. In these instances, cystoscopy with retrograde pyelography is necessary to differentiate hydronephrosis from tumor. Arteriography pictures the blood supply of the mass. Both extremely vascular renal masses and avascular ones are seen. Over 90% display some degree of vascularity. Neovascularities are described as appearing like creeping-vines or spider legs. Ultrasonography and CT scans are used to differentiate avascular tumors from cysts.

Pathology. Nephroblastomas consist of three components—epithelium, stromal, and blastematous cells. In general, the epithelial and stromal components predominate. All stages of epithelial cells, ranging from undifferentiated to partially differentiated ones, mingle with muscle cells, connective tissue, cartilage, and bone.

Treatment. Surgical removal of the kidney is the basic treatment. Radiotherapy and chemotherapy have some influences on nephroblastoma, but there is little evidence to prove that preoperative radiotherapy and chemotherapy prevent metastases.

Nephrectomy is performed via a transabdominal or transthoracoabdominal approach. Ligation of pedicle vessels is accomplished prior to manipulation of the renal mass or tumor mobilization. Afterwards, dissection of tumor including surrounding tissue is carried out. Radiotherapy is used postoperatively in combination with chemotherapy. Over 3 to 4 weeks, approximately 2,000 rads are given. Actinomycin

D is effective when begun on the day of surgery. Vincristine and Cyclophosphamide can be prescribed alone or in combination with Actinomycin D. The combination of postoperative radiotherapy and chemotherapy improve the prognosis of early stage nephroblastomas. The survival rate becomes 90% to 100%. However, the prognosis is closely related to age, with older children having a worse prognosis.

Carcinoma of Renal Pelvis

Carcinoma of renal pelvis is second to renal cell carcinoma in frequency. It occurs also between 50 years to 70 years of age, and involves more males than females. The ratio is 2:1 to 3:1.

Symptoms. Hematuria is the most common symptom, seen in 75% to 90% of victims. Gross hematuria is the rule, but only microscopic hematuria is noticed in 10% of cases. It is probable that discovery of microscopic hematuria permits earlier discovery of the lesion. Pain occurs in 20% to 50% of patients when blood clots pass through the ureters. Rarely, a palpable mass is discovered when the tumor causes ureteral obstruction and hydronephrosis.

Diagnosis. IVP is important diagnostically with the tumor tissue appearing as a radiolucent defect in the renal pelvis or calyx. (Fig. 2). However, any radiolucent defect must be differentiated from uric acid stones or blood clots. A unilateral nonfunctioning kidney on IVP is a common presentation. With gross hematuria, cystoscopy can localize the kidney with the lesion. In addition, cytological examination may be performed on the urine collection. When the tumor outline is not clear on IVP, retrograde pyelography (RP) is helpful. RP can outline the tumors clearly. Radiolucent calculi and clots are mobile on examination. RP can fill a defect produced by a vascular impression.

Pathology. The histological classification of renal pelvis carcinoma is transitional cell carcinoma (91%–92%), squamous cell carcinoma (8%), adenocarcinoma and undifferentiated carcinoma (<1%).

Treatment. Nephroureterectomy and removal of a bladder cuff is the principle treatment for tumors of the renal pelvis. With simple nephrectomy alone, local recurrence is common. To prevent local recurrence post operatively, chemotherapy and radiotherapy are added to the regimen. The latter are also used for inoperable tumors. More than 50% of squamous cell carcinomas of the renal pelvis are associated with a calculi. The prognosis of squamous cell carcinoma is worse than for transitional cell carcinoma.

Carcinoma of the Prostate

Symptoms. Symptoms may be entirely absent early in this disease. Later, patients may develop symptoms of urinary obstruction, i.e., dysuria, slow stream, urinary frequency and even complete retention. Bone pain, a symptom next in order of frequency, suggests metastases. He-

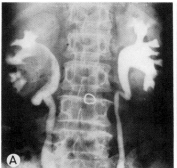 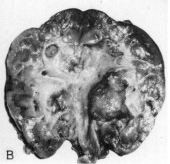

Fig. 8-2. (a) IVP shows radiolucent mass in renal calyx-pelvis; (b) Gross specimen of the mass

maturia and lower extremity edema are uncommon symptoms of prostatic carcinoma.

Diagnosis. Normally the prostate is the size of the chestnut and can be palpated easily on digital rectal examination. Prostatic carcinoma characteristically has a hard "stony" consistency. Digital examination has 50% to 80% accuracy in diagnosing prostatic carcinoma. Serum acid phosphatase activity is the most important biochemical test. Now, acid phosphatase of prostatic origin can be measured by a radioimmunoassay.

Skeletal radiographs are used to determine bone metastases. Bone metastases from prostatic carcinoma are the most commonly osteoblastic lesions (Fig. 3A) which occur most frequently in the pelvis, the lumbar vertebrae, and the proximal femurs. Radionuclide bone scans are even more sensitive than the skeletal radiograph in detecting early metastases of prostatic carcinoma (Fig. 3B).

Pathology. More than 95% of prostatic carcinomas are adenocarcinomas; transitional cell carcinoma and squamous cell carcinoma of the prostate are exceedingly rare.

Treatment. Radical prostatectomy is performed often for cure of prostatic carcinoma.

There are two routes for radical prostatectomy, the perineal and retropubic approaches. Radical prostatectomy should be limited to those patients whose prostatic carcinoma is clinically confined to the prostate. Radiation therapy for prostatic carcinoma is also used.

Endocrine therapy for prostatic carcinoma was introduced in 1941. This is effective, because prostatic cells are dependent upon androgens for maintenance. Bilateral orchiectomy ablates androgen sources. Estrogens suppress pituitary LH hormone release and inhibit the action of androgens.

Studies concerning non-hormonal cytotoxic chemotherapy have not advanced far enough to determine their efficacy.

CYSTIC DISEASE OF THE KIDNEY

Characteristically, symptoms of renal cystic disease include flank mass, hematuria, hypertension and pain. With bilateral involvement, deterioration of renal function is also evident. The following congenital cystic diseases i.e., polycystic kidney disease, medullary sponge kidney, simple cysts, congenital unilateral multicystic kidney, and the cystic lesions of mutilocular cystic kidney will be discussed.

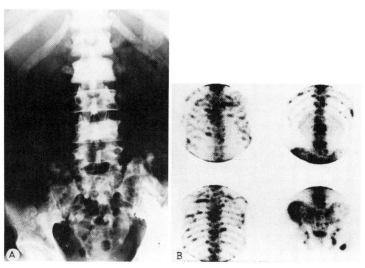

Fig. 8-3. (a) Bone metastases from prostatic carcinoma are most commonly osteoblastic; (b) Radionuclide bone scans detecting early metastases from prostatic carcinoma.

Polycystic Kidney Disease (PcKD)

Symptoms. Infantile PcKD, which manifests mainly as a flank mass, is associated with early death. In adult PcKD, flank masses, gross hematuria, urinary tract infection, lumbar pain, hypertension, weakness, polydipsia, polyuria, anorexia, nausea, constipation and anemia are observed frequently. Hematuria is seen in 30% to 50%; urinary tract infection in 32% to 94%, and hypertension in more than 70%.

Forty five % of patients with PcKD have cerebral aneurysms, while 3% develop hepatic cysts. (Fig. 4-C). Cysts can also develop in the bladder, epididymis, lungs, ovaries, pancreas, spleen, testes, thyroid gland, and uterus.

Diagnosis. Infant-form PcKD is transmitted by autosomal recessive inheritance. Differently, adult PcKD is transmitted by an autosomal dominant inheritance. A positive family history is important, PcKD is usually bilateral, and the kidneys are palpable bilaterally in more than 50% of cases. The IVP is essential. Radiographic findings are enlargement of kidneys, irregular renal outlines, disappearance of psoas muscle shadows, and elongation, irregular enlargement and distortion of calyces (Fig. 4-A).

If there is depression of renal function, retrograde pyelography may be helpful. Ultrasonography and CT scan are useful imaging techniques (Fig. 4-B).

Pathology. The characteristic feature of infantile PcKD is ductal ectasis. In newborn children, ductal dilatation occurs in the medullary pyramids; but in older children cysts of homogeneous size are scattered throughout the cortical areas. In the adult PcKD, cysts from several millimeters to several centimeters in size, replace cortical and medullary tissue. Colors of cyst contents vary from clear yellow to turbid yellow, from white to opaque dark brown, and are even blue from intracystic bleeding.

Treatment. There is no specific treatment for PcKD. Therapy is directed toward hypertension, infections, and other symptoms.

Medullary Cystic Diseases

Symptoms. The disease usually manifests during adolescence or early childhood. Terminal renal failure commonly occurs by the third decade. Medullary cystic disease is noted for

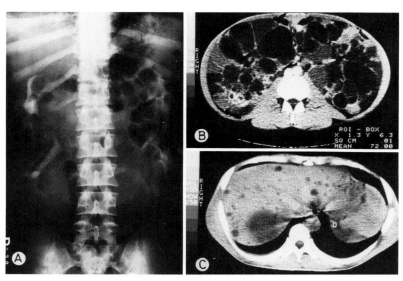

Fig. 8-4. (a) IVP shows enlarged kidney, irregular renal outline, disappearance of psoas muscle shadow and elongated, irregular enlargement and distorted calyces in PCKD; (b) CT scan is useful to portray cysts; (c) CT scan showing hepatic cysts.

polyuria and salt wasting. Hypertension is not uncommon.

Diagnosis. Diagnosis is made by the findings of severe salt and water loss in a young individual, associated with the characteristic IVP findings, especially after tomography.

Pathology. Medullary cystic disease is a rare disorder which seems to have a familial tendency. Cysts form primarily at the corticomedullary junction, and there is evidence of interstitial inflammation and fibrosis. More females are affected than males. Red hair is an association.

Treatment. No specific therapy exists. Water and salt loss and hypertension are treated.

Medullary Sponge Kidney

Symptoms. For the most part, this is a radiological diagnosis with no apparent effect on longevity. However, a large portion of patients with medullary sponge kidney suffer eventually from nephrolithiasis. Renal colic occurs occasionally. Hypertension, hematuria, and urinary tract infection are infrequent associations.

Diagnosis. During excretory urography, the contrast medium can be seen to concentrate in the ectatic tubules at the pyramidal apices. Ultrasonography, retrograde pyelography, and arteriography are not helpful or necessary for diagnosis of medullary sponge kidney.

Pathology. Males are more commonly affected than females, and both kidneys may be involved. Eight to 10 millimeter cysts are present in the pyramids; and in 40% to 60% of cases, calcareous deposits in the cysts are present.

Treatment. The treatment of medullary sponge kidney is directed toward infection, pain and hematuria.

Simple Cysts

Symptoms. Simple cysts are usually asymptomatic. The majority are discovered accidentally by excretory urography. Symptoms of simple cysts include abdominal masses, ab-

dominal or lumbar pain, hypertension, and hematuria.

Diagnosis. Simple cysts can be solitary or multiple, and are usually unilateral. Occasionally, a KUB film (plain abdominal) is useful; but definitive diagnosis is more often made by some combination of excretory urography, ultrasonography, CT scan, arteriography, and percutaneous aspiration.

Pathology. Cysts may occur anywhere in the renal parenchyma, but are most common in the cortex. They are frequently round, thin-walled and translucent. Over 90% contain clear, thin, straw-colored fluid.

Treatment. Treatment is unnecessary unless symptoms appear. Surgical treatment is excision of the cyst wall.

Congenital Unilateral Multicystic Kidney

Symptoms. A large, unilateral, lobulated, and nontender movable mass is discovered in the flank of an infant. Pain can be felt in the renal area, but very rarely.

Diagnosis. Infants are most frequently affected. There is no predilection for right or left kidney, for male or female. By excretory urography, complete absence of contrast medium excretion is observed on the involved side. The opposite kidney is roentgenographically normal. Ultrasonography and CT scan aid an accurate diagnosis.

Pathology. The kidney appears like a bunch of grapes. Normal renal tissue is replaced by a mass of cysts. The diameter of cysts measures 0.5 to 8 centimeters. The ureter is either atrophic or absent partially or completely (Fig. 5-A, B).

Treatment. The treatment of multicystic kidney is nephrectomy, and the prognosis is good.

Multilocular Cystic Kidney

Symptoms. Multilocular cystic disease is observed in patients of all ages, even infants.

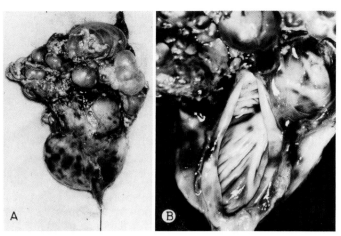

Fig. 8-5. Example of congenital unilateral multicystic kidney (a) Kidney appears like a bunch of grapes; (b) The ureter is either atrophic or partially absent.

Symptoms include flank mass, hematuria, and flank pain.

Diagnosis. It is difficult to differentiate multilocular cystic kidney from simple cysts by excretory urogram. CT scan and arteriography are helpful in diagnosing multilocular cysts.

Pathology. Large cysts are divided into a number of separate smaller cysts by septa. Multilocular cysts are unilateral and localized. Uninvolved normal renal tissues is present alongside the cysts.

Treatment. No specific therapy, short of tissue removal, is available.

HYDRONEPHROSIS

Symptoms. Symptoms of hydronephrosis are subtle. In infants under 3 years old, nearly 50% of patients have urinary tract infection. Adults may complain of abdominal or lumbar pain.

Diagnosis. Upper common ureteral lesions producing hydronephrosis include (1) segmental dysfunction, (2) fibrotic ureteral stricture, and (3) functional obstruction.

The status of the contralateral kidney, the degree of hydronephrosis, and the degree and location of the stricture are estimated by intravenous pyelography. Retrograde pyelography is sometimes necessary to visualize the entire obstructed ureter.

Arteriography can rule in or out aberrant vessels. Ultrasonography and CT scan are essential to rule out cystic lesions.

Pathology. Hydronephrosis is separated into extrarenal and intrarenal hydronephrosis. In the case of extrarenal hydronephrosis, dilatation of renal pelvis is extensive, while damage to renal parenchyma and calyces is light. With intrarenal hydronephrosis, atrophy of renal parenchyma and calyceal dilatation are great.

Treatment. Ureteropelvioplasties are the best treatment. When kidneys are badly damaged and severe chronic pyelonephritis and hypertension are present, nephrectomy is indicated. For infants and elderly patients, percutaneous nephrostomy is performed as an emergency procedure.

VESICOURETERAL REFLUX

Vesicoureteral reflux is present in 30%–50% of children with urinary tract infections. Table 2 shows a classification of vesicoureteral reflux by cause.

Table 8-2 Classification of the causes of reflux

A. Non-obstructive reflux

   a. Congenital abnormalities

      (i) Primary reflux (Weakness of the ureterotrigonal muscle, or short submucosal ureter)

      (ii) Ureteral abnormalities (Complete ureteral duplication, ureterocele, or ectopic orifice of ureter)

   b. Cystitis

   c. Iatrogenic procedures (Operations on the ureter, bladder, or prostate)

B. Obstructive reflux

   a. Organic obstruction of lower urinary tract (Urethral valve, urethral stricture, or prostatic hypertrophy)

   b. Neurogenic bladder

Symptoms. Symptoms of urinary tract infections are frequently seen in patients with reflux. Low-grade pyelonephritis is more common than acute pyelonephritis with high fevers and flank pain. In children, vague pain is felt in the flanks.

Diagnosis. Urinalysis is the most important screening test since the presence of a urinary tract infection with pyuria and bacteriuria may be the first sign of vesicoureteral reflux.

Excretory urography is helpful when reflux is suspected or when there is persistent or recurrent infection. Some degree of hydroureteronephrosis is usually found in patients with reflux. Cystoureterography, especially voiding cystoureterography, is important for diagnosing and classifying the grades of reflux. The grades of reflux are depicted in Figure 6.

Treatment. It is reported that the infants' short intravesical ureter approaches normal length by puberty. Accordingly, medical management is based upon knowledge that the natural tendency is improvement or cessation. Conservative management includes administration of continuous low dose chemoprophylaxis until the disappearance of reflux is confirmed by cystoureterography or voiding cystourethrography.

Surgical management eliminates the primary vesicoureteral reflux in over 95% of the patients. Considerations for surgical correction are: 1) the grade of reflux, 2) the age of patients, 3) abnormalities of the ureterovesical junction, 4) the position of the ureteral orifice, 5), the response to antimicrobial agents, and 6) the length of the intravesical ureter.

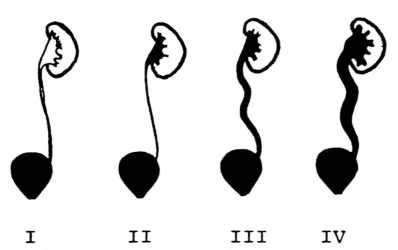

I   II   III   IV

Fig. 8-6. Depiction of the grades of reflux in vesicoureteral reflux.

SELECTED READINGS

1. Kleist H, Jonsson O, Lundstam S, Naucler J, Nilson AE, and Pettersson S.: Quantitative lipid analysis in the differential diagnosis of cystic renal lesions. Brit J Urol, 54-441-445, 1982

2. McDonald MW.: Current therapy for renal cell carcinoma. J Urol, 127:211–217, 1982

3. McNicholas DW, Segura JW and DeWeerd JH: Renal cell carcinoma: Long-term survival and late recurrence. J Urol, 127:17–23, 1981

4. Spence HM: Congenital unilateral multicystic kidney: An entity to be distinguished from polycystic kidney disease and other cystic disorders. J Urol, 74:693–706, 1955

5. Surfrin G and Murphy GP: Renal adenocarcinoma. Urological Survey, 30:129–144, 1980

Alexander C. Chester
Jeffrey P. Harris

9

Pregnancy-Related Nephrology

ANATOMICAL CHANGES OF PREGNANCY

The size of the kidney increases approximately 1 cm in length with pregnancy. Increased interstitial and intravascular volume represent the likely causes, although hormonal causes may contribute. The renal collecting system (renal pelvis and ureters) dilates because of mechanical (partial ureteral obstruction due to the gravid uterus) and endocrinological causes (hormonally induced smooth muscle relaxation). Greater dilation occurs on the right due to the tilt of the gravid uterus. These changes may continue to the third postpartum month, and therefore, require caution in interpreting roentgenological changes before this time. Dilated ureters also serve as a "dead space" reservoir for urine, thereby interfering with accurate urine volume determinations. This is minimized by assuming the lateral recumbent position for one hour prior to start of the urine collection.

PHYSIOLOGICAL CHANGES OF PREGNANCY

Changes in perfusion. Glomerular filtration rate (GFR) and renal plasma flow (RPF) increase 30%–50% in pregnancy. This adaptation starts soon after conception, and reaches its peak by the fourth month. Both gradually decline: the renal plasma flow returns to baseline by the end of the eighth month while the GFR remains elevated until term. Consequently, the normal range of creatinine clearance for the gravida is 105 ml-210 ml per minute, rather than 65 ml-145 ml per minute in the non-pregnant state.

Laboratory alterations. The enhanced renal clearance is reflected in the laboratory values. The serum urea nitrogen (SUN) concentration in pregnancy is lower (6–13 mg/dl), as is the serum creatinine (0.3–0.6 mg/dl) (Figures 1 and 2). A "normal" SUN of 20 mg/dl, or creatinine of 1.2 mg/dl, in pregnancy, may reflect sustantial renal compromise. The serum uric acid concentrations are generally lower than 5.5 mg/dl. This change is not only due to the increased glomerular clearance associated with pregnancy, but also to increased tubular secretion of uric acid.

Glycosuria is common in pregnancy, due to the increased renal load accompanying the higher GFR, and the decrease in the tubular reabsorption to 150 mg per 100 ml from 190 mg per 100 ml in the non-gravida. Additional causes include hormones and vasoactive amines, which antagonize insulin activity. If closely observed, 70% of women will have one episode of glycosuria during pregnancy (Figure 3). Diabetes will develop within 5 years in 28.5% of those with a definitely abnormal glucose tolerance test. If followed for 12 years, 60% will be diabetic. Conversely, in those who are overt diabetics, the insulin requirement during the first half of

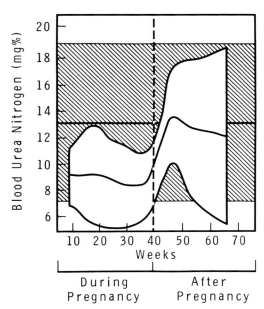

Fig. 9-1. The clear area depicts the range of BUN during normal pregnancy and after delivery. The hatched area depicts the range in the nonpregnant woman. (Adapted with permission from the Journal of Clinical Investigation 37: 1764–1774, 1958.)

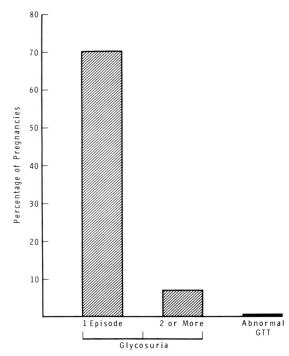

Fig. 9-3. If closely observed, 70 percent of women may have glycosuria on a single random determination. Those with two positive urine tests include only 7 percent, and only 1 percent will have an abnormal glucose tolerance test. (Adapted with permission from the American Family Physician:16: 94–101, 1977.)

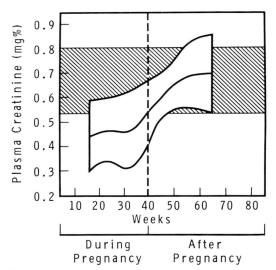

Fig. 9-2. The clear area depicts the range of serum creatinine during normal pregnancy and after delivery. The hatched area depicts the range in the nonpregnant woman. (Adapted with permission from the Journal of Clinical Investigation 37: 1764–1774, 1958.)

pregnancy may decrease due to increased urinary glucose losses. Lactosuria is not infrequent because of the presence of this sugar in the mother's blood and its poor renal reabsorption.

Miscellaneous findings during pregnancy are: an increase in plasma volume, decreased peripheral vascular resistance, increased renin and aldosterone concentrations despite volume expansion, decreased serum protein and plasma osmotic pressure which may account for the augmented GFR toward term, and orthostatic proteinuria which has been reported in as many as 20% of pregnant women.

SIGNS AND SYMPTOMS

Polyuria and nocturia. Polyuria and nocturia are common complaints of pregnancy. The symptoms are in part explained by compression of the bladder by the gravid uterus. Plasma osmolality decreases 5 mOsm to 10 mOsm per Kg H_2O, and is "reset" at that level. No abnormality in the renal concentration mechanism is noted. Nocturia can be abolished by the lateral recumbent position. This suggests that compression of the venous system in the upright position by the gravid uterus causes leg edema. The edematous fluid is gradually mobilized during the night, resulting in nocturia.

Acid-base regulation. Acid-base regulation is altered in pregnancy. Hyperventilation is noted in pregancy due to hormonal influences, with the PCO_2 averaging 30 mm Hg. Metabolic compensation results in a plasma bicarbonate concentration decrease, averaging 4 mmol/l.

Weight gain and edema. The average first pregnancy is associated with a 12.5 kg (27.5 pound) weight gain, and subsequent ones with 1 kg less. The total water increases 6L–8L (liters), 4L–6L of which are extracellular. By term, 200–900 mEq of additional sodium (about 53 grams of NaCl) are acquired. Edema in the absence of hypertension is not necessarily reason for concern, since edema is evident in 80% of normal gravidas. In up to one-third of normal pregnancies, edema may be generalized. Hypervolemia and increased red blood cell volume are noted in the gravida. Because of the large increase in GFR, more sodium is presented to the kidney daily. A host of humoral and physical factors preserve homeostasis.

Proteinuria. Physiological proteinuria in pregnancy may include values of 300 mg per 24 hours, in contrast to the usual upper limit of 150 mg per 24 hours, in females. Again, this reflects in part the increased GFR, and associated increase in filtered protein. Additional causes of proteinuria beyond normal include orthostatic proteinuria, and proteinuria associated with the lordotic posture.

Bacteriuria. The prevalence of asymptomatic bacteriuria ranges between 4% and 7%, which is similar to that of healthy nonpregnant, sexually active women. In 75% to 90% of cases, the organism is E. coli. However, the incidence of symptomatic infection, usually pyelonephritis, following, may be as high as 40%, indicating the need to treat all cases of bacteriuria in

pregnancy. The increased incidence of acute pyelonephritis begins around the fourth month and continues into the puerperium: the latter may be associated with catheterization. When unilateral, it is usually on the right side.

RENAL DISEASE IN PREGNANCY

Renal insufficiency in pregnancy. In general, successful pregnancy is jeopardized by renal insufficiency. The ability to conceive and maintain pregnancy decreases with rising creatinine, and is unusual with values exceeding 3 mg/dl. Associated hypertension is an additional risk factor. Occasionally, pregnancy is observed in advanced renal disease, and has been reported as successful in women on hemodialysis. Even with underlying renal disease, renal function increases with pregnancy.

Renal biopsy. Pregnancy is generally considered to be a relative contraindication to renal biopsy because of reports of excessive bleeding and the general desire to avoid any unnecessary risk to the fetus and the mother. An exception would be a case prior to the 34th gestational week, when the exact diagnosis would be crucial to assessment.

TYPES OF KIDNEY DISEASE

Acute renal failure. Acute renal failure in pregnancy is usually associated with septic abortion and hemorrhage. Additional causes include acute renal failure associated with preeclampsia, and a type of hepato-renal syndrome, termed acute fatty liver of pregnancy. Although acute tubular necrosis is the usual explanation for renal failure, acute cortical necrosis may also occur in pregnancy for similar reasons. Finally, idiopathic postpartum renal failure is described, resembling both hemolytic uremic syndrome and thrombotic thrombocytopenic purpura. It usually occurs one day to a few days postpartum in a setting of an otherwise uneventful pregnancy. The loss of renal function is usually irreversible.

Acute glomerulonephritis. The experience is very limited in post-infectious glomerulonephritis. In the few reported cases, outcome is generally successful.

Chronic glomerulonephritis. Pregnancy is generally successful in patients with a creatinine clearance exceeding 50% of normal. Most authors agree that there is no evidence of deterioration of the primary disease with pregnancy.

Systemic lupus erythematosus. Reports of both improvement and deterioration of the disease with pregnancy are noted.

Nephrotic syndrome. The most frequently observed cause of heavy proteinuria in advanced pregnancy is preeclampsia. Other diseases associated with the nephrotic syndrome are not generally worsened by pregnancy. The increased GFR of the gravida may increase the proteinuria. Infants born of nephrotic mothers are often small for gestational dates.

Diabetes. Renal function in diabetes is not adversely affected by pregnancy. However, an increased incidence of preeclampsia and edema is noted.

Chronic interstitial nephritis. An increased incidence of toxemia in these patients is noted when compared to comparable renal insufficiency secondary to glomerular disease.

Polycystic kidney disease. No increased risk is noted in the absence of hypertension or renal insufficiency. The ability to carry to term with renal insufficiency is less impaired than in other causes of renal disease.

Renal Transplantation

Pregnancy has been observed after transplantation. However, immunosuppressive medication does increase the risk of fetal malformation.

Hypertension in Pregnancy

Normal changes. Blood pressure decreases in early pregnancy, with a diastolic drop of approximately 10 mm Hg to 15 mm Hg by the 16th gestational week. Blood pressure gradually increases after that, approaching the prepregnancy values by term (Figure 4). The hypertensive blood pressure may normalize in early pregnancy.

Preeclampsia. This is a form of hypertension that occurs only in pregnancy, and is as-

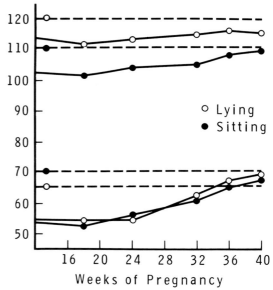

Fig. 9-4. Solid lines depict mean systolic and diastolic blood pressures during normal pregnancy. The broken lines depict the mean blood pressures in normal, nonpregnant women of the same age. During the first and second trimesters, the mean systolic blood pressure is 5 mm. Hg lower and diastolic blood pressure is 10 mm. Hg lower than in the nonpregnant state. In the third trimester, blood pressure returns to nonpregnant levels. (Adapted with permission from Clinical Science and Molecular Medicine 37: 395–407, 1969.)

sociated with proteinuria, edema, and occasional coagulation disturbances. It occurs generally in nulliparas after the 20th gestational week. Blood pressure greater than or equal to 140/85 mm Hg, or an increase of 30 mm Hg in systolic and 15 mm Hg in diastolic readings, is considered abnormal. Severe preeclampsia is characterized by: a diastolic blood pressure greater than 110 mm Hg, systolic blood pressure greater than 160 mg Hg, proteinuria of more than 5 g per day, and oliguria. An increased serum uric acid concentration is generally noted (Figure 5). All patients with any suggestion of preeclampsia require aggressive treatment. Primagravidas who have had preeclampsia have no increase in mortality rate compared to the general gravid population. Preeclamptic multiparas have a four-fold increase in mortality (Figure 6).

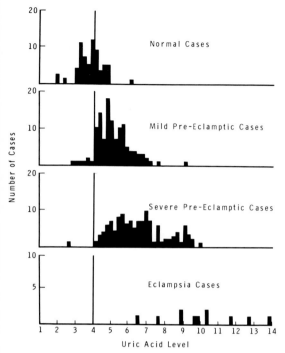

Fig. 9-5. The serum uric acid level is lower during normal pregnancy, due to increased filtration and secretion of uric acid. A rising serum uric acid level may be one of the earliest manifestations of preeclampsia and correlates with its severity. (Adapted with permission from the British Journal of Obstetrics and Gynaecology 70: 63–68, 1963.)

Women who are preeclamptic with their first pregnancy but are normotensive with subsequent pregnancies have actually, a lower probability to developing chronic hypertension then do age-matched controls. Recurrent hypertension with subsequent pregnancies predicts a higher incidence of eventual chronic hypertension.

The principal renal lesion associated with preeclampsia-eclampsia is glomerular capillary endotheliosis. It is characterized by endothelial and mesangial cell swelling. Electron microscopy reveals fibinoid material in the capillary basement membrane on the endothelial side. Immunofluorescence shows fibrin in the mesangial and endothelial cells. The findings generally resolve within a few weeks postpartum, and rarely leave any permanent damage.

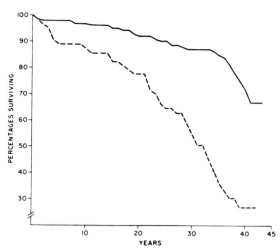

Fig. 9-6. Survival following eclampsia. The solid line represents women who had eclampsia in the first pregnancy. The broken line represents those who had eclampsia as multiparas. (Adapted with permission from the American Journal of Obstetrics and Gynecology 124: 446, 1976).

Chronic hypertension of any cause. Hypertension may be essential or arise from a known secondary cause. Patients with secondary hypertension are more likely to develop preeclampsia. The course is similar to other preeclamptics, with the exception of pheochromocytoma, where high maternal mortality rates are noted.

Chronic hypertension with superimposed preeclampsia. Increasing hypertension noted during the third trimester is observed in some multiparas with chronic hypertension. Oliguria, proteinuria, and diffuse intravascular coagulation may be observed. Chronically hypertensive females who develop preeclampsia have a 70% probability of developing preeclampsia with subsequent pregnancies.

Transient hypertension. Some women develop hypertension late in pregnancy, with a return to normal blood pressure within ten days after delivery. The pattern usually is repeated in future pregnancies. Unlike preeclampsia, it is not associated with heavy proteinuria or an elevated serum uric acid level.

Hypertensive Therapy in Pregnancy

It remains controversial whether human uterine blood flow is autoregulated. In some species, a reduction of the maternal blood flow through the use of antihypertensives results in a comparable drop in utero-placental blood flow with the attendant risk to the fetus. In other species, utero-placental blood flow remains constant over a wide range of mean arterial pressures. Until these data are available in humans, disagreement will persist over what is the optimal level at which a hypertensive gravida's blood pressure should be treated.

A woman with a diastolic pressure of greater than 80 mm Hg any time during the 12th through 36th week of gestation is above the 95th percentile of blood pressure in pregnancy. A mean arterial pressure of 90 mm Hg or greater during the second trimester of pregnancy is associated with an increased rate of stillbirths and intrauterine fetal growth retardation. Milder elevations in pressure do not appear to pose a risk. In the third trimester, the gravida's blood pressure normally rises towards non-pregnant baseline levels. Thus, a higher blood pressure is deemed "hypertensive" during the last trimester compared to the first two.

Diastolic blood pressures of greater than 100 mm Hg are associated with a risk of serious cardiovascular complications including intracerebral hemorrhage, which is the most common cause of maternal deaths in hypertensive pregnancies. Therefore, a diastolic pressure greater than 100 mm Hg warrants drug therapy. Medications are only used for diastolic pressure less than 100 mg Hg if the pressure is rising rapidly or if the mother is experiencing adverse effects from the blood pressure. Diastolic pressures in the 90–100 mm Hg range are generally treated with bed rest and possibly sedation.

When antihypertensives are required, Methyldopa appears to be the safest in terms of its effects to the fetus. Methyldopa significantly decreases the incidence of mid-trimester abortions and successfully controls maternal blood pressure. In a recent 7-1/2 year follow-up of children born to hypertensive mothers receiving Methyldopa, there appeared to be no significant long-term adverse effects on the neonate or child compared to an untreated group.

There is also extensive experience with Hydralazine, but its vasodilatory properties exacerbate some of the physiological effects of the high cardiac output of pregnancy. Patients complain of flushing tachycardia, headaches, and palpitations. Therefore, the drug is used less often than Methyldopa as a long-term oral antihypertensive. Hydralazine is quite useful, however, for short-term parenteral therapy.

Diazoxide appears to be the treatment of choice for hypertensive emergencies. I.V. boluses of 75 mg every 10 minutes may avoid precipitous drops in maternal blood pressure. However, Diazoxide may also decrease uterine contractions and thus halt labor.

Sodium Nitroprusside has been associated with thiocyanate and cyanide toxicity in the fetus. There have been reports of an increased incidence of fetal growth retardation and neonatal deaths with Propranolol. Prazosin, Clonidine, and Minoxidil have not been studied adequately to determine their safety in pregnancy-related hypertension. Limited studies of Atenolol indicate that it is effective in lowering the blood pressure of hypertensive pregnant women with apparently no deleterious effects on the fetus. In these patients, Labetalol therapy has been successful in maintaining uterine blood flow. Neither beta blockers, calcium channel blockers, or angiotensin converting enzyme inhibitors has been studied as extensively as Methyldopa or the diuretics.

Diuretics are generally reserved in pregnancy for patients with pulmonary edema or for those, who despite bed rest, sedation, 2 g of Aldomet and 200 mg of Hydralazine, remain unacceptably hypertensive. These limits have been imposed on diuretic usage out of concern over their associated decrease in plasm volume and cardiac output, along with a rise in peripheral resistance. With thiazides, there is the further concern of their occasional association with thrombocytopenia in newborns.

SELECTED READINGS

1. Essex N, Pyke DA: Brundell JM: Diabetic Pregnancy *Brit Med J,* 1973, 4:89–93
2. Gugliucci CL, O'Sullivan MJ: Intensive Care of the pregnant diabetic. *Am J Ob Gyn,* 125:435–441, 1976
3. Harris JP and Chester AC and Schreiner GE: The Kidney and Pregnancy. *Am Family Physician,* 18:98–102, 1978

4. Lindheimer MD and Katz AI: *Kidney Function* and *Disease in Pregnancy*. Lea and Febiger, 1977

5. Lindheimer MD and Baylis C: Symposium on Renal Function and Disease in Pregnancy. *Am J Kid Dis,* 9:243–375, 1987

6. O'Sullivan JB, Mahan C: Medical Treatment of the Gestational Diabetic. *Obstet and Gynec 43*:817–821, 1974

7. Romney B: Hypertension in Pregnancy. Cardiovascular Review and Reports, 1:632–640, Nov 1980

8. Strauch B and Hayslett JP: Kidney Disease and Pregnancy. *Brit Med J,* 4:578–582, 1974

9. Studd J: The Origin and Effects of Proteinuria on Pregnancy. *J Obstet. Gynaecol* Br Commonw, 80:872–883, 1973

10. Sullivan J: The Hypertensive Diseases of Pregnancy and Their Management. *Adv Int Med,* 27:407–433, 1982

Pedro Jose
Antonia C. Novello
Jean Robillard

10

Pediatric Nephrology

Pediatric nephrology is concerned with the young, developing, and maturing individual. Special characteristics must be dealt with during each stage of development. These include:

1. Intrauterine period
2. Birth and neonatal period (first four weeks of life). Babies born before 38 weeks are considered *preterm*, those born between 38 and 42 weeks are *term*, and those born after 42 weeks are *post-term*.
3. Infancy period (first two years)
4. Preschool period (2–6 years)
5. Mid-childhood period (6–10 years for girls and 6–12 years for boys)
6. Prepubescent period (10–12 years for girls and 12–14 years for boys)
7. Adolescent period (12–18 years for girls and 14–20 years for boys)

This chapter will focus mainly on the renal physiology and problems in the newborn and infancy stages because special needs are most apparent at these stages.

DEVELOPMENTAL ASPECTS OF RENAL FUNCTION

Renal Blood Flow

During fetal life, renal blood flow (RBF) and glomerular filtration rate (GFR) measured in various animal species are low, about 4–5% of cardiac output; but after birth, RBF and GFR increase significantly when renal vascular resistance (RVR) decreases (about 25%). However, RBF is still low and RVR is still high compared to adults, despite these initial changes.

Glomerular Filtration Rate

During the first 24 hours of postnatal life, measurements of GFR closely reflect the status of renal function during intrauterine life. Newborn infants take at least 24 hours to adapt their GFR to the extrauterine environment. After the first day of life, the increase in GFR is disproportionately higher than the concomitant increase in body weight, kidney weight or body surface area.

In a clinical setting, one should remember that the mean values for GFR related to surface area do not reach adult values before 1 to 2 years of age (Table 1). However, it should be pointed out (Table 1) that there is a great deal of variability between infants. The clinician should be aware of the difficulty in determining an accurate GFR during the newborn period.

Renal Na$^+$ Excretion

Premature infants have a relatively high fractional excretion of Na$^+$ (1–5%) which decreases progressively to term values of less than 1% during the first month of life. A negative Na$^+$ balance accompanied by a definite fall in

Table 10-1   Effect of Age on Glomerular Filtration Rate

Age	Glomerular Filtration Rate (ml/min/1.73 m²) and Range	Age	Glomerular Filtration Rate (ml/min/1.73 m²)
Preterm (1–1.5 Days) (Gestational Age)		Infant	
27 weeks	6 (2–10)	2 months	244 (203–321)
28 weeks	8.7 (4–11)	3 months	71 (46–125)
29 weeks	4.5 (4–5)	4 months	88 (56–120)
30 weeks	8.4 (8–10)		68 (47–89)[++]
31 weeks	8.8 (7–11)	6 months	110 (89–144)
32 weeks	8.0 (4–12)	8 months	99 (58–160)
33 weeks	15.6 (12, 18, 17)	12 months	119 (63–150)
34 weeks	10.2 (5–18.5)	18 months	140 (104–235)
35 weeks	15.8 (6–28)		
36 weeks	17.9 (12–26)	Preschool	
37 weeks	17.9 (12–26)	2 years	127 (105–172)
38–40 weeks	18.6 (6.5–33)	3 years	122 (101–179)
		4 years	147 (100–184)
Term Newborn		5 years	143 (120–184)
1–2 days			
Appropriate for Gestational Age (AGA)	23 (8–42)	School	
		6 years	134 (97–170)
		7 years	136 (100–156)
		8 years	124 (90–148)
Small for Gestational Age (SGA)	24 (14–34)	9 years	123 (99–166)
		10 years	127 (95–162)
		11 years	123 (110–146)
Neonate			
4–7 days	34 (20–53)	Adolescence	
8–12 days	50 (40–60)*	12 years	123 (110–136)
15–20 days	54 (30–90)	13–19 years	123 (110–136)
		Adult	
		Male	131 (110–152)
		Female	117 (101–133)

*Premature

serum Na^+ has been observed in premature infants during the first week of life when maintained on Na^+ intakes adequate for term newborns. Accordingly, premature infants require more Na^+ in their diet than full-term infants to maintain a positive Na^+ balance. This increased need for Na^+ is probably due to the interaction of such factors as continuing growth, coprecipitation of sodium in bone, insufficient gastrointestinal sodium absorption, and, most importantly, a high rate of Na^+ excretion by the kidney due to decreased renal response to aldosterone and/or insufficient rise in aldosterone secretion.

Increased urine flow secondary to increased fluid intake contributes to this loss.

Factors that characterize the renal handling of Na^+ in term *newborn infants* are somewhat different than the ones in premature infants. There are two well established characteristics of Na^+ metabolism in term newborn infants: a) the limited ability of the kidney to excrete a Na^+ load, and b) the existence of a positive Na^+ balance to satisfy the needs for growth and bone formation. It has been demonstrated that the limited ability of the kidney to excrete a Na^+ load in term newborn infants is not secondary to low

GFR but to an increased avidity of the distal nephron to reabsorb Na^+ and to high plasma aldosterone concentrations.

Renal Water Metabolism

Premature infants fail to concentrate their urine as well as older children or adults. During dehydration, the maximal urine osmolality achieved (600 mosm/kg H_2O) is about half that achieved in the adult. Similarly, term newborn infants also have limited ability to concentrate. The maximum osmolar concentration achieved at term is about 800 mosm/kg H_2O compared to the adults (1300 mosm/kg H_2O).

Acidifying Capacity

The ability of the newborn kidney to secrete hydrogen ions is also limited. In both term and preterm newborns, urine pH less than 5.5 is not achieved until the first week of life. After one month of age, the ability of the newborn to excrete an acid load is similar to that noted in older children. The serum bicarbonate level in preterm infants may be normally as low as 14 mEq/L but rises to about 21 mEq/L after the first week of life, similar to that seen in term newborns. The lower serum bicarbonate levels in infants has been ascribed to a lower renal threshold for bicarbonate.

RENAL PERTURBATIONS IN NEWBORNS

The major manifestations of urinary tract disease in the newborn are anuria and oliguria, edema, hypertension, abdominal masses, and hematuria.

Anuria or Oliguria

Onset of Micturition. Ninety-five percent of all infants void within the first 48 hours. A history of delayed micturition in the first 24–48 hours is most likely due to inadequate perfusion of the functioning kidneys in an otherwise normal newborn. Other causes are listed in Table 2. The volume of urine voided as a function of age is listed in Table 3.

Table 10-2   Failure of Urine Formation in the Immediate Newborn Period

Causes
Hypoxia
Postnatal intravascular hypovolemia
Restriction of fluids
Bilateral renal agenesis
Tubular necrosis
Bilateral renal vein thrombosis
Congenital nephrotic syndrome
Congenital pyelonephritis
Congenital nephritis
Obstructive uropathy

(Modified from Moore ES and Galvez MB: J Pediatr 80:867–873, 1972)

Prenatal History. The relative amount of amniotic fluid may provide some information on the status of neonatal renal function. Oligohydramnios not due to loss of amniotic fluid may be suggestive of renal agenesis, hypoplasia, dysplasia, or obstructive uropathy.

Physical Examination. Abnormal facies, including low-set ears, flattened nose, hypertelorism and micrognathia may indicate bilateral renal agenesis as seen in Potter's syndrome, characterized by large, floppy low set ears, flattened nose, receding chin, widely separated eyes, and looking like an "old person." Chromosomal abnormalities such as Down's syndrome are also associated with several forms of congenital renal anomalies. Absent abdominal musculature may be suggestive of Eagle-Barrett syndrome (Deficient abdominal wall, hydronephrosis and often cryptorchidism). The presence of a single umbilical artery has been associated with urinary tract abnormalities. Palpation of the abdomen may reveal enlarged kidneys as seen in congenital hydronephrosis, polycystic and multicystic kidney diseases, renal venous thrombosis, and rarely, tumors. The urinary bladder may be enlarged due to outlet obstruction. Abnormalities in testicular descent as well as the penis may be associated with congenital renal anomalies as well.

Bilateral Renal Agenesis. An uncommon abnormality (one in 3,000 births) is often as-

Table 10-3   Volume of Intake and Urine Volume*

Age interval, months	0–1	1–2	2–4	4–6	6–12	12–18	18–24	24–32
Body weight, kg	3.58	5.00	5.82	6.97	8.26	10.70	12.01	13.90
Volume of intake ml/day	657	998	935	1,128	1,309[1]	1,566	1,549	1,625
	(137)	(178)	(238)	(241)	(221)	(342)	(323)	(342)
Volume of intake ml/kg/day	184.1	199.1	160.5	161.8	158.9	146.5	131.1	116.9
	(38.5)	(32.6)	(34.2)	(30.2)	(23.2)	(26.7)	(29.3)	(23.2)
Urine volume ml/day	378	556	496	505	610	873	782	863[2]
	(77)	(140)	(145)	(150)	(172)	(287)	(213)	(300)
Urine volume ml/kg/day	106.6	110.7	85.2	73.3	74.1	80.6	66.2	61.7
	(2.18)	(24.6)	(21.5)	(23.4)	(19.4)	(19.9)	(18.9)	(19.9)
Urine volume % of volume of intake	59	56	53	45	47	55	51	52
	(13)	(11)	(10)	(10)	(11)	(10)	(11)	(10)
Number of voidings	20.1	20.4	19.5	18.7	20.1	15.9	13.5	10.8
	(4.6)	(2.4)	(5.6)	(6.6)	(4.4)	(3.7)	(5.1)	(3.1)
Voiding size ml/voiding	19.3	27.1	25.8	28.4	30.9	57.3	63.1	79.3
	(4.1)	(5.5)	(5.8)	(7.1)	(8.3)	(21.6)	(19.9)	(14.9)
Voiding size ml/kg/voiding	5.4	4.4	4.4	4.1	3.7	5.2	5.2	5.7
	(1.1)	(1.0)	(0.7)	(0.9)	(0.8)	(1.3)	(1.1)	(1.0)

*Mean values are given with standard deviations in parenthesis. Age intervals used: 0–1 = birth to 30 days, 1–2 = 31 to 60 days, etc.
[1]Subject-weighted mean = 1.383 ml/day
[2]Subjected weighted mean = 934 ml/day

(reprinted from Goellner MH, Zeigler EE, and Fomon SJ. Urination During the First Three Years of Life Nephron 28:174–178, 1981 with permission)

sociated with Potter's facies. If ultrasonography does not reveal the presence of kidneys, diagnosis could be established by umbilical arterial angiography. Bilateral renal agenesis is usually associated with pulmonary hypoplasia, and pulmonary dysfunction is a frequent cause of death. Unilateral renal agenesis is a more common anomaly (1 in 500 births). It is associated with anomalies of the genital system, scoliosis and gastrointestinal anomalies including imperforate anus. Other congenital anomalies include duplication of the urinary system and abnormalities of rotation and position.

Acute Renal Failure in the Newborn.
Acute renal failure in the newborn or the adult is a clinical syndrome that occurs following a sudden reduction in renal function. In the new-

born period, this may be the first manifestation of severe renal dysplasia or bilateral agenesis.

The diagnostic criteria for acute renal failure used in the adult including oliguria and azotemia may not be applicable to the newborn period. The influence of gestational age, postnatal age and concomitant disease, usually that of acute respiratory distress syndrome, on renal function presents special problems inherent in the term and preterm newborn. Acute renal failure is usually suspected when oliguria (less than 0.5 ml/kg/hour) or azotemia (SUN greater than 20 mg/dl) are noted. As in the adult, acute renal failure can occur even with normal urine flow rates. It may represent 30% of all acute renal failures during this period.

A SUN greater than 20 mg/dl may not always signify acute renal failure. High protein intake in the preterm infant, hypercatabolic states, sequestered bleeding, large areas of tissue necrosis, hemoconcentration and inborn errors of urea excretion may result in elevated urea levels despite normal renal function (Chap. 1). In our studies azotemia due to hypercatabolic states would only be distinguished from true non-oliguric renal failure by the determination of a creatinine clearance. Because creatinine levels reflect mainly maternal values in the immediate post-natal period, determination of plasma creatinine concentration is not as useful in the diagnosis of renal dysfunction as in the adult. In the newborn the daily increment in SUN occurring with acute renal failure (5 mg/dl/day), rise in serum creatinine (0.5 mg/dl/day), the rise in serum potassium (0.4– 0.8 mEq/L/day) and in serum phosphorus and magnesium and fall in serum calcium and CO_2 are less rapid in the newborn as compared to the adult. This has been related to the higher anabolic states in the newborn.

The diagnosis of acute renal failure caused by acute tubular necrosis is arrived at after the elimination of other diagnostic possibilities. In general, the history, physical examination, urinalysis, and other laboratory tests will usually categorize the cause of the renal failure, whether it is prerenal, renal parenchymal, tubular necrosis or obstructive uropathy. Laboratory aids have been used to help differentiate the entities causing renal failure in the adult. In the newborn the values are quantitatively different. They are listed in Table 4. Additionally, the presence or absence of kidneys should be determined using ultrasonographic studies or by using radionuclide techniques (Chapter 3).

The establishment of urine flow may be used as a diagnostic as well as a therapeutic maneuver in distinguishing prerenal failure from oliguric acute tubular necrosis. The first step is to assure adequate volume repletion if there is no evidence of circulatory overload and the central venous pressure is not elevated. A fluid challenge of 10% dextrose in water with 30 mmol/L NaCl at 20 ml/kg in 1–2 hours may be undertaken. In the premature newborn, plasma or albumin infusions have also been used. If ade-

Table 10-4   Laboratory Values in Various Forms of Acute Renal Failure (9).

	Pre-renal Oliguria		Oliguric Acute Tubular Necrosis	
	Adult	Infant*	Adult	Infant
Urine Na (mmol/L)	< 20	< 10	> 25	> 40
Urine Osmolality (mOsm/L)	> 500		< 350	
U/P osmolality	> 2	> 2	< 1.1	< 1.1
U/P creatinine	> 40	> 20	< 10	< 10
U/P urea	> 20	> 5	< 10	< 10
FEx Na%	< 1	< 2	> 3	> 3**
Renal Failure Index (UNa/UCr/PCr)	< 1	< 2	> 1	> 3**
Urine sediment (Casts)	hyaline & granular		cellular	

*For infants >32 weeks gestational age and preterm infants older than 2 weeks
**Values greater than 10 in 1 week old preterm infants <32 weeks gestational age

U = urine
P = plasma
FEx = fractional sodium excretion
Cr = creatinine

(Modified from Jose PA, Tina LU, Papadopoulou ZL, and Calcagno PC. in Neonatology. Pathophysiology and Management of the Newborn. Avery GB(ed.), Philadelphia J.B. Lippincott Co. 1981, p 677–700.

quate urine output is not established in 1–2 hours, a trial of mannitol, furosemide, or both, may be initiated. In the case of prerenal failure 60 ml/m^2/hour of 12.5% mannitol solution usually results in a urine output of at least 12 ml/m^2/hour within one hour of infusion. It should be noted that the use of mannitol is contraindicated in the presence of circulatory overload. Furosemide at a dose of 1–2 mg/kg intravenously has also been used, but controlled studies are not available for the newborn period. There should be an increase in urine flow 50% or greater within 1–2 hours of the injection of furosemide. In non-oliguric renal failure, fluid and electrolyte losses should be replaced to avoid dehydration. Once oliguric renal failure is diagnosed, fluid intake should be restricted to that required to replace insensible loss, urine, and any other extrarenal water and electrolyte losses. Insensible losses of water vary greatly depending upon gestational age and environmental conditions. For example, preterm infants weighing less than 1000 grams have an insensible loss of about 3.8 mg/kg/hour. Between 1000 and 1250 grams, insensible loss is about 2.5 ml/kg/hour. This decreases to about 1.8 ml/kg/hour for those weighing between 1251–1500 grams and decreases to about 1 ml/kg/hour for those weighing between 1501–1750 grams. Those weighing 1751–2000 have an insensible loss of about 0.8 ml/kg/hour. With the use of radiant warmers and phototherapy there is a 50% increase in insensible water loss. The use of relatively high humidity would reduce insensible water loss by about 30%. Nutritional status should be monitored carefully to provide a minimal exogenous caloric intake of 40 KCal/kg/day as carbohydrate and fat. Recent studies in infants and adults suggest that the addition of essential amino acids may be of benefit.

In the well managed patient, hyperkalemia is rarely a problem. In the first ten days of life, potassium may be normally as high as 7 mmol/L. As in adults with severe hyperkalemia, serum potassium greater than 7.5 mmol/L with major EKG abnormalities should be treated with calcium gluconate, bicarbonate and glucose administration; and the patient should be prepared for dialysis.

In oliguric renal failure in the newborn as in the adult the duration of the oliguria is quite variable, ranging from hours to weeks, 1–2 weeks being the usual period. Oliguria lasting more than 4 weeks is suggestive of cortical necrosis. In ap-proximately two-thirds of patients, glomerular filtration rate may remain 20%–40% below normal for a year or more after the episode of oliguria. Non-oliguric renal failure tends to have a shorter period of significant azotemia. In the newborn period, 40% of mortality is due to concurrent illness, usually due to respiratory distress syndrome.

Edema of the Newborn. Edema of the newborn constitutes a major clinical problem. In the newborn period, 75% of newborn bodyweight is water and just about adult values of 65% at the end of the first year of life. Extracellular water in skin and subcutaneous tissue accounts for 16% of the infant's body water compared with 8% in the adult. *In utero* and immediately after birth, the extracellular fluid mass is greater than that of the intracellular fluid. Weight loss within the first few days of life to as much as 10% would indicate recovery from physiological edema and has not been associated with adverse renal function. Edema of the preterm infant is usually associated with increased capillary permeability. It may also be related to asphyxia, hypotension, poor perfusion, and failure to maintain appropriate body temperature. Edema has also been associated with Vitamin E deficiency, Rh incompatibility, and the congenital nephrotic syndrome. Rarer causes of edema include hereditary hypoparathyroidism, hypomagnesemia, and hypocalcemia. The management should be based upon the etiology. Diuretics, such as furosemide, may occasionally be indicated at 1 mg/kg/dose. The use of diuretics in the newborn period presents special problems. The thiazide diuretics are not usually indicated because of their tendency to reduce glomerular filtration rate. Athough some studies have suggested that the diuretic response to furosemide given parenterally was unrelated to age, other studies have suggested that the furosemide response in stressed term infants may be less intense but more prolonged when compared to the adult. In infants with fluid overload, the plasma clearance of furosemide was slower and volume of distribution greater in preterm and full-term neonates as compared to the adult.

Hypertension. Hypertension in the newborn has been defined as systemic blood pressure greater than 90/60 in term infants and greater than 80/45 in preterm infants. A percentile of blood pressure distribution through one year of age is shown in Figure 1. An incidence of 2.5% has been reported in intensive care nursery admissions. Over 75% may be caused by renal artery thrombosis. The next most common cause is renal artery stenosis (18%). Rare causes include congenital renal anomalies, adrenal hyperplasia, hypoplastic aorta, and coarctation of the aorta. In some cases, no clear etiology could be found. Signs and symptoms are nonspecific. Heart failure may be present.

Therapy should be directed at identifying and correcting the etiology. In one series, 85% of the infants had an indwelling umbilical artery catheter prior to or at the onset of hypertension. Mild hypertension (10 torr greater than the upper limits of normal) may respond to salt restriction or diuretics. Greater elevations of blood pressure may be treated with hydralazine (1–6 mg/kg/day) and furosemide (2–5 mg/kg/day) in four divided doses. When pulmonary and heart disease are not present, propranolol (2–4 mg/kg/day) may also be used. Captopril at 0.2 to 2 mg/kg/day may be used if bronchopulmonary dysplasia is aggravated by propranolol. Extreme elevations of blood pressure may be managed with diazoxide (2–5 mg/kg/dose IV). Nitroprusside may be used, starting at a dose of 2 μg/kg/minute. Thiocyanate levels should be monitored if nitroprusside is used for more than 3 days. Uncontrollable hypertension caused by unilateral renal disease may necessitate nephrectomy.

Renal artery thrombosis has been associated with umbilical artery catheterization, patent ductus arteriosus, cardiac arrhythmias, trauma, sepsis, hypovolemia, and hypercoagulable states. Hypertension is common. The kidneys are not usually enlarged. Urinalysis may be normal but more commonly reveals hematuria and proteinuria. Renal function may be diminished and irreversible renal cortical necrosis or infarction may occur. Peripheral renin activity is elevated. Nephrosonography should be first performed to ascertain the size of the kidneys. Radionuclide studies are usually sufficient to establish the di-

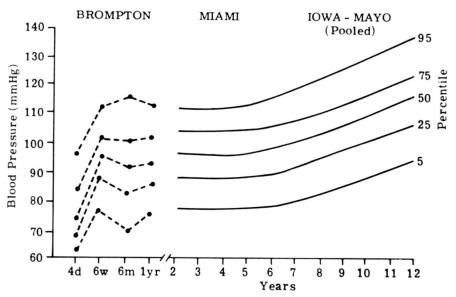

Fig. 10-1. Percentiles of blood pressure in infants awake (both sexes pooled) at age 4 days to 1 year (Brompton study). The percentiles for ages 2 to 14 years have been taken from the values for 29 to 45 boys from the Miami study and from 453 to 592 boys from the Muscatine and Rochester studies (Iowa-Mayo pool) as summarized by the Task Force for Blood Pressure Control in Children: (de Swiet, M., Fayers, P., and Shinebourne, E. A. Systolic Blood Pressure in a Population of Infants in the First Year of Life. Pediatr 56:1028–1035, 1980, with permission).

agnosis. The treatment is entirely symptomatic with aggressive treatment of the hypertension. Thrombectomy and anticoagulant therapy remain to be evaluated.

Abdominal Mass

Hydronephrosis. Unilateral hydronephrosis is usually due to ureteropelvic obstruction. Bilateral hydronephrosis should call attention to posterior urethral valves in the male. Urinalysis is usually normal. Serum chemistries are variable. Diagnosis is confirmed by sonography. Anatomical localization could be made by renal scan. A voiding cystourethrogram is indicated if posterior urethral valves are suspected. Treatment requires a pediatric urologist.

Bilaterally enlarged kidneys with enlarged bladder is characteristic of obstructive uropathy most commonly due to posterior urethral valves. Since vesicoureteral reflux is present in about 50% of all cases, a voiding cystourethrogram is often of value in outlining renal size and bladder size as well as the site of obstruction.

Cystic Disease of the Kidney. The presence of bilaterally enlarged kidneys should call attention to the possibility of renal cystic disease. Multicystic kidney disease may be bilateral but is more commonly unilateral and is as frequent as a cause of abdominal mass of renal origin in the newborn as hydronephrosis. Adult type polycystic kidney disease, which is transmitted as an autosomal dominant trait, could present in the newborn. The cysts can be demonstrated by ultrasonography in the kidney and may also be present in the spleen and in the liver. Because of the frequent association with intracerebral aneurysms, a careful search for a bruit should be undertaken.

Infantile polycystic kidney disease is inherited as an autosomal recessive trait, usually associated with hepatic fibrosis, in contrast to multicystic kidney disease and adult type of polycystic kidney disease. Ultrasonographic study will just reveal enlarged kidneys with increased echogenecity but without cysts.

Renal Tumors. Renal tumors are exceedingly rare.

Renal Venous Thrombosis. This condition is seen in the newborn period in association with asphyxia, hypoxia, vomiting, diarrhea, and dehydration, hypovolemia, hyperosmolality, disseminated intravascular coagulation, cyanotic heart disease, following contrast angiography, and in infants of diabetic mothers. In the newborn period, the babies affected are predominantly males. The kidneys may be palpably enlarged in 60% of cases. Blood pressure is usually normal. Oliguria may be noted; hematuria is usually present. The presence of hematuria, enlarged kidneys and intravascular clotting is suggestive of renal venous thrombosis. Nephrosonography and renal scans are usually sufficient to establish the diagnosis.

Oliguric infants should be treated in a fashion similar to those with acute renal failure in the newborn. Hypovolemia and intravascular clotting should be corrected. Heparinization is usually not necessary unless there is evidence of continued intravascular coagulation with abnormally low platelet counts. Late sequella is variable and may be a cause of neonatal hypertension later on.

Neonatal Ascites. Causes include obstructive uropathy, congenital nephrosis and hydrops fetalis.

Hematuria

Red urine in the newborn may indicate gross hematuria, hemoglobinuria, myoglobinuria. If dipstick is negative for blood, urates should be suspected. Hematuria may be associated with renal vascular accidents such as renal venous thrombosis, trauma to a normal or more commonly abnormally enlarged kidney, hypoxic kidney or that associated with acute tubular or cortical necrosis and urinary tract infection.

ENURESIS

Enuresis, or bedwetting, characterized by the involuntary passage of urine during sleep more than once a month, is subdivided into *primary* or *secondary* bedwetting. The former refers to a patient who has never been dry, the latter to a patient previously toilet trained who starts wetting again.

PREVALENCE

The prevalence of enuresis is similar in industrial and nonindustrial societies. It has been known to occur in 30% of children at age 4, 10% at age 6, 3% at age 12, and 1% at age 18. Enuresis carries a spontaneous cure rate of 15% per year. It is more prevalent in boys than girls, and has often been associated with lower socioeconomic groups, smaller families, and broken homes.

ETIOLOGY

Most patients have neither primary nor secondary emotional or organic problems, but instead have a small functional bladder capacity. Thus, enuresis should be considered a normal variation in bladder control rather than a disease state. Nonetheless, genetic predisposition exists, since the symptom can be uncovered in other siblings or at least one parent in 40% of the cases.

ASSESSMENT AND EVALUATION

A systematic approach will avoid any unnecessary manipulations and allow for the prompt differentiation between true enuretic episodes and commonly confused entities. A complete physical examination is of the utmost importance to screen out any relevant abnormalities or irritative lesions. The exam should include: observation of the urinary stream, good abdominal and genital examination, inspection of the lower spinal area, perineal sensation, anal tone, and neurological screening.

Given a normal history and physical exam, the laboratory evaluation should be limited to: (1) urinanalysis for both males and females (including specific gravity and osmolality); (2) culture and sensitivity in females. Radiographic studies; (A) IVP (Intravenous Pyelogram); (B) Voiding Cystourethrogram; and/or urologist's examination, but only after a urinary tract infection has been documented 2 or more times in females; or at least once in males; with or without abnormal urinary stream.

ASSOCIATED FINDINGS

In the past, sleep disorders have been associated with enuresis, including longer periods of deep sleep, sleep terrors, confusional arousals, and increased duration of sleep latency. Enuresis has also been associated with stress during toilet training, allergies, and confused with polyuric episodes such as those found in diabetes insipidus, sickle cell anemia, and diabetes mellitus. But recent studies at the NIH have shown that enuretic events are not associated with

a particular sleep stage. Likewise their results do not support the hypothesis that enuresis is an arousal disorder. Most of the enuretic children have neither organic problems nor emotional problems. Organic etiologies are present in no more than 1 to 2% of patients, with urinary tract infections being the most frequent problem. Even when these are documented, there are few radiological abnormalities.

TREATMENT

Scientists and physicians have not agreed on a treatment; however, they do accept a general approach to resolving enuresis. This approach includes motivation, full responsibility, and active participation in the treatment process by the patient. Several treatment modalities have been advocated, with motivational counseling, utilized as an adjuvant to all modalities. With counseling, the patient starts to play an active role, becomes reassured, and receives positive reinforcement about improvement.

Counseling. It is important to meet with the patient separately and to reassure him or her of the high prevalence of enuresis, its spontaneous cure rate, and the familial incidence. Dry nights are to be praised, wet nights downplayed.

Bladder Exercises. In those children with small bladder capacities, bladder stretching exercises should be used. The primary goal is to increase bladder capacity by holding urination as long as possible. These exercises are aimed at expanding the previous functional levels of the bladder as well as encouraging the child to be in control of his or her level of bladder response. During this phase, a child can also be encouraged to do stream interruption exercises, which will aid in withstanding bladder spasm. Motivational counseling also works well in children with normal bladder capacities. When bladder exercises are the mode of treatment, an increased capacity of one ounce per month of urine should be considered successful, and cure can be attained in at least 35% of the cases.

Enuresis Alarms. This is the most widely used technique when everything else has failed, and the child has a small bladder capacity. The alarm works particularly well with primary enuretics. With the newest sets of alarms, only few drops of urine will trigger the mechanism. Although alarms are a slow process of cure, a child eventually will awaken by a full bladder sensation rather than by the sound of the buzzer. The alarm should be continued for at least 3 more weeks past the dry period. The cure rate is 70%.

Medications. At this time, no drug is 100% safe and effective for children with small bladder capacities. However, Imipramine (Tofranil) has been the most extensively studied. Imipramine seems to work because of its anticholinergic effect. Larger doses do not seem to increase the success rate, although plasma concentrations shows a significant correlation with clinical effect. Imipramine can be utilized for the short-term management of enuresis, and successful response is usually seen in the first week. The drug has not been approved for children under 6 years of age, and when utilized in children with secondary enuresis, the cure rate is 25%. Some caution has to be exercised when using Imipramine since it is potentially lethal. Physicians should prescribe just enough for 2 weeks, not give the medication to smaller children, and obtain an EKG before the treatment starts, for Imipramine is known to cause arrhythmias and raise the resting pulse rate and diastolic blood pressure. The normal dose is 50 mg at bedtime up to 12 years and 75 mg over 12 years. Withdrawal should be gradual to prevent relapse. Thus, with only 25% cure rate and a 50% relapse rate Imipramine has to be prescribed only for cases where the success outweighs the risk.

Two other drugs frequently used are oxybutynin (Ditropan) and Desmopressin (DDAVP). Ditropan differs from Imipramine in its antispasmodic effects and its use in children under 8 years of age. It has no cardiac complications and works in nocturnal, diurnal enuresis and daytime bladder spasms. DDAVP allows for the temporary relief of enuresis secondary to its water retention capacity. But the place of this vasopressin analog in the treatment of enuresis remains to be determined.

SUMMARY OF TREATMENTS

1. Motivation and Counseling
   (a) For all ages, alone or as an adjuvant
2. Bladder Exercises, (Interruption of Stream and Increased Fluid Intake and Retention)
   (a) For all ages
   (b) First line of treatment from age 6 to 8
   (c) Especially for children with small bladder capacities
3. Enuretic alarms
   (a) Successful with primary enuretics
   (b) For children older than 8 years and older teenagers with enuresis
   (c) Not recommended as the first line of treatment for children with normal bladder capacity, or who are deaf, emotionally disturbed or share bed or room with siblings.
4. Medications
   (a) Not for children under 6 years
   (b) For secondary enuretics
   (c) For only short-term effect
   (d) Only to be used in conjunction with motivational techniques

Relapses and Failures. The relapse rate varies from 10% with the alarm to 50% with drugs. If there is a relapse, one must reinitiate the successful treatment program. If there is no success after 2 to 3 months, the patient needs reassurance that the problem will improve eventually as well as advice to continue the last successful program for at least 6 months to 1 year. Constant motivation is crucial.

Although a frustrating problem, enuresis is usually harmless and self-limiting. In the long run most cures occur with maturity rather than with medical treatment.

SELECTED READINGS

Aperia A, Broberger O, Herin P, Theodenius K, and Zetterstrom R. Postnatal control of water and electrolyte homeostasis in pre-term and full term infants. Acta Pediatr. Scand. (Supp). 305:61, 1983

Jose PA, Tina LU, Papadopoulou ZL, and Calcagno PL. Renal Diseases in Neonatology. Pathophysiology and Management of the Newborn. Avery GB, (Ed), J. B. Lippincott, Co., Philadelphia, p. 661, 1981

McLain LG: Childhood Enuresis. Current Problems in Pediatrics 9:1–36, 1979

Meadow SR, Enuresis. In Edelman CM (ed); Pediatric Kidney Disease, Vol. 11. Boston, Little, Brown and Company, 1978 pp. 1176–1181

Robillard J, and Matson JR. The premature nephron: Physiologic characteristics and clinical implications. Pediatric Update. Review for Physicians. Mass AJ (Ed.) Elsiever, N.Y. (1980), p. 167–191

Schmitt BD: Nocturnal Enuresis: an Update on Treatment. In Symposium on Persistant Signs and Symptoms. Pediatric Clinics of North America. Vol. 29 No. 1: 21–36, 1982

Bernard B. Davis, M.D.
Terry V. Zenser, M.D.
Robert D. Lindeman, M.D.

11

Geriatric Nephrology

BACKGROUND

The approach to renal, fluid and electrolyte problems must be modified for elderly patients as kidney function decreases with age. Kidneys have a remarkable physiological reserve and aging is associated with a loss of this reserve. Fluid, electrolyte and acid-base chemistries are usually reported as "normal" in the elderly, but the capacity to modulate these values during physiological stress is diminished. For example, serum pH and bicarbonate may be normal under basal conditions, but when an acid challenge is given lowering the pH and serum bicarbonate, it takes longer for these parameters to return to baseline.

Physicians frequently are faced with solving problems in this potentially "brittle" population. The purpose of this chapter is to describe the anticipated changes in kidney anatomy, function and capacity to regulate fluid, electrolyte and acid-base balance that occur with age.

ANATOMY

Morphological changes specifically related to the aging process are difficult to separate from those resulting from insults occurring throughout lifetime as a result of inflammatory, degenerative and mechanical (hypertension) perturbations. Nonetheless, there are definitive changes in renal structure primarily related to aging listed in Table 1. Prominent are age-related renal vasculature changes including intimal thickening and reduplication of the lamina elastica interna. There

also is an age-related deposition of hyaline material seen first in the afferent arteriole and later in the efferent arteriole.

The number of functioning glomeruli decreases with age by a process known as ischemic obsolescence whereby the vasculature to individual glomeruli is compromised. Although it is widely assumed that age-related changes in the kidney are vascular in origin, involuted glomeruli often retain patent afferent arterioles (cortical glomeruli) or forms shunts between the afferent and efferent arterioles (juxtamedullary glomeruli). Thus the major changes may occur at the capillary level, and glomerular regression could be initiated by either vascular or tissue factors. By the seventh decade, only one-half of the early glomerular complement remains. Glomerular obsolescence is accompanied by a parallel loss of renal tubules and subsequent replacement with interstitial tissue. Total renal size, as measured by x-ray or ultrasound, remains relatively constant despite decreased renal parenchyma because an increase in mesenchymal tissue with age takes place. Since kidney size is frequently utilized to assess chronicity of renal impairment, this discrepancy between renal size and function in the elderly should be borne in mind.

PHYSIOLOGY

The clinically important age-related changes in renal function are listed in Table 2. Glomerular filtration declines progressively with age.

Table 11-1 Anatomical Changes in the Kidney Associated with Aging

Arterial	Intimal thickening Reduplication of lamina elastica interna
Arteriolar	Hyaline deposition
Glomerular	Hyalinization Decreased number of functional glomeruli
Tubular	Decrease in number
Interstitial	Increase in interstitium Cellular infiltrate

Table 11-2 Physiological Changes in the Kidney Associated with Aging

Decreased glomerular filtration rate and renal blood flow.
Decreased capacity to concentrate the urine.
Decreased capacity to conserve sodium
Decreased capacity to excrete an acid load.

Although a number of formulae have been proposed to predict aging changes in GFR, a good rule of thumb is that the GFR decreases 1% per year after age 40. This correlates well with the age-related decrements in the nephron population.

In most elderly individuals, there is a progressive decrease in muscle mass even though total body weight may increase. Because the production of creatinine is directly related to muscle mass (chapter 1), there is an age-related decrease in creatinine production. In the absence of acute renal failure or rhabdomyolysis where serum creatinine concentrations are rapidly changing, the rates of creatinine production and excretion are equal. The decrease in creatinine production is matched by a decrease in GFR resulting in very little change in serum creatinine concentration. In severe muscle wasting associated with nutritional deficiencies and/or catabolic disease in the elderly, the decrease in muscle mass may be greater than the loss of GFR resulting in a fall of serum creatinine concentration despite loss of renal function. Factors normally used to correct creatinine clearances such as body mass or surface area can be misleading in the elderly. If the clinician is not aware of these relationships, significant miscalculations can be made using serum creatinine concentrations alone in elderly patients to modify the dosages of drugs eliminated by the kidney.

An age-related decrease in capacity to concentrate urine is not uncommon. The defect appears to be primarily renal in origin rather than secondary to alterations in vasopressin secretion. The renal defect in the elderly person is probably due to an inability of the countercurrent system to generate the same medullary hypertonicity as the younger individual. A decreased responsiveness of the collecting tubule cells to the hydroosmotic effects of vasopressin is not apparent. Elderly patients require a larger urinary volume to excrete the daily mandatory solute load of approximately 500–600 mOsm. If the older person does not compensate for this defect by increasing fluid intake, he will more readily develop dehydration than a younger person. Obviously, water deprivation can involve more risk in the elderly, especially after such diagnostic maneuvers as water deprivation in preparation for intravenous urography or in such infirmities as central nervous system or musculoskeletal disease which impairs easy access to water. This decreased capacity to conserve water also predisposes to hypotonic fluid losses and hypernatremia.

In addition to poor water conservation, the elderly are limited in their ability to react to sodium deprivation with effective conservation. One reason for this is that on both restricted and unrestricted sodium intakes, plasma renin activities and urinary aldosterone excretions are decreased in elderly individuals compared to younger subjects under matching conditions of sodium intake. Another factor may be an increased solute excretion per surviving hypertrophied nephron which creates a relative solute diuresis.

Care should be exercised when prescribing low sodium diets for geriatric patients, because they more easily become sodium and volume-depleted. Both the decreased capacity to conserve sodium and water make the defense of the extracellular fluid volume precarious. A reduced extracellular volume may be insufficient to support adequate perfusion of all organ systems. Specific clinical findings depend upon the existence of underlying vascular pathology, e.g., the presence of cerebral vascular pathology predisposes to central nervous system symptomatology in dehydrated elderly.

Decreased aldosterone excretion often leads to hyperkalemia in older persons especially when subjected to additional potassium loads. Among men hospitalized in acute care hospitals, 25% of those over 70 had serum potassium concentrations exceeding 4.5 mEq/L. and 15% had potassiums above 5.0 mEq/L. In patients with relative hyperkalemia, serum bicarbonate concentrations are slightly depressed and serum chlorides slightly increased.

Elderly individuals have decreased ability to excrete acid in the urine, although serum pH and bicarbonate under basal conditions are not different in young and old subjects. Furthermore, after acid loading with ammonium chloride, the urine pH decreases comparably in the old and the young. However, augmentation in production and excretion of ammonia and, to a lesser extent, titratable acid are less in the elderly. This results in a delay in the return of serum pH and bicarbonate to basal levels after an acid challenge. The loss of physiological reserve in acid-base homeostasis has the same implications as it does in altered salt and water metabolism. Accordingly, this reduced capacity to respond to environmental stress should be recognized by the clinician when dealing with older patients.

PATHOPHYSIOLOGY

How kidney function decreases with age in the individual normal subject remains unclear. Is there a progressive involutional change with loss of nephron units during life or does renal function remain stable until intervening acute or chronic disease processes lessen renal function? Examples of such destructive events might be vascular occlusion with resultant ischemic injury and tubulointerstitial damage secondary to drug toxicity, infection or immunological injury. The observation that many young and old subjects can be followed over periods of many years with no decline in renal function suggests the latter.

Localized functional defects consistent with ischemic injury were identified by scintillation scanning techniques in two-thirds of one patient

population studied with ages ranging from 60–93 years. A high incidence of urinary tract infections, evidenced by chronic pyuria and bacteriuria, is found in both elderly males and females with the incidence reaching 50% in women in the eighth decade. Approximately one-third of patients over age 70 have pyuria when urinary sediment is examined. Importantly, renal clearances are decreased in this group compared to patients of comparable age without pyuria.

The clinical picture in many elderly patients simulates a tubulointerstitial nephritis (chapter 14) which could be due to ischemic changes or chronic infectious, inflammatory and/or immunological processes. There is a greater tendency with this histologic picture to develop decreased capacity to concentrate urine and a tendency toward renal salt wasting, hyperchloremic acidosis, hyperkalemia and hypoaldosteronism. In its most complete form, it is referred to as a type IV renal tubular acidosis. Urinary infections are common in such patients.

CLINICAL

Tables 3 and 4 illustrate misconceptions that can be perpetrated by using only serum creatinine concentrations in elderly patients to determine dosages of drugs cleared primarily or partially by the kidney. As mentioned earlier, mean serum creatinine concentrations are similar in old and young subjects, yet creatinine production and

Table 11-3 Mean values for serum creatinine concentrations, 24 hour urinary creatinine excretions, and creatinine clearances in young and old subjects*

Mean Values	Young 20–40 years	Old 60–80 years
Serum creatinine (mg/dl)	0.80	0.84
24-hour urine creatinine (g)	1.5	0.8
Creatinine clearance (ml/min)	130	66

*Based on data from Rowe, et al (5).

Table 11-4 Kinetics of digoxin and gentamycin clearances and modifications in maintenance therapy necessary to maintain appropriate therapeutic blood levels.

Digoxin Kinetics	Serum Half Life (days)	Daily Mtce. dose (% of loading dose)
Normal renal function	1.6	40
Anuric patient	4.4	14
Reported patient (Cl_cr 48 ml/min)	2.4	25

Gentamycin Kinetics	Serum Half Life (days)	Dose Fraction*
Normal renal function	2.3	1.0
Anuric patient	51.0	0.05
Reported patient	4.6	0.5

*A nomogram for dose modification has been provided by Bryan and Stone (see under Selected Readings) A formula commonly used for calculating gentamycin dosage is 1 mg/kg body weight every eight hours times the serum creatinine concentration. In the above-reported case, the patient received nearly twice the dose required to maintain therapeutic blood levels. It is common for such patients to develop nephrotoxicity increasing further the serum concentrations of administered medications.

excretion are only one-half compared to the young. The impact of this is illustrated in the following case report.

An 86 year old white male with congestive heart failure and urinary tract infection secondary to klebsiella was admitted. A decision was made to treat with digoxin and gentamycin (digoxin is metabolized by the liver and cleared by the kidney; gentamycin is cleared by the kidney). His SUN was 16 mg%, and serum creatinine concentration was 1.0 mg%. Because these were considered normal, he received the usual recommended initial and maintenance doses of each drug, (a 24-hour urine creatinine excretion was 0.7 g, and the creatinine clearance was calculated to be 48 ml/min). Ten days later, serum creatinine increased to 4.5 mg/dl (gentamycin nephrotoxicity), and his electrocardiogram showed paroxysmal atrial tachycardia with 2:1 atrioventricular block (evidence of digoxin toxicity). It was felt that the impairment of renal function due to gentamycin nephrotoxicity further diminished the clearance of these two drugs. Table 4 shows the clearance kinetics of digoxin and gentamycin in a normal young subject, an anuric patient, and this patient at the time his medications were started.

SELECTED READINGS

1. Adler S, Lindeman RD, Yiengst MJ, Beard E, Shock NW: Effect of acute acid loading in primary acid excretion by the aging human kidney. J Lab Clin Med 72:278–289, 1968.
2. Bryan CS, Stone WJ: Antimicrobial dosage in renal failure: A unifying nomogram. Clin Nephrol 7:81–84, 1977.
3. Epstein M: Effects of aging on the kidney. Fed Proc 38:168–171, 1979.
4. Goldman R: Aging of the excretory system: Kidney and Bladder. In: Finch CE, Hayflick L (eds), Handbook of the Biology of Aging. New York: Van Nostrand Reinhold, p. 409–431, 1977.
5. Murray T, Goldberg M: Chronic interstitial nephritis: Etiologic factors. Ann Intern Med 82:453–459, 1975.
6. Rosen R: Renal disease in the elderly. Symposium on geriatric medicine. Med Clin North Am 60:1105–1119, 1976.
7. Rowe JW, Andres R, Tobin ID, Shock NW: The effect of age on creatinine clearance in man: A cross-sectional and longitudinal study. J. Gerontol 31:155–163, 1976.

John P. Johnson, M.D.
Jack Moore, Jr., M.D.

12

Primary Glomerular Diseases

INTRODUCTION

The purpose of this chapter is to provide the reader with a practical approach to the diagnosis and management of primary glomerular diseases. This heterogenous group of diseases shares a common feature in that the major site of pathologic involvement is the glomerulus. The etiology of most primary glomerular diseases is unknown, thus they are defined by their dominant morphological characteristics. Accordingly, individual disease entities are described by the natural history of patient groups whose renal biopsies disclose similar morphologies. In secondary glomerular diseases, many of the same morphological expressions are seen, herein usually associated with a well-defined clinical illness.

Primary glomerulopathies may therefore be defined as those not clearly associated with identifiable systemic processes. These entities are dominated clinically by renal dysfunctions: proteinuria, hematuria, presence of urinary casts, variable decline in renal function, and consequent edema and hypertension.

The approach to primary glomerulonephritis (PGN) which we outline here is reasonably straightforward. The clinician initially utilizes the medical history, physical examination and laboratory studies to include or exclude the possibility of systemic disease and to define the degree of renal involvement. If this information indicates a systemic illness, the need for morphologic diagnosis and therapy tends to be guided by what is known of the renal abnormalities associated with the systemic disease. Conversely, if systemic illness appears unlikely, the information gathered as above should allow the clinician to place the patient into one of the major syndromes associated with PGN. Knowledge of the morphologies associated with the major clinical syndromes allows one to decide to follow the patient or to proceed to renal biopsy for definitive morphologic diagnosis and therapeutic guidance. Since the general assumption of the literature is that morphology predicts natural history and response to therapy, it is our belief that wherever possible in adults, treatment should be based upon definitive morphologic diagnosis. Since so much depends upon morphology, a description of the major patterns of glomerular involvement will assist the reader in assessing studies of the treatment of PGN.

MORPHOLOGIC CLASSIFICATION

The major glomerular responses of glomeruli to injury illustrated in Figures 1 and 2. *Minimal* changes refer to variably subtle increases in the number or amount of mesangial

The opinions contained herein are the private views of the authors, and are not to be construed as representing the official views of the Department of the Army or the Department of Defense.

cells or matrix on light microscopy (LM). Immunofluorescence microscopy (IF) is negative, while electron microscopy (EM) demonstrates fusion of the epithelial cell foot processes. These changes describe minimal change GN, also known as lipoid nephrosis or nil disease. Clinically patients with this lesion present with heavy proteinuria and normal or slightly increased renal function.

Membranous changes refer to thickening of the capillary loops with minimal cellular increase on LM. IF demonstrates diffuse, granular deposition of immunoglobulin (Ig), usually IgG, and the third component of complement (C3) along the walls of the capillary loops. EM demonstrates that electron-dense deposits, representing immune complexes, are located within the basement membrane. Homogeneity of glomerular involvement and a paucity of deposits other than within the basement membrane suggest primary GN. These changes describe membranous GN, which is clinically expressed as heavy proteinuria and a variable, but progressive decline in renal function. Similar, albeit more heterogenous glomerular involvement is seen with systemic diseases, including systemic lupus erythematosus, heavy metal injury, and in association with chronic viral (hepatitis) infection and certain tumors.

Endocapillary proliferative changes refer to mesangial or inflammatory cell (acute or chronic) proliferation within the glomeruli. Proliferative responses are further classified as to whether they are diffuse, in which greater than 50% of glomeruli on biopsy are involved, or focal, in which less than 50% of glomeruli are involved. Diffuse proliferative changes on LM may be accompanied by deposition of IgG, IgA, and C3 on IF, with EM demonstrating deposits primarily in the subepithelial portions of the basement membrane. These changes are referred to as idiopathic diffuse proliferative GN, and may represent post-infectious syndromes in which the inciting antigen is unknown. These disorders often present as acute nephritis, with cellular elements and protein in the urine, hypertension, edema, and a decline in renal function.

Focal proliferative changes noted on LM may be accompanied by mesangial deposition of IgA and lesser amounts of IgG, or IgM on IF. In either variety EM demonstrates electron dense deposits located in the mesangial areas. These changes, when associated with IgA and IgG on IF, describe IgA nephropathy (Berger's disease), which is clinically associated with recurrent hematuria and a generally benign course. These changes, accompanied by IgM on IF, describe IgM nephropathy, which is clinically expressed as heavy proteinuria. When expressed as a systemic illness, IgA deposition can be seen in forms of lupus and in Henoch-Schoenlein Purpura, while IgM can sometimes be seen in varieties of focal glomerulosclerosis.

Extracapillary proliferative changes refer to the formation of fibroepithelial crescents from proliferation of the parietal epithelium of Bowman's capsule and incorporation of vascular macrophages. Crescents may circumferentially compress the glomerulus on LM, and demonstrate fibrin when examined by IF. The glomeruli themselves may be involved with linear deposition of IgG, granular deposition of IgG and C3, or absence of staining for any Ig on IF. With substantial involvement of the kidney crescenteric lesions present as rapidly progressive GN, in which renal function is destroyed in days to weeks. Crescents may also be seen in many forms of systemic illness, including lupus, post-streptococcal GN, HSP, Wegener's granulomatosis, and polyarteritis nodosa.

Membranoproliferative changes refer to the generally diffuse mixed thickening of capillary loops and endocapillary (mesangial) cell proliferation seen on LM. There are two main types of membranoproliferative GN (MPGN). IF may reveal granular deposition of IgG and C3 (Type I MPGN), or smooth linear deposition of C3 without Ig (Type II MPGN). The former lesion is associated with subendothelial and mesangial deposits on EM, with splitting of the basement membrane of the capillary loop by mesangial extensions. The latter lesion is associated with deposition of massive amounts of electron dense material in the basement membrane on EM. Both types present with an active urinary sediment, proteinuria, and progressive loss of renal function.

Primary sclerosing changes tend to initially be focal, and may be missed by biopsy since deeper, juxtamedullary glomeruli are often first affected. Such changes are often seen on LM to involve only segments of glomeruli. IF and EM are unremarkable in most cases. These lesions tend to present with proteinuria or abnormalities of the urinary sediment, and progress inexorably to heavy proteinuria and loss of renal function.

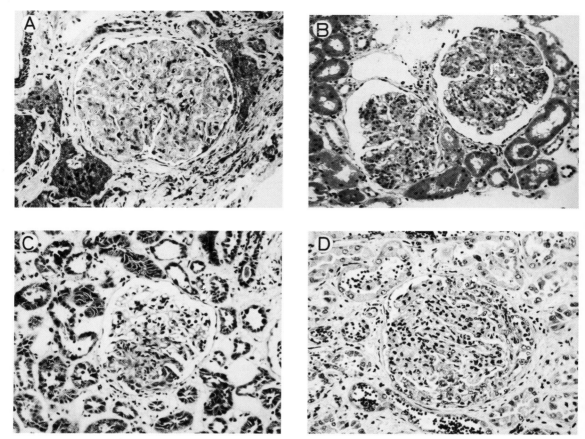

Fig. 12-1. Major Morphological Patterns of Primary Glomerulonephritis Under Light Microscopy. (a) Membranous GN: Glomerular capillary loops are diffusely thickened and glomerulus fills Bowman's space. There is essentially no increase in cellularity; (b) Diffuse Proliferative GN: Both glomeruli are involved with a marked increase in cell number throughout with some intense foci. Mesangial cells are increased in number and some acute inflammatory cells are present. Capillary loops on the periphery, where not obscured by increased cellularity, are thin and delicate; (c) Focal Proliferative GN: One segment of this glomerulus has marked increase in cellularity with early adhesion to Bowman's capsule. Other glomeruli within this biopsy specimen are normal. The capsular adhesion may be an early sign of crescent formation; (d) Crescentic or Rapidly Progressive GN: Within the glomerulus there is increased cellularity. Inside the surrounding Bowman's capsule can also be seen a proliferation of "extracapillary" cells roughly in a crescent surrounding and compressing the right side of the glomerulus in this picture. This proliferation involves both epi-

Clinical Diagnosis

Since the clinical manifestations of PGN are few and nonspecific, the clinician's history and physical examination should be geared to elicit evidence of an associated systemic disease. This requires some knowledge of those diseases which may manifest themselves as GN. These include vasculitides, a number of acute and chronic infectious illnesses, some neoplastic processes, exposure to toxins, and some infiltrative processes such as amyloidosis. Although uncommon, at times the GN may be the only clinical manifestation of systemic disease, and renal biopsy may serve as a definitive diagnostic procedure.

The clinical findings in PGN are useful in that they allow the patient to be placed into one of several relatively well-defined clinical syn-

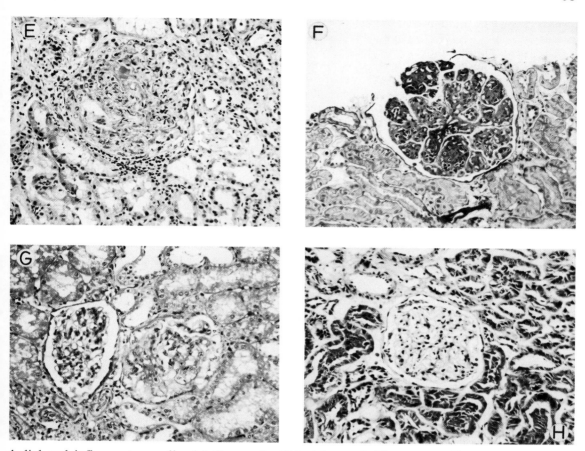

thelial and inflammatory cells; (e) Crescentic GN, Advanced: The extracapillary proliferation or crescent seen in D has progressed to compression and distortion of the glomerular tuft which is reduced to a small area in the middle of Bowman's space. There is marked inflammation in the interstitium surrounding Bowman's space; (f) Membranoproliferative GN: There is a marked tendency to lobular simplification of the glomerular architecture. This is a relatively advanced lesion, and all glomeruli will be involved. Capillarly loops are thickened and obscured by increased mesangial matrix, and there is increased number of cells throughout; (g) Focal Sclerosing GN: The glomerulus on the left is relatively normal with perhaps mild increase in cellularity. That on the right is markedly distorted by a scaring lesion with minimal increased cellularity; (h) Minimal Change Disease: This glomerulus is normal by light microscopy. Nevertheless this patient presented with severe nephrosis similar to the membranous GN patient whose biopsy is pictured above (A). In this specimen, the capillary loops are thin and delicate; and there is no increase in cellularity.

dromes, and allow the severity and rapidity of clinical renal involvement to be estimated. In terms of historical features, the patient should be questioned for the duration, severity, and signs of progression of hematuria, hypertension, and edema. Similarly, a history of remote or antecedent infections should be sought. With severe or rapidly progressive loss of renal function, symptoms may vary from fatigue, anorexia, and nocturia, to nausea, vomiting, and other symptoms of uremia. The physical examination may reveal evidence of the duration or severity of hypertension, pallor and other signs of anemia, and evidence of nephrosis with or without volume overload.

Laboratory tests obtained initially are used to evaluate whether systemic disease is present, and to evaluate the renal syndrome. A complete blood count and multiphasic chemistry screen are useful. However, the single most useful test is the urinalysis, including a screening dipstick to detect both hemoglobin pigment in red blood cells and protein and a properly performed microscopic analysis of the urinary sediment. The urinalysis is so important that it should be performed by the physician evaluating the patient. An early morning urine has the most concentrated sediment, and is preferred. Several urine samples should be examined, as the excretion of casts may not be constant.

The presence of red blood cells in the urinary sediment may or may not reflect renal parenchymal disease. Phase contrast microscopy of the sediment to determine whether red cells are isomorphic or polymorphic can be useful if the observer is properly trained, since polymorphic red cells connote glomerular bleeding. When the urinary sediment contains granular, cellular, or waxy casts, the parenchymal nature of the renal lesion is confirmed. Other indicators of parenchymal disease include white cell or renal tubular epithelial casts, although these are uncommon in most forms of PGN. Red blood cell casts can be seen in GN, but their absence does not eliminate the diagnosis. A sediment which is filled with cellular casts is said to be nephritic, and signifies a more inflammatory lesion in the glomerulus. Conversely, a sediment with waxy casts and fine or coarse granular casts, with evidence of proteinuria and lipiduria, is said

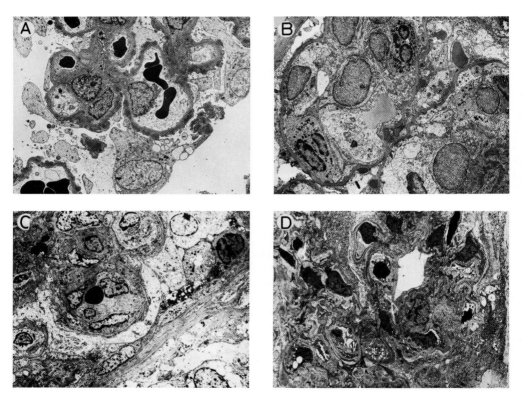

Fig. 12–2. Major Morphological Patterns of Primary Glomerulonephritis Under Electron Microscopy. (a) Membranous GN: Red cells may be seen in the capillary lumens. Surrounding the capillaries is the dark line of basement membrane which is studded with electron dense deposits appearing as humps. These are primarily located on the outside or epithelial cell side of the capillary basement membrane. There is a suggestion of increased cellularity in this section which is not typical of membranous GN; (b) Proliferative GN: Capillary lumens are largely obscured by an increased number of cells (many nuclei) in this sample. Discrete electron dense deposits can be seen along the basement membrane; (c) Membranoproliferative GN: Type 1. Increased numbers of nuclei are seen. Both subendothelial and mesangial deposits are present and mesangial matrix can be seen

to be nephrotic, and suggests less inflammatory lesions. A sediment which contains nephritic and nephrotic elements is said to be telescoped, and indicates an aggressive glomerular lesion.

Quantitation of daily protein excretion provides the opportunity to properly assign the patient to the proper renal syndrome, and assists in following the patient's illness. Such quantitation is conventionally done by collecting a 24 hour urine for protein and creatinine. When analyzed in conjunction with a concurrent plasma creatinine, both the adequacy of the urine collection and endogenous creatinine clearance can be calculated. Once the relationship between the calculated creatinine clearance and the plasma creatinine have been established, the patient can ordinarily be followed with the less cumbersome plasma creatinine concentration as an index of renal function. The quantity of proteinuria has important clinical connotations. Given an adequate collection of urine and an essentially normal plasma albumin concentration, excretion of ≥ 3.5 g/24 h signifies the nephrotic syndrome, while excretion of < 3.5 g is described as non-nephrotic proteinuria. Proteinuria in this latter category is often in the 1–1.5 g/d range. Qualitative descriptions of proteinuria have limited utility with the exception of the evaluation of patients with paraprotein disorders.

Serologic testing in PGN may suggest systemic disease. A broad array of tests for collagen vascular diseases, chronic infections, complement components and paraprotein disorders are frequently ordered. In the absence of any suggestion of systemic disease on history or physical examination, the value of such studies is conjectural, and they serve mainly to reassure the clinician. The single direct diagnostic serologic test is the demonstration of circulating antiglomerular basement membrane antibody (anti-GBM Ab) by radioimmunoassay. Its presence correlates well with linear immunofluorescence of IgG on glomerular capillary loops and is diagnostic of anti-GBM nephritis. However, this test is not widely available, and its utility as a screening test in the absence of clinical indications is limited due to the infrequent incidence of this disease.

Imaging procedures of the kidney consume a great deal of time and money. Clear thought is necessary to determine the indications for intravenous urography, renal scans, arteriograms, ultrasounds and cystoscopy. Once the presence of parenchymal renal disease has been established by the history, physical examination, basic laboratory data, and the urinalysis, only two pieces of information are required of imaging studies: does the patient have two kidneys, and what is their size? A renal untrasound provides

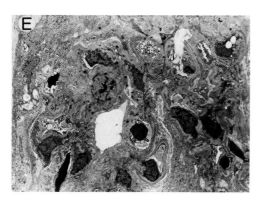 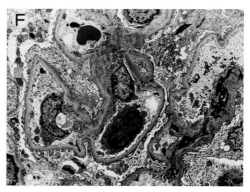

extending around and into the basement membrane; (d) Membranoproliferative GN: Type 2. Dense Deposit Disease: Redundant basement membrane coils throughout this specimen. In some areas it appears extremely dark (electron dense) without discrete deposits; (e) Glomerulosclerosis. Capillary loops are compressed and partially collapsed; (f) Minimal Change Disease. Both RBC and WBC may be seen inside capillary loops. The surrounding basement membrane appears normal without deposits. Some relatively normal epithelial foot processes may be seen on the outer edge of the basement membrane to left and below center. Further along this basement membrane, the foot processes are fused together.

this information without the risk of radiocontrast, and will serve to eliminate the possibility of urinary tract obstruction. This information also affects the decision to perform renal biopsy. In the presence of reduced renal function, small kidney size suggests chronic disease with scarring and atrophy; treatable lesions in this situation are unlikely.

Thus the clinical and laboratory evaluation of the patient with suspected PGN should lead rapidly to a decision as to whether renal biopsy is indicated for definitive diagnosis. The problem confronting the clinician concerns whether the likelihood of discovering a treatable lesion or gaining prognostic information are equivalent with the risk of renal biopsy. This is an area of some controversy, since decision analysis techniques suggest that *a priori* treatment with corticosteroids and biopsy are essentially of equal utility. The premises on which these techniques are based assume prevalence rates of categories of PGN and their response rates to corticosteroids in adults which are not universally accepted. In experienced hands, renal biopsy is a relatively safe procedure, with a morbidity rate of 1–3% and a mortality rate of < 0.1%. Nonetheless, the decision to biopsy requires careful thought, and should be made in consideration of the clinical syndrome which best describes the patient's condition.

Major Clinical Syndromes

The major clinical syndromes associated with PGN and their associated morphologic diagnoses are listed in Table 1. A scheme for consideration for biopsy is listed in Table 2. We will discuss each syndrome, reviewing the evidence that associated conditions respond to specific therapy (Table 3).

Syndrome of Isolated Urinary Abnormalities with normal renal function. The two major presentations of this syndrome are isolated hematuria and non-nephrotic proteinuria (<3.5 g/d). In each of these entities, renal function is normal, there are few symptoms, and hypertension and edema are absent.

Isolated hematuria may be accompanied by recurrent loin or flank pain, along with exacerbation of the hematuria in close temporal proximity to an upper respiratory infection. If these two latter features are present, either alone

or in combination, IgA nephropathy is the likely diagnosis. In the absence of any symptoms, isolated hematuria should be evaluated once with cystoscopy and urography, to rule out a mass or inflammatory lesion in the urinary tract. It is our view that renal biopsy is not generally indicated for isolated hematuria, as most of the associated entities are benign or there is no known effective therapy. Since isolated hematuria may herald serious glomerular disease, close followup is indicated, with biopsy performed if the sediment becomes active, proteinuria becomes significant, or renal function deteriorates.

Isolated proteinuria is usually asymptomatic, and is comprised of two clinical entities: orthostatic proteinuria and true isolated proteinuria. The evaluation of orthostatic proteinuria includes collection of sequential 12 hour urines, one while upright and one while supine. The diagnosis is made when all proteinuria is excreted in the upright position. This condition has a benign course, and when diagnosed, the patient can be reassured. The prognosis of true isolated proteinuria, in which proteinuria is constantly present, is unclear, although there is suggestion in the literature of a small increment in renal morbidity over decades. In both types of proteinuria, close followup initially is indicated, in case the syndrome represents an early form of a potentially treatable glomerular lesion.

Nephrotic syndrome. This syndrome, which may be abrupt or insidious in onset, is defined by heavy proteinuria (>3.5 g/d), and may be accompanied by edema, hypoalbuminemia, lipiduria, and hyperlipidemia. Patients generally present with edema, which may be mild or massive, the severity of which is related to the degree of protein loss, salt intake, and renal function. The urinalysis is invariably abnormal, with hyaline and granular casts. Red blood cells are frequent, and cellular casts may be present, although red blood cell casts are uncommon. Lipiduria is seen under polarized light examination of the sediment in the form of oval fat bodies. Renal function may be normal or depressed, the latter case often due to prerenal azotemia due to decreased renal blood flow with subsequent sodium retention. Hypertension is not commonly present, and patients may only complain of back pain, which is probably due to the distention of the renal capsules by renal edema.

Salt restriction and diuretics, in addition to

Table 12-1   Classification of Primary GN by Syndrome

I. Syndrome of Isolated Urinary Abnormalities with Normal Renal Function
   A. Isolated Hematuria
      1. Focal Proliferative GN: IgA Nephropathy
      2. Membranoproliferative GN
      3. Crescentic GN, early in course
      4. Membranous GN, Focal Sclerosing GN, or Minimal Change GN, rarely

   B. Isolated Non-nephrotic Proteinuria
      1. Focal Proliferative GN: IgM Nephropathy
      2. Minimal Change GN
      3. Membranous or Focal Sclerosing GN, early
      4. Orthostatic Proteinuria
      5. True Isolated Proteinuria

II. Nephrotic Syndrome
   A. Minimal Change GN
   B. Membranous GN
   C. Focal Sclerosing GN
   D. Membranoproliferative GN
   E. Proliferative GN

III. Rapidly Progressive (Crescentic) GN
   A. Proliferative with immune complexes
   B. Proliferative without immune complexes
   C. Anti-GBM antibody mediated GN

IV. Acute Nephritis
   A. Proliferative GN, focal or diffuse, with crescents
   B. Membranoproliferative GN
   C. Focal Proliferative or Sclerosing GN, occasionally

V. Chronic Glomerulonephritis

appropriate protein intake, are the mainstays of therapy for nephrotic syndrome. The hyperlipidemia which may be present has been difficult to treat, although newer anti-lipid drugs recently available hold promise.

It is our practice to biopsy most adults with nephrotic syndrome since there is evidence that some of the histologic entities respond to specific therapy, and the goals of therapy may be different depending upon the diagnosis.

Adults with minimal change disease run courses similar to children, with a long-term benign prognosis and variable course of spontaneous remissions and exacerbation. Adults are typically initially steroid responsive, but may become steroid dependent or resistant. The goal of therapy is to induce the longest possible remission. Initial therapy is with oral prednisone or prednisolone at 1–2 mg/kg/d for 4–8 weeks. Steroids are tapered to alternate day schedule

when remission occurs, and are tapered off after several weeks. If relapse occurs, a second course of steroids is indicated. Early relapse, eg, less than 6 months from remission, suggests that the lesion may be steroid dependent and cytotoxic drugs may be considered. The use of cyclophosphamide (2–3 mg/kg/d for eight weeks) or chlorambucil (0.2–0.3 mg/kg/d for eight weeks) is associated with more sustained remission in steroid dependent patients, and may assist in the induction of remission in steroid resistant patients. Although the long term consequences of cytotoxic therapy in this disease are unknown, such therapy is probably indicated when the nephrotic syndrome is uncontrollable by conservative measures, and severe complications of nephrotic syndrome, such as thromboemboli or severe hyperlipidemia, are present.

Adults with membranous GN present in a similar fashion to those with minimal change

Table 12-2 Renal Biopsy in Primary GN

Use history, physical examination and laboratory to exclude indentifiable systemic disease, then classify by syndrome.

  I. Isolated Urinary Abnormalities
    A. Isolated Hematuria
    B. Isolated Proteinuria

Indication for biopsy: at time of initial diagnosis biopsy rarely indicated. Biopsy if evidence on followup of decreased renal function, substantial change in activity of urinary sediment, or development of nephrotic syndrome.

  II. Nephrotic Syndrome

Indication for biopsy: biopsy for identification of potentially treatable lesion

  III. Rapidly Progressive Glomerulonephritis

Indication for biopsy: urgent biopsy for accurate diagnosis to assist in therapy

  IV. Acute Nephritis

Indication for biopsy: should be performed if any question of rapidly progressive GN

  V. Chronic Glomerulonephritis

Indication for biopsy: almost never indicated

Table 12-3 Therapy of Primary Glomerulonephritis

  I. Minimal Change GN:
    Daily corticosteroids, 1–1.5 mg/kg, for 8 weeks; frequent relapses may respond to short courses of oral cyclophosphamide, 2–3 mg/kg/d, or chlorambucil, 0.3 mg/kg/d.

  II. Membranous GN:
    A. Alternate day steroids, 2 mg/kg/qod for 8 weeks
    B. Intravenous methylprednisolone boluses followed by alternating monthly courses of prednisone and chlorambucil.

  III. Rapidly Progressive (Crescentic) GN, with or without Immune Complexes:
    Intravenous methylprednisolone, 15–30 mg/kg/d for 3–5 days, followed by tapering oral steroids and oral cytotoxic agents.

  IV. Rapidly Progressive (Crescentic) GN with anti-GBM Antibody:
    Oral steroids, 2 mg/kg/d, for 3 weeks, then taper to alternate day, with oral cyclophosphamide, 2–3 mg/kg/d. 4 liter plasma exchange every 2–3 days for severely active disease with viable tissue on renal biopsy. High dose intravenous methylprednisolone for pulmonary hemorrhage.

Little evidence that specific therapy uniformly effective in other forms of primary GN.

Control of hypertension and volume, adequate nutrition, and control of calcium and phosphate levels important in all forms of primary GN.

disease, although the former is commonly associated with less severe proteinuria and edema. Several recent studies suggest that this lesion responds to therapy. In this case, the goal of therapy is long-term preservation of renal function, since the effects of therapy on proteinuria are not remarkable. One course of therapy involves eight weeks of alternate day steroids (80 mg). A more promising effort involves six months of therapy with intermittent intravenous methylprednisolone and alternating monthly course of oral prednisone and chlorambucil. This latter course is more aggressive than the former, and may require further proof of efficacy before being widely accepted.

The remaining pathologic entities associated with nephrotic syndrome lack impressive evidence for therapy other than conservative measures. In severe, debilitating nephrosis a course of steroids may be justified, but long-term steroid therapy is probably not rational.

Rapidly progressive glomerulonephritis. This syndrome is associated with evidence of acute nephritis on urinalysis and rapid loss of renal function over weeks to months. Patients present with constitutional symptoms and hematuria or an otherwise abnormal urinalysis. The syndrome should be suspected when there is acute deterioration of renal function, proteinuria, and an active urinary sediment. It is our view that renal biopsy should be performed urgently when this syndrome is suspected, even with relatively severe renal failure, since there is good evidence to support the concepts that effective therapy exists for many associated disorders, and the type of therapy depends upon the morphologic diagnosis. Without therapy, most patients will progress to end stage renal failure in a short period of time.

The hallmark of this syndrome is the presence of crescents on renal biopsy. Three categories of rapidly progressive GN have been described on the basis of immunofluorescence patterns. Patients with granular immunofluorescence or absent immunofluorescence should be treated with high dose intravenous methylprednisolone (15–30 mg/kg/d) for three to five days, followed by a six to eight week course of prednisone (1 mg/kg/d), in association with cyclophosphamide or azathioprine. Response rates of 75% are probable, and may occur even in patients with severe pathologic involvement and

renal failure requiring analysis.

Patients with linear immunofluorescence usually have circulating anti-GBM antibody, and do not respond to high dose steroids. Therapy should include oral prednisone (2 mg/kg/d) for one to two weeks, followed by a taper to 1 mg/kg/d for four weeks. Cyclophosphamide (2–3 mg/kg/d) is used in conjunction. Plasmapheresis has been extensively used and reported to be of value in these patients. In contrast to other forms of rapidly progressive glomerulonephritis, patients with anti-GBM disease have a treatment outcome more tightly coupled to their degree of functional and morphologic impairment at time of initial therapy. Patients with mild disease (creatinine <3.0 mg/dl, <30% crescents on biopsy) seem to do well on oral therapy, with or without plasmapheresis. Patients with severe disease (creatinine >5.0 mg/dL, >70% crescents), do not seem to respond to any form of therapy. Although it is our view that the value of plasma exchange in this disorder is conjectural, it may be utilized in mild to moderately severe disease, and can be show to result in a more rapid elimination of anti-GBM antibody than is seen with drugs alone. Three 4-liter exchanges per week, using at least 2 liters of fresh frozen plasma as replacement fluid, are associated with minimal complications.

When pulmonary hemorrhage occurs in anti-GBM nephritis, a short course of high dose intravenous methylprednisolone (1 g/d for 2–3 days) is the most effective therapy. Hemorrhage is often associated with infection or volume overload, and should not be used as an indication to conduct plasmapheresis, the major suggested benefit of which is preservation of renal function.

Acute nephritic syndrome. This syndrome is characterized by an active urinary sediment, frequently with edema and hypertension. The onset is often abrupt, and if renal insufficiency is present, this syndrome may be indistinguishable from rapidly progressive nephritis. Many patients present several weeks after, or with, an active infection. Experience gathered in the care of patients with post-streptococcal GN, the prototype of acute nephritis, argues for a search for infection and definitive treatment of it if present. Treatment of hypertension is usually indicated. Renal biopsy of these patients is often performed to eliminate rapidly progressive GN or for prognostic reasons. The morphologic entities associated with this syndrome are associated with little convincing evidence of benefit from therapy if the lesion does not resolve spontaneously. For those patients with histologic proof of membranoproliferative glomerulonephritis, alternate day steroid therapy, or combined therapy with aspirin and dipyramidole may be associated with reduction in proteinuria or reduction in the rate of renal function loss. Each type of therapy is relatively benign, but should be considered unproven at this time.

Chronic glomerulonephritis. Since the signs and symptoms of PGN may be quite insidious, many patients will not present until the disorder is quite advanced and significant degrees of renal insufficiency are present. Patients may present with non-specific symptoms, or may be detected in the course of evaluating other medical problems. When significant renal failure has developed over many years there is little hope of reversal, whatever the cause, and renal biopsy is not indicated. The major clinical problem is to determine whether newly detected renal insufficiency is due to an acute or chronic deterioration.

The medical history should be focused to elicit evidence of progressive fatigue, diminished activity, change in appetite or weight, or episodic hematuria. Nocturia is often a sign of loss of renal function accompanying chronic GN. Hypertension is frequently present, as is evidence of physiologic adaptation to pronounced anemia. Evidence of chronic adaptation is the key to determining whether renal insufficiency is acute or chronic. Thus, severe anemia (Hct < 30 vol%) with a paucity of symptoms, moderately compensated metabolic acidemia without hyperkalemia, and hyperphosphatemia and hypocalcemia with or without radiographic evidence of renal osteodystrophy are characteristics of long-standing renal disease. The single most useful feature is renal size, since with progressive GN the kidneys will be small and scarred. Renal biopsy in this situation is not only difficult, but non-diagnostic, and should be avoided. These patients should be managed with conservative therapy commensurate with their degree of renal dysfunction, since primary therapy for their glomerular disease is unlikely to be effective.

Management of Chronic Glomerulonephritis

Although it is apparent that there is no specific therapy for many of the morphologic types of PGN, new approaches are constantly emerging, and are being evaluated with large scale collaborative studies which may allow conclusions about therapy in many forms of PGN.

Even more important is the realization that adequate conservative therapy may significantly prolong survival in progressive GN. The judicious use of salt restriction, diuretics, and anti-hypertensive agents allows for successful treatment of most patients. New evidence is emerging to suggest that some anti-hypertensive agents are more efficacious than others even with equal control of systemic arterial pressure.

The clinician should always be alert for reversible complications which may hasten the decline of renal function. Serial assessment of renal function by measurement of the serum creatinine, in conjunction with calculation of the reciprocal of the serum creatinine concentration, are most helpful. The latter calculation provides a measurement of the rate of loss of renal function, which is roughly linear over the time course of progressive GN. If the patient deviates from this line, this may suggest problems such as volume depletion from diuretics or heart failure from volume overload, urinary tract infections, the effects of uncontrolled hypertension, exposure to nephrotoxic drugs or agents, or renal vein thrombosis, to which nephrotic patients are susceptible.

Finally, dietary therapy may play an important role in future management strategies. Evidence suggests that protein restriction and phosphate restriction, both alone or in combination, reduce the rate of progressive renal damage. Although the ultimate value of dietary therapy is under study, it is clear that close and careful followup of the patient with otherwise untreatable renal disease provides the patient with a reasonable lifestyle and may delay or obviate the need for dialysis or transplantation.

SUGGESTED READINGS

General
1. Skorecki K, Nadler S, Badr K, Brenner B. Renal and Systemic Manifestations of Glomerular Disease. In *The*

Kidney, Vol. 1. Brenner and Rector, eds. New York: WB Saunders, 1985; 891–928.
2. Glassock R, Cohen A, Adler S, Ward H. Primary Glomerular Diseases. Ibid, 929–1013.

Membranous GN
1. Collaborative Study of the Adult Idiopathic Nephrotic Syndrome. N Eng J Med 1979; 301: 1302–1306.
2. Ponticelli C, et al. Controlled Trial of Methylprednisolone and Chlorambucil in Idiopathic Membranous Nephropathy. N Eng J Med 1984; 310:946–950.

Membranoproliferative GN
1. Donadio J, et al. Membranoproliferative Glomerulonephritis. N Eng J Med 1984; 310:1421–1426.
2. West C. Childhood Membranoproliferative Glomerulonephritis: An Approach to Management. Kidney Int. 1986; 29:1077–1093.

Rapidly Progressive Glomerulonephritis
1. Couser W. Idiopathic Rapidly Progressive Glomerulonephritis. Am J Nephrology 1982; 2:57–69.

2. Johnson JP, Moore J, Austin HA, et al. Therapy of Anti-Glomerular Basement Membrane Antibody Disease. Medicine 1985; 64:217–227.

Minimal Change Disease
1. Hoyer J. Idiopathic Nephrotic Syndrome with Minimal Glomerular Changes. In, Nephrotic Syndrome. Brenner and Stein, eds. New York: Churchill Livingston, 1983; 145–174.

Progression of Renal Disease
1. Maschio G et al. Effects of Dietary Protein and Phosphorus Restriction on the Progression of Early Renal Failure. Kidney Int 1982; 22:371–376.
2. Brenner B, Meyer T, Hostetter T. Dietary Protein Intake and the Progressive Nature of Kidney Disease. N Eng J Med 1982; 307:652–659.
3. Meyer T, Anderson S, Rennke H, Brenner B. Converting Enzyme Inhibitor Therapy Limits Progressive Glomerular Injury in Rats with Renal Insufficiency. Am J Med 1985; 79:31–37.

James E. Balow
Howard A. Austin, III

13

Systemic Glomerulopathies

I. SYSTEMIC LUPUS ERYTHEMATOSUS

Systemic lupus erythematosus (SLE) is considered the prototype of autoimmune disease. The disturbances of immunoregulation which underlie this disease have not been adequately defined but appear to involve multiple components of the immune system. Genetic, hormonal, and viral factors are considered to have possible contributory roles in the pathogenesis of SLE. The preponderant immunological disturbance is the presence of highly activated B lymphocytes which secrete immunoglobulin and cause hyperglobulinemia, autoantibodies and circulating immune complexes. It is considered that qualitative and quantitative properties of these immunoreactants determine the expression of SLE.

Essentials of Diagnosis

The clinical features of SLE are protean. The criteria for diagnosis and classification of SLE are shown in Table 1. As noted, the criteria for renal involvement are persistent proteinuria (>0.5 gms/day or 3+ dipstick quantitation) or the presence of cellular casts.

Renal Syndromes

The spectrum of involvement of the kidney in SLE is as broad as that of the other clinical manifestations. Renal involvement is clinically evident in at least two-thirds of patients with SLE and approaches 100% in studies of renal biopsies. Low grade hematuria and/or proteinuria may be unnoticed by the patient and can be easily overlooked by the clinician in evaluation of patients with SLE. The clinician should search for subtle evidence of renal involvement, such as changes in urination patterns and early abnormalities of urinary sediment. It is important that the clinician personally continue to monitor the urinary sediment in patients with SLE, since it can be an important indicator of change in status of glomerular disease. Asymptomatic hematuria/proteinuria are typical features of mild disease, but may be simply the earliest expression of evolving lupus nephritis. Nephrotic syndrome is a common feature of both proliferative and membranous forms of lupus nephritis. Interestingly, nephrotic syndrome has been recognized as the initial expression of SLE in some patients with the membranous form of lupus nephritis. In the severe proliferative forms of lupus nephritis, nephrotic syndrome is usually accompanied by additional renal complications such as nephritic urinary sediment, hypertension, and azotemia. Rapidly progressive renal failure due to crescentic glomerulonephritis is seen in a relatively small subset of patients with lupus nephritis. The differential causes of declining renal function in patients with lupus nephritis are as varied as those of any other form of complicated renal disease. However, in lupus nephritis deterioration of renal function is most commonly due to worsening proliferative and inflammatory

Table 13-1 Revised Criteria for Classification of SLE*

1. Malar rash
2. Discoid rash
3. Photosensitivity
4. Oral ulcers
5. Arthritis
6. Serositis (pleuritis or pericarditis)
7. Renal disorders (proteinuria >0.5 gm/ day or cellular casts)
8. Neurologic disorder (seizures or psychosis)
9. Hematologic disorder (hemolytic anemia or leukopenia or lymphopenia or thrombocytopenia)
10. Immunologic disorder (Le prep or anti-DNA or anti-Sm or false-positive syphilis serology
11. Antinuclear antibody

*Adapted from: Arthritis Rheum 25:1271–1277, 1982

Table 13-2 World Health Organization Classification of Lupus Nephritis

I. Minimal disease
II. Mesangial
III. Focal proliferative GN
IV. Diffuse proliferative GN
V. Membranous GN
VI. Sclerosing nephropathy

glomerular disease, decreased renal perfusion due to severe nephrotic syndrome, or complications of medical therapy. Renal vein thrombosis and severe crescentic glomerulonephritis are relatively rare but must be considered causes for sudden deterioration of renal function. The vast majority of patients with lupus nephritis have slowly progressive or persistent chronic azotemia. Remissions and exacerbations of SLE may be presaged by changes in urinary sediment, level of urinary protein excretion, and sometimes by major changes in lupus serologies, such as serum complement and anti-DNA antibody. It should be underscored that changes in urinary sediment activity are generally the most readily obtained and dependable indices of disease activity, which may be supplemented by clinical and other laboratory features. Residual uncertainty may prompt the careful clinician to recommend a repeat renal biopsy to define the nature of the renal involvement.

Renal Pathology

Because essentially the entire spectrum of renal histologic changes can be seen in SLE, it is often difficult to categorize the biopsy among a small number of classes. The goal of identifying uniform prognostic groups by using various classifications of lupus nephritis has been considered to be limited by the use of conventional classification systems. Certain approaches which denote the type and extent of specific pathologic lesions have been proposed as modifications of conventional classification systems. At the present time, renal biopsies are generally assigned to one of six categories proposed by the World Health Organization based primarily on light microscopy criteria (Table 2). In Category 1, biopsy specimens have minimal or no changes by light microscopy, even though mesangial deposits are often present on immunofluorescent and electron microscopy. Category 2, mesangial nephritis, exhibits widening of mesangial regions caused by immune complex deposition, increased matrix formation and/ or hypercellularity of the mesangial region. By definition, mesangial disease indicates that most capillary loops are patent and no active lesions, such as karyorrhexis, fibrinoid necrosis, hematoxylin bodies, wire loops, hyaline thrombi, cellular crescents or electron dense deposits are present. Patients with mesangial lupus nephritis typically have low grade urinary sediment abnormalities, mild proteinuria, and minimal, if any, decrease in renal function. Category 3, focal proliferative lupus nephritis, is the least precisely defined class. Glomerular lesions in focal disease are qualitatively similar to those of diffuse lupus nephritis. Focal disease is commonly defined by the presence of glomerular solidification (loss of capillary space due to hypercellularity and other active lesions) in less than 50% of glomeruli. Characteristically, focal disease also exhibits highly irregular, segmental involvement within glomeruli. Category 4, diffuse proliferative lupus nephritis, encompasses a broad spectrum of pathologic changes. Basic to the definition is the presence of hypercellularity and/ or sclerosing changes which obliterate circulatory space in more than 50% of glomeruli. Electron dense deposits are typically seen in mesangial, subendothelial and subepithelial locations in both focal and diffuse proliferative lupus nephritis. Membranoproliferative and crescentic subsets of diffuse proliferative lupus nephritis are occasionally seen.

The breadth of the spectrum of pathology in diffuse proliferative lupus nephritis relates to the extent of solidification and the variable numbers of active lesions listed above which are also present. Moreover, there is a highly variable degree of tubulointerstitial disease, particularly tubular atrophy and interstitial fibrosis, seen in patients with diffuse proliferative lupus nephritis. The heterogeneity of pathologic changes in diffuse proliferative lupus nephritis probably accounts for the discrepancies among different studies which have sought to define a uniform prognosis in this category of patients. It has recently been determined that a semi-quantitative assessment of the individual pathologic features (Table 3) provides an improved basis for assessing prognostic outcome in lupus nephritis. In general, the changes listed as active lesions were relatively weak prognostic indicators suggesting that they have the potential to reverse with effective therapy, except under the most extremely severe circumstances. On the other hand, the presence of chronic irreversible changes, particularly tubular atrophy and interstitial fibrosis, identifies patients with high risk of developing end stage renal disease. In addition to the utility of the semi-quantitative scoring system in identifying prognosis at a single point in time, this system provides a means to assess the evolution of renal pathologic changes.

Category 5, membranous lupus nephritis, is characterized by a uniform thickening of capillary loops in glomeruli which otherwise lack signs of active lesions. Immune complex deposits are predominantly formed in subepithelial locations, along with variable amounts in the mes-angium. Membranous lupus nephritis is usually accompanied by mesangial hypercellularity, and occasionally a mixed membranous and proliferative nephritis is seen. Moreover, certain patients with proliferative forms of lupus nephritis undergoing treatment appear to "heal" their glomerular disease by reducing the number of subendothelial, and increasing the number of subepithelial deposits which may then resemble membranous lupus nephritis.

Category 6, advanced sclerosing glomerulonephritis, may represent the final common pathway of injury in any of the forms of glomerulonephritis. It may be also secondary to nonglomerular disease, such as hypertension, vasculitis, or tubulointerstitial nephritis. This category of lupus nephritis has recently been separated as a way to identify situations in which little or no active disease is present and in which glomerular sclerosis dominates in the majority of glomeruli. It should be underscored that some degree of glomerular sclerosis is regularly seen in Categories 3, 4 and 5 listed above.

Indications for Therapy

There are a multitude of factors which impact on therapeutic decisions in lupus nephritis. It is clear that the prognosis of lupus nephritis has steadily improved over the past three decades. There is general acknowledgement that immunosuppressive drug therapy has contributed to the improvement of the outcome, particularly in diffuse proliferative lupus nephritis. However, it is evident that there is no simple way to assess the degree of risk in lupus nephritis. Several clinical, pathological and immunological factors must be balanced against the risk of development of iatrogenic complications of treatment. An ordering of the strength of indications for therapy is shown in Table 4. Progressive azotemia in the face of worsening ne-

Table 13-3   Special Renal Biopsy Features of Relevance in Assessing Lupus Nephritis

Active Lesions	Chronic Lesions
1. Proliferation/hypercellularity	1. Glomerular sclerosis
2. Necrosis/karyorrhexis	2. Fibrous crescents
3. Hyaline thrombi	3. Tubular atrophy
4. Cellular crescents	4. Interstitial fibrosis
5. Interstitial inflammation	

phritic urinary sediment is clearly an indication for therapeutic intervention. Diffuse proliferative disease, extensive fibrinoid necrosis, cellular crescents, and extensive immune complex deposition in a subendothelial location on renal biopsy are also major indications. Several clinical, pathological and laboratory features are of less certain value but are generally taken into consideration in a therapeutic decision. These factors include worsening proteinuria, falling serum complement values and increasing anti-DNA antibody levels. Mesangial and focal proliferative lupus nephritis may indicate intrinsically low grade forms of lupus nephritis; alternatively, they may represent relatively early stages of disease with the probability of evolving to a more severe form of lupus nephritis (can be suspected on the basis of deterioration of urinary findings or proven on repeat renal biopsy). Similarly, membranous lupus nephritis is considered to indicate a relatively favorable prognosis but the therapeutic decision may need to be modified by the degree of accompanying clinical factors. The presence of scattered subendothelial deposits on electron microscopy, as well as interstitial mononuclear cell infiltrates, is suggestive of the presence of active nephritis and the need for therapy. There are several poor

Table 13-4 Indications for
Treatment in Lupus Nephritis

I. Major indications
  A. Clinical features
    1. Rapidly progressive GN
    2. Highly active, worsening urinary sediment
  B. Pathological features
    1. Active diffuse proliferative or crescentic GN
    2. Extensive subendothelial deposits
II. Intermediate indications
  A. Clinical features
    1. nephritic urinary sediment
    2. Slowly progressive azotemia
    3. Worsening proteinuria
    4. Falling serum complement
    5. Rising levels of anti-DNA
  B. Pathological features
    1. Focal proliferative GN
    2. Scattered subendothelial deposits
    3. Membranous GN

indications for therapeutic intervention in lupus nephritis including fixed azotemia, proteinuria, abnormal anti-DNA, and abnormal complement. Comparable morphologic features include predominant glomerulosclerosis, fibrous crescents, tubular atrophy, interstitial fibrosis, and intramembranous deposits. Overall these guidelines are designed to assist the clinician in treating patients with the highest likelihood of progression and, at the same time, the greatest potential for reversal of the disease process. Recent evidence suggests that nonimmunological factors may contribute to progressive renal insufficiency and can be easily mistaken for active lupus nephritis. Verification by repeat renal biopsy of the activity of lupus nephritis may be warranted if the other indications for therapy are not compelling.

Therapeutic Options

The major forms of therapy used to alter the course of progressive lupus nephritis are outlined in Table 5. The therapeutic options include corticosteroids, cytotoxic drugs, and experimental therapies. Aggressive induction therapy for major indications include high dose prednisone (1.0 mg/kg/day) for approximately four to six weeks. Continuation of daily therapy for longer periods of time greatly increases the risk of iatrogenic complications which can be avoided by tapering to alternate day therapy within eight weeks. Alternative therapies may be considered if there is inadequate response of the objective signs of lupus nephritis, excessive dose dependency, or flair of the lupus nephritis while tapering to alternate day therapy.

Pulse methylprednisolone (1.0 gm/m^2) is a widely used alternative form of aggressive induction therapy. Intravenous methylpredniso-

Table 13-5 Induction and
Maintenance Treatment Options
in Lupus Nephritis

1. Conventional, high-dose prednisone
2. Pulse methylprednisolone
3. Cyclophosphamide
4. Azathioprine
5. Experimental
   a. Pulse cyclophosphamide
   b. Plasma exchange

lone is typically given on three consecutive days and followed by moderate doses of prednisone (e.g. 0.5 mg/kg/day) for approximately four weeks followed by tapering to alternate day therapy. There have been no objective comparisons between oral high dose prednisone and methylprednisolone pulse therapy, but it is considered that pulse therapy is at least as effective and has fewer short term side effects than conventional oral prednisone. Cyclophosphamide, azathioprine or combinations of these oral agents have been tested. At the present time, there is no consensus regarding the use of these agents, although there have been some favorable trends in therapeutic trials which have compared these agents to conventional prednisone therapy.

Certain experimental therapies have been studied in patients with major indications for treatment of lupus nephritis. Plasmapheresis therapy, which included supplemental prednisone and cyclophosphamide therapy, was not shown to be more effective or safer than conventional drug therapy in lupus nephritis in a recently reported controlled study. Experimental pulse cyclophosphamide is under evaluation in NIH protocols. A recent report indicated that this therapy is well tolerated and appears to be effective for treatment of severe lupus nephritis. Intermittent cyclophosphamide pulse therapy appears to reduce the risk of chronic bone marrow depression, bladder complications, and malignancy seen with conventional oral cyclophosphamide therapy.

The decision of when and which cytotoxic agent to employ in lupus nephritis is difficult and cannot be based on a wide consensus regarding the superiority of any one of these alternative choices. Indeed, patients and physicians are likely to assign different weights to the various risk factors involving corticosteroids and cytotoxic drugs. In general, it is considered imperative that the physician repeatedly attempt to taper corticosteroids to the minimal dose required for disease activity, preferably in an alternate day regimen. Consideration should be given to the addition of cytotoxic drugs if flares of nephritis occur during the tapering process, excessive maintenance doses are required, or unsatisfactory therapeutic responses are established.

Although certain patients will progress to end-stage renal failure in spite of one's best therapeutic efforts, the risk of developing renal failure even in patients with diffuse proliferative lupus nephritis ranges between 25 and 50% at ten years in most contemporary series. Interestingly, clinical activity of SLE generally subsides if the appearance of uremia is gradual. However, clinical remission is not universal, especially if renal failure occurs rapidly. Indeed, deaths from complications of extrarenal SLE have been noted and patient survival is less than for demographically comparable patients on dialysis as a result of renal failure from other causes. Transplantation is certainly a viable therapeutic alternative for the patient with end stage renal disease due to lupus nephritis. There has been a gratifyingly low incidence of reactivation of SLE following renal transplantation, with only rare instances of recurrence of lupus nephritis in the engrafted kidney.

II. SYSTEMIC VASCULITIS

Few medical conditions present with such diversity as systemic vasculitis. This diversity presumably emanates from systemic vasculitis being comprised of a family of conditions of multiple etiologies which affect vessels of various sizes and locations. Classic polyarteritis nodosa is rarely seen in modern times, as it probably represents late stage, untreated vasculitic disease causing nodular swelling of large vessels. At the other end of the spectrum of systemic vasculitis is microscopic polyarteritis which is mainly expressed as glomerular capillary disease. More typically encountered however, are patients with so-called overlap syndromes of systemic vasculitis with a broad spectrum of involvement of large and small vessels.

The immunological basis of systemic vasculitis remains elusive. Circulating immune complexes have been described but tissue deposits of immune complexes are rarely impressive in the organs involved. Recent studies have noted autoantibodies to neutrophil cytoplasmic antigens but the role of these antibodies in the pathogenesis of vasculitis is uncertain.

Diagnostic Considerations

The majority of clinical manifestations of systemic vasculitis are vague and nonspecific.

The extrarenal manifestations of classic and microscopic polyarteritis are comparable. A vasculitis "syndrome" is characterized by weight loss, fever, malaise, and vague arthralgias and myalgias. The clearest diagnostic features include vasculitic skin lesions, mononeuritis multiplex, gastrointestinal involvement with ischemia and/or hemorrhage and renal disease. Diagnosis of systemic vasculitis is confirmed by organ biopsies and/or demonstration of typical lesions on arteriography such as aneurysms, vessel tapering, or beading. Blind tissue biopsies are generally considered to be of low yield, while arteriography should be strongly considered in patients in which there is a high suspicion of classic polyarteritis even without obvious evidence of specific organ dysfunction.

Renal Syndromes

Hypertension is a relatively common expression of classic polyarteritis nodosa apparently due to relative renal ischemia and/or the presence of glomerulonephritis. Prolonged ischemia may be associated with thrombosis and renal cortical infarcts. Loss of renal function may occur due to ischemic and atrophic change, often in the absence of glomerulonephritis. In cases where glomerular involvement occurs (microscopic polyarteritis), the clinical expressions may range from asymptomatic hematuria and/or proteinuria to rapidly progressive and crescentic glomerulonephritis.

Renal Pathology

Gross infarcts of the renal parenchyma leading to lobular scars of the cortex are commonly observed in classic polyarteritis nodosa. Attendant atrophy and sclerosis due to nephron ischemia are observed microscopically. Vasculitic changes including arterial thickening in association with fibrinoid necrosis and leucocytic invasion of the vessel wall may be seen with open renal biopsies but less commonly in needle biopsy specimens. Aneurysms may be associated with spontaneous rupture causing parenchymal hemorrhage. Arterial thrombosis with recanalization is a late complication of classic polyarteritis nodosa, a complication causing vascular insufficiency which may be difficult to distinguish from persistent vasculitis. Glomeru-

lonephritis due to microscopic polyarteritis is typically focal and necrotizing, often complicated by crescentic glomerulonephritis. Studies of renal biopsies by immunofluorescence and electron microscopy generally demonstrate sparse or absent immunoreactants in involved areas.

Clinical Course and Indications for Therapy

The hallmark for systemic vasculitis is the variability and unpredictability of clinical course. Approximately one half of patients exhibit an early aggressive and complicated course with a high mortality due to complications of serious extrarenal vasculitis. Survivors of the acute phase of the disease may subsequently experience an entirely self limited course while others may develop chronic or relapsing disease. A certain percentage of patients may exhibit a smoldering course of chronic systemic disease without major organ systemic involvement, a situation which often contributes to late diagnosis of systemic vasculitis. Morbidity and mortality in the late phases of systemic vasculitis are often due to vascular catastrophies resulting from complications of hypertension and healed vasculitic lesions or from side effects of prolonged high dose corticosteroid therapy. Documentation of the appearance of renal ischmia, aneurysms, renal dysfunction or active glomerulonephritis are certain indications for initiating therapy. Static renal functional or anatomical lesions are often an expression of old injury, and therefore weak indications for initiating or continuing therapy.

Therapy

There are no prospective data upon which to base treatment of systemic vasculitis. Cumulative survival figures derived from several published series involving patients mainly with classic polyarteritis nodosa or overlap syndromes indicate at two years the risk of mortality is greater than 70% in untreated patients, while the risk is reduced to 25 to 40% in corticosteroid treated patients. These historical comparisons form the basis for the standard use of early high dose corticosteroid therapy in systemic vasculitis. Typically patients with active disease are treated with prednisone (1 mg/kg/day) for six to eight weeks followed by careful tapering to alternate day therapy and/or discontinuance. Considerable anxiety is usually engendered during this period when soft clinical findings may suggest recrudescence of disease activity, prompting retreatment or stabilization at a high corticosteroid dosage level. Corticosteroid complications commonly begin to overshadow the concern for persistent disease activity. Consideration of cytotoxic drug therapy with azathioprine or cyclophosphamide generally arises because of a need for therapeutic alternatives with increased efficacy and ultimately with reduced complications compared to prolonged (even if effective) corticosteroid therapy. In short, it has not been proven whether or not early institution of cytotoxic drugs provides an advantage over corticosteroid therapy. In general, corticosteroids are considered the first line of treatment but the astute clinician should be ready to add cytotoxic drugs to the therapeutic regimen if inadequate responses are seen, particularly in those patients with unusually aggressive, progressive or persistent disease and those with corticosteroid complications or prolonged steroid dependency. Conventional cyclophosphamide therapy started at 2 mg/kg/day is the most widely favored approach. It is imperative that careful monitoring of white blood counts is performed to avoid serious complications of leukopenia. In patients treated with cyclophosphamide therapy, the drug is maintained for six to twelve months after clinical remission is achieved.

The renal complications of microscopic polyarteritis often warrant some modification of the foregoing therapeutic approach. Pulse methylprednisolone or plasma exchange are commonly used for severe necrotizing and crescentic glomerulonephritis. The final perspective on the role of these adjunctive therapies in systemic vasculitis cannot be formulated from available data.

Patients progressing to end stage renal failure often experience complications of severe hypertension requiring very aggressive antihypertensive therapy. Bilateral nephrectomy is rarely necessary with currently available antihypertensive drugs. Chronic dialysis and/or transplantation therapy may be undertaken in patients with renal failure due to systemic vasculitis. Patients appear to experience no unusual problems except for somewhat increased risk of vascular complications. The recurrence of systemic vasculitis in renal allografts does not appear to present a serious risk.

III. WEGENER'S GRANULOMATOSIS

Wegener's granulomatosis is a subset of systemic vasculitis with a characteristic profile of clinical and pathologic features. Its pathogenesis is unknown but the recent description of autoantibodies to neutrophil cytoplasmic antigens is intriguing. These antibodies are consistently present in patients with active disease and usually fall with remission. The clinical syndrome includes chronic inflammation of the upper and lower airways, along with glomerulonephritis and variable involvement of vasculitis in other organs. Pathologic diagnosis includes the presence of necrotizing granulomas and vasculitis on biopsies within the respiratory tract as well as necrotizing glomerulonephritis on renal biopsy. Extrarenal disease typically dominates the clinical picture, including chronic nasopharyngitis, sinusitis, otitis media and laryngotracheitis. These symptoms may divert attention from evaluation and monitoring for renal involvement; the latter may be complicated by sudden acceleration to a severe necrotizing and crescentic glomerulonephritis with renal failure.

Renal Syndromes

Limited Wegener's granulomatosis may be present in the absence of any renal involvement. Asymptomatic hematuria/proteinuria may be the only renal manifestations, but when present should be considered to indicate a high risk for accelerated glomerulonephritis. Morphologically, early glomerulonephritis is manifested by focal, segmental proliferative (often necrotizing) glomerulonephritis. Nephrotic range proteinuria is unusual in Wegener's granulomatosis. Rapidly progressive glomerulonephritis is a major risk in patients with clinical evidence of renal involvement and is considered an urgent indication for intervention with immunosuppressive drug therapy. Granulomatous lesions are rarely seen in renal biopsy material. As is typical of most forms of vasculitis, deposition of immune reactants in involved renal tissue is generally unimpressive by immunofluorescence or electron microscopy studies.

Indications for Therapy

Historically, patients with Wegener's granulomatosis and glomerulonephritis have a greater than 60% one year mortality even when treated with corticosteroid therapy. Current actuarial survival analysis in patients with renal involvement treated with immunosuppressive drug therapy shows that mortality has been reduced to approximately 15% at one year and approximately 30% at five years. Essentially any evidence of renal involvement, other than fixed azotemia without active urinary sediment, is considered to be an indication for initiation and maintenance of immunosuppressive drug therapy.

Therapy

Cyclophosphamide therapy has become the mainstay of treatment in Wegener's granulomatosis. Other cytotoxic immunosuppressive drugs appear to be efficacious but have been less well characterized. Conventional oral cyclophosphamide (initiated at 2 mg/kg/day) is used in most patients but certainly in patients with evidence of glomerulonephritis. High dose prednisone therapy (1 mg/kg/day) is often administered in the early phases of Wegener's granulomatosis, in patients with aggressive granulomatous inflammation, vasculitis, and particularly in those with necrotizing and/or crescentic glomerulonephritis. This approach is undertaken because of the anti-inflammatory effect of corticosteroids and the expected one to two week delay in therapeutic effect of cyclophosphamide. Prednisone is usually tapered after approximately one month, first to an alternate day regimen and finally discontinued, unless debilitating constitutional symptoms remain which have been responsive to corticosteroid therapy. The avoidance of serious complications of cyclophosphamide requires complete understanding and diligent observation by the patient and the physician. In all patients who are able to tolerate prolonged cyclophosphamide, treatment is continued for a minimum of one year after induction of remission of Wegener's granulomatosis. Patients who are unable to tolerate or who are experiencing complications of cyclophospha-

mide have been successfully maintained on azathioprine therapy. Plasma exchange may be therapeutically effective in Wegener's granulomatosis. Plasma exchange has been utilized as a rapid stop-gap measure until cytotoxic drugs could be expected to become effective; it is occasionally used in patients who are unable to tolerate adequate doses of cyclophosphamide or in those who are refractory to cyclophosphamide therapy.

Fulminant glomerulonephritis may prompt the need for dialysis intervention. Reversal of renal failure depends on the degree of crescent formation and the extent of chronic irreversible changes. There is gratifying experience that the majority of patients recover from the initial episode of serious glomerulonephritis with adequate therapy. On the other hand, patients experiencing major relapses of glomerulonephritis exhibit a high risk of persistent renal failure. Complications of extrarenal Wegener's granulomatosis may persist and require immunosuppressive therapy in patients requiring maintenance dialysis or transplantation. Recurrence of glomerulonephritis apparently due to Wegener's granulomatosis has been documented but appears to be rare following renal transplantation.

IV. HENOCH-SCHONLEIN NEPHRITIS

Essentials of Diagnosis

Henoch-Schönlein purpura (HSP) is a generalized vasculitis which most often affects children from 2 to 12 years of age, and is usually recognized by typical constellations of clinical features which may affect, in any order, skin, joints, kidneys and/or gastrointestinal tract. Of note, only approximately 6% of reported cases of Henoch-Schönlein nephritis have occurred in individuals over 16 years of age. Thus consideration should be given to the other, more common, forms of systemic vasculitis before accepting the diagnosis of Henoch-Schönlein nephritis in adults.

Rash eventually occurs in nearly all cases; when not a component of the presenting syndrome, the disease may be difficult to recognize. Typically, recurrent crops of purpuric skin lesions appear over the extensor surfaces of the lower legs, arms and buttocks, but in severe cases, any area may be affected. Skin biopsies reveal leukocytoclastic vasculitis with granular deposition of IgA along dermal vessels of purpuric and unaffected skin. Of note, urticarial or erythematous lesions may emerge infrequently and confound the diagnosis.

Transient arthralgias and/or arthritis, most often affecting ankles, knees, wrists and fingers, occur in about 75% of patients. The nondeforming joint involvement may be the first sign of HSP in one-quarter of cases. Diagnostic difficulties may arise in the occasional patient who presents with colicky abdominal pains, vomiting, gastrointestinal hemorrhage and/or intussusception prior to the onset of rash. Particularly in the face of intussusception, exploratory laparotomy may be difficult to avoid. Neurologic manifestations including seizures, pulmonary disease, hepatomegaly, parotitis, orchitis, as well as hemorrhage into scrotum, testes and muscles have also been described.

Estimates of the prevalence of renal involvement vary from 22% to 92% depending on patient selection and diagnostic approach. Typically, Henoch-Schönlein nephritis presents as hematuria plus proteinuria within 3 months after the initial skin and/or visceral manifestations. Infrequently, the nephritis may precede (or follow by months to years) other features of the syndrome. Renal involvement ranges from transient, isolated microscopic hematuria to rapidly progressive glomerulonephritis and uremia. The severity of extra-renal disease is an unreliable predictor of the risk of progressive renal insufficiency.

Renal Syndromes

Hematuria is evident in nearly all cases of Henoch-Schönlein nephritis and is usually accompanied by various degrees of proteinuria. Approximately 6% of cases in series from referral centers have presented with uncomplicated microscopic hematuria and three-quarters of those patients have remitted without evidence of residual renal dysfunction. Progressive azotemia was not reported among these patients.

Approximately 50% of reported cases manifest hematuria plus proteinuria without nephrotic syndrome. Typically the proteinuria is nonselective and the overall prognosis is favorable. On long term follow-up, 80% remit, while 10% develop progressive azotemia and another 10% have evidence of persistent nephropathy, defined as proteinuria (>1 gm/day), hematuria, hypertension and/or mild renal insufficiency. The unusual patients with highly selective proteinuria tend to have relatively mild renal disease.

While the prevalence of nephrotic syndrome in referral centers approximates 40%, the rate of occurrence is uncertain in the general population with Henoch-Schönlein nephritis. Renal outcomes for patients with uncomplicated nephrotic syndrome are similar to those for patients with hematuria plus proteinuria without nephrotic syndrome; progressive azotemia emerges in only 10%. On the other hand, the nephrotic syndrome may be complicated in two-thirds of cases by various combinations of hypertension, azotemia, oliguria and/or hypoproteinemia. Unfortunately more than 40% of these patients develop moderate to severe degrees of renal insufficiency on long term follow-up.

The acute nephritic syndrome may be defined as hematuria complicated by combinations of hypertension, azotemia, and/or oliguria. While the overall risk of the acute nephritic syndrome among HSP patients is unknown, this occurred in 40% of children in a large referral center. Typically the acute nephritic syndrome became manifest within 6 weeks of disease onset and in most cases, was associated with the nephrotic syndrome. Acute nephritis may be further complicated by potentially devastating rapidly progressive glomerulonephritis. The risk of end stage renal disease (ESRD) is high in these patients and may best be defined by the percentage of glomeruli affected by crescents as described below.

Uremia is an unusual consequence of Henoch-Schönlein nephritis. Based on available data from literature reviews, terminal renal failure appears more frequently in adults (13%–14%) than children (5%). Among children it is unclear whether increased age is associated with more severe renal complications. Renal failure tends to occur relatively early in the course of follow-up; approximately two-thirds of patients destined for ESRD have failed within 3 years of disease onset. On the other hand, renal failure after 15 years has been recorded, emphasizing the importance of long-term observation.

Pathology

Similar to the diversity of clinical presentation, the renal histology ranges from minimal lesions to severe crescentic glomerulonephritis. Frequently seen are relatively mild lesions such as mesangial proliferation alone or focal segmental proliferative glomerulonephritis. On electron and immunofluorescent microscopy, granular deposits are predominantly mesangial and most often contain IgA. Granular deposits of C3, fibrin, IgG, properdin and IgM are also seen in that order of frequency. The early complement components are rarely detected. These pathologic observations as well as evidence of circulating IgA immune complexes in HSP suggest an immune complex pathogenesis with predominantly alternative pathway complement activation. At present it is unclear whether the IgA originates from mucosa stimulated by upper respiratory infection or from peripheral blood lymphocytes associated with altered T-cell regulatory functions.

Within the more severe range of the histologic spectrum, diffuse proliferative or membranoproliferative glomerular lesions may be seen, associated with more widespread subendothelial and subepithelial granular deposits. The more proliferative glomerular lesions tend to be associated with an increased incidence of crescents which are of considerable prognostic significance. Pooled data from long-term follow-up studies reveal that only 4% of patients with a minority of glomeruli affected by crescents progressed to chronic renal insufficiency. In the context of 50–75% crescents, the risk of uremia increased to 25%, and two-thirds of patients with more than 75% crescents subsequently failed.

Therapy

General. Recognizing that various infections and numerous drugs, including antibiotics, have been implicated as causal factors in HSP, it is appropriate to reserve antimicrobial therapies for specifically identified infections. Although certain foods have also been incriminated, there is little evidence to support the efficacy of dietary modifications. Joint and soft tissue symptoms appear to be alleviated by nonsteroidal anti-inflammatory drugs including as-pirin. On the other hand, antihistamines are probably not beneficial.

Uncontrolled observations suggest that corticosteroids may favorably affect soft tissue swelling, joint and gastrointestinal symptoms but are less likely to alter the course of skin or renal abnormalities. Abdominal colic and gastrointestinal hemorrhage have responded dramatically. Furthermore, corticosteroids may prevent but certainly cannot treat intussusception. Thus, surgical consultation may be of critical importance in these cases.

Renal Disease. Lacking data from prospective randomized therapeutic trials, current recommendations must be regarded as tentative at best. Of concern is the unpredictable nature of Henoch-Schönlein nephritis, which may frequently spontaneously remit, rendering interpretation of uncontrolled studies very difficult.

Decisions regarding therapeutic interventions should be based on careful considerations of prognostic factors. The risks of aggressive therapies can be avoided in individuals with mild renal disease. On the other hand, increased risk of ESRD has been associated with the presence of greater than 50% crescents as well as acute nephritis and/or nephrotic syndrome complicated by combinations of hypertension, azotemia, oliguria, and hypoproteinemia. For patients with such ominous prognostic indicators, a trial of coticosteroids and immunosuppressive therapy is probably warranted, although of unproven benefit.

Efforts to improve therapeutic outcomes have led to trials of experimental approaches including quadruple therapy (corticosteroids plus immunosuppressive drugs, anticoagulants and antiplatelet agents) and plasmapheresis. At present, the former does not appear to offer a therapeutic advantage over corticosteroids and immunosuppressives alone and may be associated with significant risk of hemorrhage. The experience with plasmapheresis is limited. While a number of favorable responses have been reported, these were uncontrolled observations and the application of multiple concurrent therapies make interpretation of these data very difficult. Thus, prospective therapeutic trials are needed to address the unresolved issues regarding the treatment of Henoch-Schönlein nephritis.

V. SCLERODERMA

Scleroderma or systemic sclerosis is a progressive disorder involving skin and essentially all internal organs with a process of connective tissue degeneration and fibrosis. Fibrotic changes are the primary causes of major organ dysfunction particularly the skin, lungs, heart and gastrointestinal tract. Vascular changes are associated with certain functional deficits, as in Raynaud's phenomenon, and also major anatomical lesions producing ischemic ulcerations. In the kidney the arterial process is morphologically similar to that induced by malignant hypertension. Although the arterial lesion of scleroderma is typically complicated by the appearance of malignant hypertension, the characteristic vascular changes are considered to be a cause rather than a result of hypertension.

The appearance of renal involvement is indicated by the presence of low grade proteinuria or emerging azotemia. The classical presentation, however, is that of superimposition of accelerated or malignant hypertension on these urinary abnormalities. Rapidly progressive renal failure occurs in a high percentage of the patients with this clinical constellation unless rapid control of hypertension can be achieved. That the process is primarily a vasculopathy is underscored by the occasional patient who develops accelerated renal failure without significant hypertension or who fails to improve renal function with early effective control of hypertension.

The renal vasculopathy is characterized by marked intimal thickening with an attendant "mucoid" appearance. Adventitial fibrosis is often observed. Fibrinoid necrosis is common but inflammatory vasculitis is not characteristic. Glomeruli typically exhibit ischemic changes but in severe cases may develop crescent formation. Deposition of immune reactants on fluorescence or electron microscopy are rarely observed. Hyperplasia of the juxtaglomerular apparatus is typically seen and appears to correlate with the presence of hyperreninemia.

Therapy

Little is known of the pathogenesis of scleroderma. No clearly effective form of therapy is currently available which adequately treats any of the primary manifestations of scleroderma. The major focus of therapy relates to control of hypertension. Intensive antihypertensive therapy has been occasionally successful in interrupting the vicious cycle of renal vascular disease, azotemia and hypertension. Angiotensin-converting enzyme inhibitors have been the most successful in treating scleroderma renal crisis. Stabilization and/or reversal of renal dysfunction has been documented in some patients. Whether or not these drugs have any salutory effect on the primary vascular lesion in the absence of hypertension has not been assessed. Bilateral nephrectomy is rarely considered in refractory and complicated hypertension.

Because of the extensive complications in other major organ systems which commonly appear in close proximity to renal crisis, patients who develop renal failure due to scleroderma have historically been considered to be poor candidates for maintenance therapy by dialysis or transplantation. Hemodialysis is particularly complicated by difficulties of vascular access. Maintenance peritoneal dialysis and renal transplantation have been undertaken to a limited degree and with some success, particularly in patients with dominant renal scleroderma. In general, survival of patients undergoing any form of treatment of end stage renal disease due to scleroderma has been poor.

VI. THROMBOTIC THROMBOCYTOPENIC PURPURA AND HEMOLYTIC UREMIC SYNDROME

Both thrombotic thrombocytopenic purpura (TTP) and hemolytic uremic syndrome (HUS) are potentially devastating disorders that result in Coomb's negative hemolytic anemia associated with marked erythrocyte fragmentation (microangiopathic hemolytic anemia), thrombocytopenia and fibrin/platelet thrombi in small arteries and arterioles. Red cell and platelet destruction apparently results from contact with abnormal endothelial cells and/or deposited fibrin. Despite several common features, TTP and HUS typically present different clinical syndromes reflecting, in part, differences in distribution of vascular lesions.

Essentials of Diagnosis

Thrombotic Thrombocytopenic Purpura. Reports of this rare disorder span a broad age range with a predominance of cases in the third and fourth decades. Common presenting complaints include weakness, fatigue, malaise, nausea, vomiting, diarrhea, and fever, as well as more specific hemorrhagic and neurologic manifestations. The diagnosis of TTP may be recognized by various combinations of the five classical features, namely: microangiopathic hemolytic anemia, thrombocytopenic purpura, neurologic abnormalities, kidney disease and fever. While all five occur in less than 50% of cases, the first three findings are reported to coexist in three-quarters of patients.

Demonstration of microangiopathic hemolysis is generally regarded as a prerequisite for the diagnosis, although it is clearly not specific for TTP. Erythrocyte fragmentation has also been associated with malignant hypertension, toxemia of pregnancy, scleroderma, renal graft rejection, carcinomatosis, hemangiomas, abnormal or prosthetic cardiac valves and disseminated intravascular coagulation (DIC), as well as HUS. Most of these conditions can be distinguished clinically, and studies of TTP and HUS usually do not provide convincing evidence of concomitant DIC.

Histologic confirmation of the diagnosis may be difficult and in some cases, blind biopsies may be helpful. Recommended biopsy sites include bone marrow, gingiva, lymph nodes, skin, muscle and kidney. An unusual diagnostic problem may emerge if TTP and SLE coexist; all of the features of TTP, including fragmented erythrocytes may be ascribable to SLE.

Hemolytic Uremic Syndrome. A clinical diagnosis of HUS may be suggested by the typical constellation of acute renal failure, thrombocytopenia and microangiopathic hemolytic anemia. First described was childhood HUS; the patients are often less than 4 years of age and frequently experience a prodromal gastroenteritis or upper respiratory tract illness. Approximately 7–10 days later patients characteristically present with hematuria, proteinuria, oligoanuric acute renal failure and evidence of skin and/or gastrointestinal hemorrhage. Hypertension, fluid overload and congestive heart failure

may evolve. Furthermore, neurologic problems, such as convulsions and coma, may occur and may be associated with increased risk of death.

The diagnosis may be further supported by knowledge of geographic locale and family history. HUS appears to be endemic in South Africa and Argentina. The occurrence of HUS among siblings is well described. In endemic areas, an environmental factor may be responsible and several siblings may be affected within a few weeks; on the other hand, in non-endemic areas, genetic predisposition may be important, and cases within a family tend to occur more than a year apart.

The various clinical settings in which adult HUS is encountered reflects the diversity of implicated etiologic factors. HUS has been described in association with pregnancy, oral contraceptive agents, metastatic carcinoma, immunization injections, thymic dysplasia and SLE.

Of particular note is postpartum HUS which may occur up to 3 months following a normal pregnancy, labor and delivery. As in childhood HUS, there may be a prodromal illness. Subsequently emerges the typical syndrome of acute oligo-anuric renal failure, hypertension, microangiopathic hemolytic anemia and severe thrombocytopenia. Heart failure and/or neurologic problems including seizures may further complicate the clinical picture. Of concern, postpartum HUS may recur following a subsequent normal pregnancy.

A similar syndrome has been described in women taking oral contraceptive agents for 1 to 10 years. Familial occurrence of this form of HUS underscores the potential role of a genetic factor. Patients who develop hypertension while on oral contraceptives may be at increased risk for this complication.

Renal Syndromes

Thrombotic Thrombocytopenic Purpura. Clinical evidence of kidney involvement has been described in three-quarters of reported cases. Gross or microscopic hematuria was the most frequent manifestation. Proteinuria, usually less than 2 gm/day, was also detected in many patients. The nephrotic syndrome has rarely been ascribed to TTP. Modest degrees of azotemia occur in a third of patients with TTP. In contrast to HUS, acute renal failure is infrequent (approximately 10%).

Hemolytic Uremic Syndrome. Typically present are hematuria, proteinuria, and acute (often rapidly progressive) renal failure. Hypertension and fluid overload are frequent complicating features. Indeed, the duration and severity of the hypertension and oligo-anuria are important prognostic indicators. Return of renal function may be evident within 2–3 weeks of disease onset or may occur after months (even a year) of maintenance dialysis. The recovery phase may be protracted, lasting 12–18 months. If incomplete, malignant hypertension and/or progressive azotemia may result. Furthermore, HUS may recur on multiple occasions, months to years after the initial event.

Renal Pathology

Similar renal histologic lesions are observed in TTP and HUS, although they tend to be more severe in the latter. Fibrin thrombi may be found in glomeruli, arterioles, and small arteries up to the size of arcuate arteries. Perfusion may be further impaired by endothelial damage and subintimal fibrin deposition. If vascular occlusion is extensive, focal or diffuse cortical necrosis can occur, and the prognosis for renal recovery will be seriously compromised. Arteriolar aneurysms may form near the glomerular hilus; once thrombosis and organization of these structures occurs, they may resemble a diseased glomerulus (the so-called "glomeruloid structure").

The consequence of a focal vascular process is highly variable glomerular alterations. Observed lesions include capillary collapse or congestion, endocapillary proliferation (usually modest), capillary thrombosis, fragmented erythrocytes, fibrinoid necrosis or total infarction of a glomerulus, and occasionally crescents. Subsequently, bland glomerular sclerosis may result in complete obliteration of capillaries.

Characteristic glomerular capillary wall thickening and double contour formation are associated with accumulation of loose fibrillar and granular material in the subendothelial space. Fibrin, fibrinogen, immunoglobulins and complement components may be detected inconsistently in the subendothelial locations by immunofluorescence microscopy. Similar subendothelial accumulations may be seen in arterioles and small arteries.

Therapy

Thrombotic Thrombocytopenic Purpura. An improved outlook for patients with TTP appears to be associated with prompt recognition of the syndrome, application of new modalities of supportive care, and introduction of therapies, such as plasmapheresis and antiplatelet agents, directed at the suspected pathophysiologic process. Patients with relatively mild disease and minimal neurologic involvement may receive a short trial (2–3 days) of high-dose oral corticosteroid therapy alone. Those who fail to respond and those with more severe disease may benefit from the addition of plasma infusion or plasmapheresis employing fresh frozen plasma as the replacement solution. Dramatic recovery following plasma therapy may occur and has been ascribed to replacement of a missing factor that may stimulate prostacyclin activity and thus prevent widespread formation of platelet thrombi. Although many reported cases have received relatively large doses of fresh plasma (6–12 units/day), the optimum dose is unknown and at present should be determined on an individual basis according to alterations in LDH, platelet count and clinical status.

The role of anti-platelet agents is unclear. While some authors combine them with plasma therapy, others do not. Of particular interest is the suggestion that maintenance anti-platelet therapy for 6 to 18 months may prevent relapses of TTP. Splenectomy may be offered to those who fail the above. Anticoagulation and/or immunosuppressive agents are unlikely to be beneficial.

Hemolytic Uremic Syndrome. General therapeutic recommendations can be offered while recognizing the need for further investigation of unresolved issues. Clearly meticulous management of fluid and electrolyte problems, acidosis, and hypertension is critically important. Some patients, particularly children, may remit following such conservative care. More severely affected patients develop anuria, rapidly progressive azotemia, acidosis, hyperkalemia, profound hypertension and/or heart failure. Prompt initiation of dialysis appears to have reduced the mortality rate associated with these complications. While peritoneal dialysis may be preferable in small children, hemodialysis is frequently employed for adults.

Controversy surrounds the role of additional therapies such as anti-coagulation, anti-platelet agents and plasma exchange. Recognizing the potential risks of these interventions and the frequently benign course of childhood HUS, the treatment of children should focus on the vigorous applications of general supportive and dialytic measures. Since adults tend to have a less favorable prognosis, they are most frequently treated with heparin and occasionally with anti-platelet agents as well. Although the experience is uncontrolled, current data suggests this approach may be efficacious.

Plasma infusion and plasma exchange have also been recommended, in part, because of the apparent response of a closely related illness, TTP. Additional experience is needed to determine the value of plasma therapy in HUS.

VII. DIABETES MELLITUS

Nephropathy is a common complication of diabetes mellitus associated with serious morbidity and mortality. Typically the earliest clinical abnormality is proteinuria which appears, in most series, over a range of 12–22 years after detection of insulin-dependent diabetes mellitus. Proteinuric patients are at risk for progressive azotemia and resultant end stage renal disease after an additional 3–5 years.

While these parameters provide an overview of natural history, there is considerable individual variation. Only approximately one-half of diabetics develop proteinuria after 20 years of observation. Glomerulosclerosis usually develops in patients with insulin dependent diabetes, but it may also appear in some patients with insulin resistant diabetes. The rate of decline of renal function may be influenced by recognition and treatment of reversible factors, such as ureteral obstruction, infection, analgesic abuse and hypertension. More controversial is the impact of "tight" glucose control on the natural history of diabetic retinopathy, neuropathy and nephropathy.

Renal Syndromes

Hyperfiltration. Prior to the onset of proteinuria in diabetic patients, typical clinical observations include nephromegaly and enhanced glomerular filtration rate which persists despite good control of blood glucose. Increased effective renal plasma flow and filtration fraction have also been observed. Evidence has been presented suggesting that diabetic kidney hyperfiltration may be related to an increase in glomerular capillary surface area, although a number of factors are likely to be contributory. At this early stage, detection of enhanced urinary albumin excretion by sensitive assays may permit identification of patients at increased risk for progressive diabetic nephropathy despite absence of proteinuria by standard laboratory tests. While this abnormality may be reversible by strict metabolic control, the long term impact of this intervention on renal function has yet to be established.

Asymptomatic Proteinuria. The evolution of proteinuria more than 10 years after the diagnosis of diabetes is a characteristic feature of diabetic nephropathy and for most patients is of ominous prognostic significance; the majority progresses to end stage renal disease within 5 years. The non-selective proteinuria of diabetic nephropathy appears to reflect loss of electrostatic barrier function due to reduction of glomerular polyanion, as well as structural membrane defects.

Nephrotic Syndrome. Clinical and laboratory features of the nephrotic syndrome typically emerge during the pre-terminal phase of diabetic nephropathy and are associated with progressive azotemia and hypertension. While unusual, significant hematuria, red cell casts or early onset nephrotic syndrome without retinopathy may be the consequence of diabetic nephropathy; concurrent superimposed renal diseases should be considered, including papillary necrosis, infection, obstruction, proliferative glomerulonephritis, and steroid responsive minimal change nephropathy.

Azotemia. Once proteinuria evolves, progressive loss of renal function is characteristic of diabetic nephropathy. While the rate of decline varies from patient-to-patient, evidence has been presented that it is nearly constant in individuals and that once azotemia emerges, there is a linear relationship between the inverse of the serum creatinine (1/cr) and time. Thus, a graph of this relationship may facilitate patient follow-up and the timing of therapeutic interventions. It is noteworthy that some patients manifest an accelerated course to terminal renal failure.

The frequency and potential mortality of arteriosclerotic cardiovascular disease among azotemic diabetic patients has prompted angiographic procedures to identify this important risk factor. Unfortunately, these investigations are not infrequently associated with x-ray contrast-induced acute renal failure which is occasionally irreversible.

Renal Pathology

Enlargement of otherwise normal appearing glomeruli appears early in the disease. Subsequently there evolves a generalized expansion of eosinophilic mesangial matrix and thickening of glomerular capillary basement membranes. This process, called diffuse intercapillary glomerulosclerosis, eventually leads to obliteration of adjacent capillary lumina and is frequently, but not invariably, associated with the evolution of proteinuria and azotemia.

The nodular form of diabetic glomerulosclerosis, described by Kimmelstiel and Wilson, occurs in approximately one-quarter to one-half of patients with the diffuse lesion and is considered to be the most distinctive form of diabetic nephropathy. Located at the center of glomerular lobules, the lesions tend to be round, eosinophilic, PAS-positive and relatively hypocellular with a peripheral rim of compressed endocapillary cell nuclei. These segmental lesions correlate poorly with clinical manifestations of diabetic nephropathy.

Also commonly seen are hyaline lesions located in Bowman's capsule ("capsular drop"), in the lumina of glomerular capillaries ("hyaline cap"), and in the intima and media of arterioles. Hyaline arteriolosclerosis typically affects both the afferent and efferent arterioles and recognition of this distribution may aid in diagnosis of diabetic nephropathy.

Immunofluorescence microscopy frequently reveals linear deposits of IgG and other plasma proteins along glomerular and tubular basement membranes as well as Bowman's capsule. This pattern of staining is felt to represent non-specific accumulation of circulating proteins attributed in part to altered capillary permeability and mesangial clearing function.

Therapy

In view of the potentially devastating complications associated with diabetic nephropathy, timely interventions may profoundly influence the patient's survival and quality of life. In relation to progressive azotemia, consideration of reversible factors (such as hypertension, infection or obstruction due to papillary necrosis or bladder dysfunction) may be rewarding. Furthermore, diabetic patients are at risk for hyperkalemia out of proportion to the degree of azotemia. Typically this is associated with hyperchloremic acidosis and is ascribed to hyporeninemic, hypoaldosterone renal tubular acidosis (Type 4 RTA). A low potassium diet, potassium wasting diuretics, and/or kayexalate may be indicated. The risks of hypertension and fluid accumulation associated with mineralocorticoid therapy are of particular concern in these patients.

Interventions aimed at slowing the progression of diabetic macrovascular and microvascular disease are under investigation. Efforts to control well recognized risk factors such as hypertension, cigarette smoking, obesity, and abnormal lipids are encouraged. Recommendations regarding angiotensin converting enzyme inhibitors and dietary protein restriction for reduction of glomerular hypertension, hyperfiltration and progressive renal failure must await results of prospective trials.

Also of interest are recent reports which support the therapeutic efficacy of "tight" glucose control in efforts to arrest progressive retinopathy, neuropathy and nephropathy. Thus, home blood glucose monitoring and pre-prandial regular insulin, in addition to long acting preparations, may be advantageous. Continuous subcutaneous insulin infusion and pancreatic islet-cell transplantation may further enhance long-term outcomes and are under investigation.

The azotemic phase of diabetic nephropathy tends to be relentlessly progressive and complicated by a vicious cycle of uremia, hypertension, congestive heart failure, retinopathy and neuropathy. Thus, early entry into dialysis/

transplantation programs (serum creatinine 5–6 mg/dl) may improve patient survival and rehabilitation.

Currently available data permit tentative observations and recommendations regarding modalities of end stage renal disease therapies. While survival of the diabetic patient on hemodialysis appears to be improving, analysis of pooled data reveals that only 40–60% of diabetics live 2 years, compared to approximately 85% for non-diabetics. The principal causes of death among hemodialyzed diabetics include cardiovascular disease, cerebrovascular accidents, infection and voluntary termination of therapy.

Survival data on peritoneal dialysis is difficult to interpret because, in general, the more complicated patients have been offered this modality. At present one year survival approximates 60%. Death is often due to the relentless progression of cardiac and vascular disease. While peritoneal infection has been troublesome, hyperglycemia may be avoided by the use of intraperitoneal insulin. It is controversial whether peritoneal dialysis is associated with reduced progression of neuropathy and retinopathy compared to hemodialysis.

Life expectancy following cadaveric renal transplantation approaches that for chronic hemodialysis; approximately 50% survive 2 years. The outlook is more favorable for diabetics undergoing living related donor transplantation—approximately 80% are alive at 2 years.

An unresolved issue is the impact of successful transplantation on the progression of retinopathy and peripheral neuropathy. If observations suggesting a favorable effect are confirmed, recommendations for relatively early renal transplantation would be warranted.

VIII. PARAPROTEINEMIAS

Numerous plasma protein derivatives which are either produced at an excessive rate, as in multiple myeloma, or characterized by unusual biochemical properties, such as amyloid, macroglobulinemia or cryoglobulinemia, are associated with distinct forms of renal disease.

Amyloidosis

Systemic amyloidosis is commonly associated with deposition of amyloid in glomeruli and renal blood vessels. Both immunoglobulin-associated amyloid (primary) and secondary amyloid have been associated with renal involvement. Glomerular deposition of amyloid protein causes nephrotic range proteinuria. Amyloid deposits are recognized by the characteristic staining with metachromatic dyes, such as Congo red which exhibits birefringence on polarized light microscopy. Electron microscopic findings of fibrillar material of characteristic morphology confirms the diagnosis of amyloidosis.

Progressive accumulation of amyloid material in renal vessels and glomeruli may lead to progressive renal insufficiency, often complicated by severe nephrotic syndrome. Control of the causes of secondary amyloidosis may prevent, stabilize and sometimes reverse this process. In cases where definitive treatment for the underlying disease cannot be adequately applied, attempts at treatment with colchicine have met with limited success. Treatment of immunoglobulin-associated amyloid with cytotoxic agents has generally not resulted in favorable long term control of the amyloidosis.

Multiple Myeloma

Malignant plasma cell dyscrasias may produce an excess of immunoglobulin components in an uncontrolled fashion. Several renal complications of this paraprotein excess have been described. Renal tubular acidosis, hypercalcemic nephropathy, amyloidosis, plasma cell infiltration of the kidney, and a special type of tubular injury called myeloma kidney have been described. In the latter case, immunoglobulin light chains precipitate in the renal tubular lumens and produce a cast nephropathy. On the other hand, light chains may precipitate along the tubular basement membrane leading to tubular injury and dysfunction; a glomerular lesion associated with precipitation of immunoglobulin light chains in a fashion analogous to amyloidosis may complicate multiple myeloma. Several of these complications of multiple myeloma may lead to progressive renal failure unless effective chemotherapy is able to contain the plasma cell malignancy. It is noteworthy that dehydration and/or x-ray contrast dyes may cause acceleration of renal failure apparently by enhanced precipitation of paraproteins in renal parenchyma.

Macroglobulinemia

This paraprotein disorder is characterized by deposition of immunoglobulin (IgM) in glomerular capillaries. The glomerular deposits reside in the subendothelial space of the capillary loops and occasionally resemble hyaline thrombi. Progressive azotemia may be seen in some patients but disorders of glomerular permeability which would induce nephrotic range proteinuria are not observed in macroglobulinemia-associated nephritis. Treatment with cytotoxic drug therapy and plasma exchange have been anecdotally reported to be beneficial.

Cryoglobulinemia

Plasma proteins with the chemical property of being cryoprecipitable have a predeliction to localize in glomerular capillaries. Cryoglobulins may represent a component of systemic diseases, such as SLE, vasculitis, or malignancies, or may represent a primary (essential) cryoglobulinemia. Typically, the cryoprecipitable material is composed of IgG, IgM, certain complement components, and in rare instances, specific antigens such as hepatitis surface antigens (HBsAg). Deposition of cryoglobulins usually occurs in the glomerular subendothelial space and these deposits exhibit a unique fibrillar appearance on the electron microscope. The glomerulonephritis is typically membranoproliferative and/or crescentic in nature. The renal disease encompasses a range from asymptomatic hematuria/proteinuria to chronic glomerulonephritis and occasionally rapidly progressive renal failure. Treatment with combinations of cytotoxic drug therapy and plasma exchange aimed at reducing the rate of production of immunoglobulin and immune complexes, as well as their bulk depletion, have been reported successful in controlling cryoglobulinemic glomerulonephritis. It appears that the prognosis in cryoglobulinemia is determined predominantly by the extrarenal manifestations and associated complications.

IX. MALIGNANCY

Glomerular lesions have been associated with various neoplastic diseases including carcinomas, Hodgkin's disease, non-Hodgkin's lymphomas, leukemias and embryonal tumors. Nephrotic syndrome is the most frequently recognized clinical manifestation, although asymptomatic proteinuria, and crescentic glomerulonephritis have also been described.

Immune complex glomerulopathies have been reported to complicate carcinomas affecting the lung, colon, stomach, breast, kidney and cervix. Investigations to date have implicated (but not proven the relevance of) tumor antigens, as well as fetal, viral and normal endogenous antigens. Membranous glomerulopathy was the histologic lesion most frequently reported (approximately two-thirds of cases). Immunofluorescent studies revealed granular deposition of immunoglobulins and complement along the glomerular capillary loops, and subepithelial electron-dense deposits were seen on electron microscopy. Infrequently, minimal change disease, as well as membranoproliferative, crescentic and focal sclerosing glomerulonephritis, have also been described in carcinoma patients.

These observations can be relevant to the adult patient with apparent idiopathic membranous glomerulopathy. Several series suggest that the incidence of occult neoplasm approaches 5–10% of cases of membranous nephropathy, particularly in the elderly. Occasionally, the nephrotic syndrome remits following successful treatment of the tumor. Unfortunately, in the majority of cases, both the tumor and the renal disease are poorly responsive to therapeutic interventions.

The pattern of renal involvement is quite different among patients with Hodgkin's disease, in which approximately 50% of reported cases have revealed minimal change nephropathy. Anyloidosis and minimal change nephropathy, while well described in early series, appear less prevalent currently, probably reflecting modern intensive tumor therapy. Membranous glomerulopathy occurs infrequently. As in carcinoma, the nephrotic syndrome may precede, coincide with, or follow recognition of Hodgkin's disease. Effective therapy of Hodgkin's disease is frequently associated with complete remission of the nephrotic syndrome, which may occasionally recur with tumor relapse.

Minimal change nephropathy occurs relatively infrequently in association with non-Hodgkin's lymphomas and various leukemias.

Membranous and membranoproliferative glomerulopathy have also been described.

X. POST-INFECTIOUS GLOMERULOPATHIES

An ever-expanding list of infectious agents has been associated with various forms of immune complex glomerulonephritis. Syndromes involving bacterial infections (e.g., occult sepsis, endocarditis, infected ventriculoatrial shunts, syphilis and leprosy) are particularly important in that prompt recognition and treatment may be lifesaving and lead to reversal of the renal abnormalities. Typically, the infections which cause nephropathy are protracted and associated with circulating immune complexes, cryoglobulins, high titer rheumatoid factor, as well as depression of complement components C_3, C_4 and $C1q$ (the latter two may be near normal if alternative pathway complement activation predominates as may occur with pneumococcal infection). A broad range of glomerular lesions has been described including membranoproliferative (infected ventriculoatrial shunts), focal proliferative and necrotizing (endocarditis), diffuse proliferative with or without crescents (endocarditis and occult sepsis), and membranous glomerulopathy (leprosy and syphilis). Immunofluorescent studies typically reveal granular deposits of immunoglobulins and complement components within glomeruli. The antigen of the offending organism has been demonstrable in some cases.

Glomerulopathies have been ascribed to various viral infections including hepatitis B, infectious mononucleosis, measles, mumps, and chickenpox. Of particular interest, chronic hepatitis B surface antigen (HBsAg) carriers are at risk for systemic vasculitis as well as for membranous and membranoproliferative glomerular lesions. High levels of circulating immune complexes and/or cryoglobulins have been detected. In this setting, nephrotic syndrome and renal failure may evolve without clinically evident liver disease. Thus, a high index of suspicion is often required for identification of the HBsAg carrier state. Parasitic infections, particularly plasmodium malariae and toxoplasmosis, have also been implicated as causal factors in glomerular disease. The former is typically associated with nephrotic syndrome and a membranoproliferative lesion, whereas the latter may result in acute proliferative glomerulonephritis.

SUGGESTED REFERENCES

Systemic Lupus Erythematosus

Austin HA, Klippel JH, Balow JE, leRiche NGH, Steinberg AD, Plotz PH, Decker JL: Therapy of lupus nephritis: controlled trial of prednisone and cytotoxic drugs. *N Engl J Med* 314:614–619, 1986

Baldwin DS, Gluck MC, Lowenstein J, Gallo G: Lupus nephritis: clinical course as related to morphologic forms and their transitions. *Am J Med* 62:12–30, 1977

Balow JE, Austin HA, Muenz LR, Joyce KM, Antonovych TT, Klippel JH, Steinberg AD, Plotz PH, Decker JL: The effect of treatment on the evolution of renal abnormalities in lupus nephritis. *N Engl J Med* 311:491–495, 1984

Balow JE, Austin HA, Tsokos GC, Antonovych TT, Steinberg AD, Klippel JH: Lupus nephritis. *Ann Intern Med* 106:79–94, 1987

Dinant HJ, Decker JL, Klippel JH, Balow JE, Plotz PH, Steinberg AD: Alternative modes of cyclophosphamide and azathioprine therapy in lupus nephritis. *Ann Intern Med* 96:728–736, 1982

Donadio JV, Holley KE, Ferguson RH, Ilstrup DM: Treatment of diffuse proliferative lupus nephritis with prednisone and combined prednisone and cyclophosphamide. *N. Engl J Med* 299:1151–1155, 1978

Ponticelli C, Zucchelli P, Banfi G, Cagnoli L, Scalia P, Pasquali S, Imbasciati E: Treatment of diffuse proliferative lupus nephritis by intravenous high-dose methylprednisolone. *Q J Med* 51:16–24, 1982

Systemic Vasculitis

Balow JE: Renal vasculitis. *Kidney Int* 27:954–964, 1985

Croker BP, Lee T, Gunnells JC: Clinical and pathologic features of polyarteritis nodosa and its renal-limited variant: primary crescentic and necrotizing glomerulonephritis. *Hum Pathol* 18:38–44, 1987

Fauci AS, Haynes BF, Katz P: The spectrum of vasculitis. Clinical, pathologic, immunologic and therapeutic considerations. *Ann Intern Med* 89:660–676, 1978

Leib ES, Restivo C, Paulus HE: Immunosuppressive and corticosteroid therapy of polyarteritis nodosa. *Am J Med* 67:941–947, 1979

Savage CA, Winearls CG, Evans DJ, Rees AJ, Lockwood CM: Microscopic polyartertis: presentation, pathology and prognosis. *Q J Med* 56:467–483, 1985

Serra A, Cameron JS, Turner DR, Hartley B, Ogg CS, Neild GH, Williams DG, Taube D, Brown CB, Hicks JA: Vasculitis affecting the kidney: presentation, histopathology and long-term outcome. *Q J Med* 53:181–207, 1984

Wegener's Granulomatosis

Fauci AS, Haynes BF, Katz P, Wolff SM: Wegener's granulomatosis: prospective clinical and therapeutic experience with 85 patients for 21 years. *Ann Intern Med* 98:76–85, 1983

Van der Woude FJ, Rasmussen N, Lobatto S, Wiik A, Permin H, Van Es LA, Van der Giessen M, Van der Hem GK, The TH: Autoantibodies against neutrophils and monocytes: tool for diagnosis and marker of disease activity in Wegener's granulomatosis. *Lancet* 1:425–429, 1985

Henoch-Schonlein Nephritis

Ogg CS, Cameron JS, Williams DG, Turner DR: Presentation and course of primary amyloidosis of the kidney. *Clin Nephrol* 15:9–13, 1981

Tarantino A, De Vecchi, A, Montagnino G, Imbasciati E, Mihatsch MJ, Zollinger HU, Barbiano di Belgiojoso G, Busnach G, Ponticelli C: Renal disease in essential mixed cryoglobulinemia. *Q J Med* 50:1–30, 1981

Malignancy

Alpers CE, Cotran RS: Neoplasia and glomerular injury. *Kidney Int* 30:465–473, 1986

Dabbs DJ, Morel-Maroger L. Mignon F, Striker G: Glomerular lesions in lymphomas and leukemias. *Am J. Med* 80:63–70, 1986

Post-Infectious Glomerulonephritis

Dormant J, Delfraissy JF: Renal involvement in various conditions: infectious diseases, In *Nephrology,* edited by Hamburger J, Crosnier J, Grunfeld JP, New York, John Wiley and Sons, Inc, 1977, pp. 767–790

Austin HA, Balow JE: Henoch-Schonlein nephritis: prognostic features and challenge of therapy. *Am J Kidney Dis* 2:512–520, 1983

Counahan R, Winterborn MH, White RH, Heaton JM, Meadow SR, Bluett NH, Swetschin H, Cameron JS, Chantler C: Prognosis of Henoch-Schonlein nephritis in children. *Brit Med J* 2:11–14, 1977

Levy M, Broyer M, Arsan A, Levy-Benoilila D, Habib R: Anaphylactoid purpura nephritis in childhood: natural history and immunopathology. *Adv Nephrol* 6:183–228, 1976

Systemic Sclerosis

LeRoy EC, Fleischman RM: The management of renal scleroderma. *Am J. Med* 64:974–978, 1978

Lopez-Overjero JA, Saal SD, D'Angelo WA, Cheigh JS, Stenzel KH, Laragh JH: Reversal of vascular and renal crises of scleroderma by oral angiotensin-converting enzyme blockade. *N Engl J Med* 300:1417–1419, 1979

Oliver JA, Cannon PJ: The kidney in scleroderma. *Nephron* 18:141–150, 1977

Traub YM, Shapiro AP, Rodnan GP, Medsger TA, McDonald RH, Steen VD, Osial TA, Tolchin SF: Hypertension and renal failure (scleroderma renal crisis) in progressive systemic sclerosis. *Medicine* 62:335–352, 1983

Thrombotic Thrombocytopenic Purpura and Hemolytic Uremic Syndrome

Goldstein MH, Churg J, Strauss L, Gribetz D: Hemolytic uremic syndrome. *Nephron* 23:263–272, 1979

Mammen EF: Management of thrombotic thrombocytopenic purpura. *Semin Thromb Hemostasis* 7:1–51, 1981

Ponticelli C, Rivolta E, Imbasciati E, Rossi E, Mannucci PM: Hemolytic uremic syndrome in adults. *Arch Intern Med* 140:353–357, 1980

Ridolfi RL, Bell WR: Thrombotic thrombocytopenic purpura. *Medicine* 60:413–428, 1981

Diabetes Mellitus

Kaplan SA, Lippe BM, Brinkman CR, Davidson MB, Geffner ME: Diabetes mellitus. *Ann Intern Med* 96:635–649, 1982

Krolewski AS, Warram JH, Christlieb AR, Busick EJ, Kahn CR: The changing natural history of nephropathy in type I diabetes. *Am J Med* 78:785–794, 1985

Mauer SM, Steffes MW, Brown DM: The kidney in diabetes. *Am J Med* 70:603–612, 1981

Mogenson CE: Microalbuminuria as a predictor of clinical diabetic nephropathy. *Kidney Int* 31:673–689, 1987

Zatz R, Brenner BM: Pathogenesis of diabetic microangiopathy. The hemodynamic view. *Am J Med* 80:443–453, 1986

Paraproteinemias

Fang LS: Light-chain nephropathy. *Kidney Int* 27:582–592, 1985

Gorevic PD, Kassab HJ, Kevo Y, Kohn R, Prose P, Franklin EC: Mixed cryoglobulinemia: clinical aspects and long-term follow-up of 40 patients. *Am J Med* 69:287–308, 1980

Hill GS, Morel-Maroger L, Mery JP, Brouet JC, Mignon F: Renal lesions in multiple myeloma. *Am J Kidney Dis* 2:423–438, 1983

Husby G, Sletten K: Chemical and clinical classification of amyloidosis 1985. *Scand J Immunol* 23:253–265, 1986

Jack Moore Jr.
Harry G. Preuss

14

Tubulointerstitial Disease

Tubulointerstitial diseases (TID) affect tubules and interstitial areas of the kidney, while initially preserving the glomeruli and renal vasculature. The tubulointerstitial area subserves many renal functions, including maintenance of sodium balance, urinary concentration and dilution, renal acidification, and divalent ion metabolism. Perturbations in these functions may be the earliest signs of TID.

Many different insults cause TID. Our understanding of these disorders has increased dramatically in recent years, and "tubulointerstitial disease" is preferred over the term "chronic pyelonephritis," which heretofore was the rubric for all non-glomerular renal disease. Chronic pyelonephritis now should be used only to identify TID which is primarily caused by recurrent bacterial urinary tract infection.

The recognition of TID is often made difficult by the poor distinction between tubulointerstitial, glomerular, and vascular injury. Such distinction is particularly difficult when renal disease is advanced. Initially however, specific tubular defects often provide useful clues to the possibility of TID and may provide an opportunity to intervene early in the pathological process. As many disorders responsible for TID progress, signs of glomerular injury, such as the nephrotic syndrome, may obscure the primary tubulointerstitial process.

TID assume particular importance for the clinician, because many of the responsible conditions are amenable to therapy. Thus, a careful history, physical examination and judicious use of routine laboratory testing in conjunction with the performance of specific laboratory tests, provide the opportunity to attenuate what may otherwise be an inexorable decline in renal function.

PATHOGENESIS

With the variety of insults capable of causing TID, it is not surprising that our understanding of the exact pathogenesis behind these disorders remains limited. TID is often secondary to a toxic effect on the tubulointerstitial area. Renal tubules are epithelia composed of metabolically active cells, and are subsequently susceptible to toxic injury. Moreover, the unique structure-function relationships of tubules and surrounding interstitium may be disrupted by any process which disturbs this relationship. For the most part, the pathogenesis of TID must be discussed in a descriptive manner until more precise mechanisms become known.

A useful way to consider pathogenesis is to examine the disorders which are known to produce TID. It has become useful clinically to divide the disorders arbitrarily into those which typically produce acute TID and those which produce chronic TID. There may be considerable overlap between the two groups, but the distinction between an acute or chronic disorder is exceedingly important.

DISORDERS USUALLY
PRESENTING AS ACUTE TID

For practical purposes, there are two conditions which regularly present as acute TID. The first is drug-induced injury, the most important cause, and the second is infection of the kidney.

Drug Induced Acute TID

Although many different drugs may cause acute TID, most documented cases occur secondary to the penicillins, sulfonamides, phenytoin, furosemide, rifampin, and thiazide diuretics, (Table 1). Drug-induced acute TID assumes particular importance because of its potential reversibility, especially if recognized early.

Occurrence does not necessarily relate to total dose. In most instances, reactions appear to be idiosyncratic and resemble allergic or hypersensitive reactions. Fever and signs of hypersensitivity such as rash, arthralgias, and eosinophiles in the blood, urine, or renal biopsy material, suggest the diagnosis (Fig. 1).

Drugs cause acute TID in several ways. First, the drug may elicit antibody formation

Table 14-1   Some Common Drugs Causing Acute Tubulointerstitial Disease

Drug Class	Example
Penicillins	Methicillin
Sulfonamides	Trimethoprim-Sulfamethoxazole
Diuretics	Thiazides
Anti-Tubercular Drugs	Rifampin

against renal tissue. Such antibodies are produced either against the drug or a drug-protein complex directly, or against renal tissue which has been altered by the drug. An example of this mechanism is methicillin nephritis. Second, the drug may act as a direct renal toxin, and injure the kidney or induce other toxic products, which subsequently injure the kidney. (ATN is discussed in Chapter 5). An example of this mechanism is the direct toxicity and intravascular hemolysis with hemoglobinuria induced by sulfonamides. Third, the drug may cause alterations in lymphocyte populations with resultant

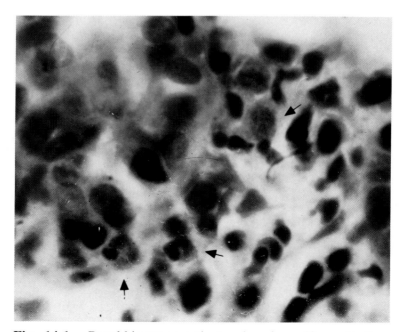

Fig. 14-1. Renal biopsy on patient undergoing sulfonamide therapy for streptococcal infection. Patient developed an acute rise in serum creatinine. Arrows point to eosinophiles.

cellular-mediated injury. An example is the injury induced by cimetidine.

Infection-Induced Acute TID

Bacterial infection of the kidney, pyelonephritis, is generally caused by gram-negative organisms which reach the renal parenchyma through an ascending route. The renal response to bacterial invasion includes edema, mobilization of inflammatory cells, and local antibody production. The swelling and inflammatory cell infiltration induce changes in the structure-function relationship in the tubulointerstitial area, with resultant acute TID.

In most cases, primary infection-induced TID is not clinically apparent, nor is it of clinical importance. When infection is added to underlying renal disease, or to obstructive injury, however, overt tubular defects may become obvious.

DISORDERS USUALLY PRESENTING AS CHRONIC TID

A multitude of conditions are capable of producing chronic TID. The identification of chronic TID, and the demonstration of the cause, may require extensive investigation. These disorders can be divided into several classes listed in Table. 2.

Endogenous toxins, e.g., hypercalcemia, hyperuricemia, and hyperoxaluria, not only precipitate in the tubulointerstitial area, but incite chronic inflammatory cell infiltrates and induce fibrosis. Thus, the normal structure-function relationship is distorted. In methoxyflurane-induced TID, oxalate as well as inorganic fluoride may be causative.

Exogenous toxins include heavy metals (lead, cadmium) and drugs. Cadmium is used in metallic plating and alkaline batteries. The cadmium-metallothionein complex is particularly toxic to proximal tubular cells. Urinary screening for B_2 microglobulin is useful in early detection. Lead is a frequent component of paints and used in stills to make moonshine. Lead nephropathy increases the excretion of lead, copraporphyrins and gamma-amino-levulinic acid. Characteristic lead inclusion bodies are often seen in renal tissue (Fig. 2). Inappropriate hyperuri-

Table 14-2   Disorders Which Cause Chronic Tubulointerstitial Disease

1. Endogenous Substances
   Hypercalcemia
   Hyperuricemia
   Hyperoxaluria

2. Exogenous Toxins
   Cadmium
   Lead

3. Drugs
   Analgesics
   Non-steroidal Anti-inflammatory Drugs
   Anti-neoplastic Agents
   (Platinum, Nitrosoureas)

4. Plasma Cell Dyscrasias
   Multiple Myeloma
   Light Chain Disease

5. Granulomatous Disorders
   Sarcoidosis

6. Vascular Disease
   Sickle Cell Nephropathy

cemia and high frequency of associated hypertension are common.

The most important drugs which cause chronic TID are analgesics. Analgesic nephropathy, in which mixtures of analgesics decrease the synthesis of vasodilatory prostaglandins, accounts for 5% to 6% of chronic renal failure. Analgesic nephropathy should be suspected in patients with unexplained renal insufficiency who complain of headaches, back pain, gastrointestinal upset, or who have a history of psychiatric problems. Analgesic nephropathy is frequently associated with papillary necrosis, which gives the characteristic "ring sign" on x-ray (Fig. 3). Documentation of excessive analgesic use is difficult, so a positive ferric chloride test on the urine or the presence of methemoglobin or sulfhemoglobin in the urine may be clues for diagnosis. A serum salicylate level may also be helpful. The non-steroidal anti-inflammatory agents are associated with interstitial nephritis and minimal change nephropathy, although a cause and effect relationship remains to be determined.

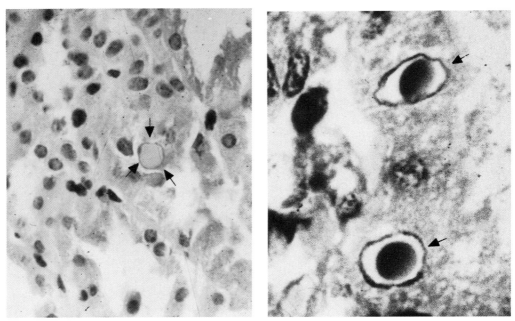

Fig. 14-2A + B. Two views of lead inclusion bodies (arrows) in renal biopsy tissue.

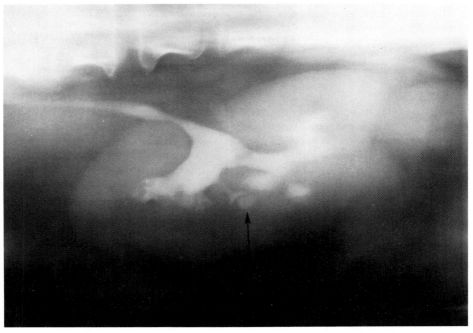

Fig. 14-3. Arrows point to ring sign secondary to sloughed papilla in patient who abused analgesics (with permission of American Family Physician).

Other drugs known to cause chronic TID include the anti-neoplastic agents cis-platinum and methyl-CCNU. Both of these drugs may cause chronic TID which is first noted after the course of therapy has been completed.

Chronic TID is particularly important as a manifestation of renal injury in the plasma cell dyscrasias. Excess light chains appear to be quite toxic to tubular epithelial cells, and may deposit in the interstitial area and glomeruli with subsequent fibrosis. The development of Fanconi's syndrome (glucosuria aminoaciduria, phosphaturia and bicarbonaturia) may appear before a definitive diagnosis has been made.

Another cause of chronic TID is sarcoidosis. Both hypercalcemia and noncaseating granuloma formation in the renal interstitium may induce renal disease.

Finally, if the tubulointerstitial area is deprived of its blood supply, as occurs when the medullary blood vessels are occluded in sickle cell nephropathy, ischemic injury may result, with subsequent fibrosis and loss of function.

Various hereditary disorders fall into the category of TID. Among them are cystic disorders such as polycystic kidney disease (PCKD), medullary cystic disease, and medullary sponge kidney. These must be distinguished from simple renal cortical cysts which are rarely associated with disease except for occasional infection.

Hereditary nephritis is associated with deafness, retinal and lenticular abnormalities, and megathrombocytopathia. Inheritence is autosomal dominant with varying penetrance. Severity is greater in males. On biopsy, lipid-filled foam cells may be seen in the interstitium. The kidney exhibits features of both TID and glomerular disease. Chronic hereditary nephritis may be seen in the absence of nerve deafness and ocular disease.

CLINICAL SYNDROME OF TUBULOINTERSTITIAL DISEASE

TID can present as acute fulminating renal failure, or in any other fashion from asymptomatic abnormalities of the urinary sediment to advanced chronic renal insufficiency. These syndromes are listed in Table 3.

Table 14-3 Clinical Syndromes of Tubulointerstitial Disease

Acute Interstitial Nephritis
  Generally drug induced; may mimic acute renal failure

Asymptomatic Urinary Sediment Abnormalities
  Hematuria
  Pyuria
  Proteinuria

Isolated Tubular Defects
  Proximal Tubular Dysfunction
  Distal Tubular Dysfunction
  Medullary Dysfunction

Chronic Renal Insufficiency or Failure

Acute tubulointerstitial nephritis is difficult to distinguish from acute renal failure of any cause, and may present as acute oliguric renal failure.

Asymptomatic urinary abnormalities include hematuria, pyuria, or proteinuria. Hematuria may be gross or microscopic, intermittent or constant. Red blood cell casts, however, signify glomerular disease. Pyuria, including white cell casts and eosinophiluria, seen most often in drug-induced diseases, is common. Urine cultures are generally sterile. Proteinuria is usually of non-nephrotic magnitude, although tubular proteinuria can, on occasion, be excessive. Both albumin and non-albumin are commonly present.

Specific tubular defects are often extremely helpful in recognizing the presence of TID. They can be localized to the proximal tubule, where one can demonstrate either proximal renal tubular acidosis, or the complete Fanconi's syndrome. The distal tubule may be primarily involved; in which case, distal renal tubular acidosis or disorders of potassium secretion may be prominent. Finally, the injury may primarily involve the medullary areas, in which case the inability to concentrate urine may be evident.

Lastly, it is not uncommon for azotemia to be the presenting problem. In this case, it may be exceptionally difficult to establish a diagnosis of TID.

DIAGNOSIS OF
TUBULOINTERSTITIAL DISEASE

The first step in the diagnosis of TID is to distinguish between glomerular diseases and TID. Some of the criteria useful in distinguishing glomerular etiologies from TID are listed in Table 4.

However, in many instances the initial manifestation of glomerular and tubulointerstitial injury may be remarkably similar; thus, further evaluation must be performed. A proposed evaluation is listed in Table 5.

The patient's history should be carefully checked for identification of TID risk factors. Particularly important is a thorough drug history, including questions designed to elucidate analgesic use. Any history of stones or infections should be obtained, as they may guide the physician to an underlying metabolic or structural abnormality. The patient should be queried specifically about symptoms of renal disease. Polyuria, nocturia, or episodic weakness may reflect tubular defects in water or K^+ handling, respectively.

The physical examination should be directed towards a search for tophi, signs of lead toxicity, bone pain, calcium deposits, or seeking evidence for the Sicca syndrome. In general, however, the physical examination is not particularly rewarding in the evaluation of TID.

The laboratory evaluation of the patient with

TID can be divided into tests obtained on a routine basis, and more specialized tests used for further delineating both the nature and the extent of tubulointerstitial injury. Routine laboratory tests are listed in Table 5.

Of particular importance is the urinalysis, which should be performed on the first specimen voided in the morning. Preferably, the specimen should be collected under mineral oil, after the patient has been kept from drinking overnight. An intact urinary concentrating ability, especially if the patient has been dehydrated overnight, is established if the specific gravity of the urine exceeds 1.020. Collection of the urine under oil allows the pH to be checked with a

Table 14-4 Distinguishing Features Between Glomerular and Tubulointerstitial Disease

	GN	A-TID	C-TID
Proteinuria >3.5 g/24 h	+	−	−
Red Cell Casts	+	−	−
Tubular Defects (Concentration) (Acidification)	−	+	+
Azotemia	+	+	+
Eosinophiluria	−	+	−
Leukocyturia	+	+	+

A = Acute C = Chronic

Table 14-5 Evaluation of Patients in Whom TID is Suspected

I. History

  A. Identification of Risk Factors

   1. Toxin Exposure
   2. Medication History
   3. Analgesic Use
   4. Urinary Tract Infections
   5. Nephrolithiasis

  B. Identification of Symptoms of Renal Disease

   1. Polyuria—Nocturia
   2. Episodic Weakness
   3. Symptoms of Uremia

  C. Identification of Extra-Renal Disease

   1. Bone Pain—Myeloma
   2. Monoarticular Arthritis—Gout

II. Physical Examination

III. Laboratory Tests

  A. Routine Tests

   1. CBC, Automated Blood Chemistry Profile
   2. Urine Sample for pH, SpGr, Microscopic, Chemistries
   3. 24-Hour Urine for Creatinine Clearance, Protein Excretion, Calcium, Uric Acid Excretion
   4. Anatomical Study—IVP or CT Scan

pH meter. A pH 5.5 or lower eliminates distal renal tubular acidosis as a diagnostic possibility. Together, evidence of normal concentrating and acidification capabilities make a diagnosis of TID unlikely. Creatinine clearance, as an index of glomerular filtration rate, and total protein excretion, should be performed. Simultaneously, the urine can be analyzed for calcium, uric acid, and oxalate. Finally, each patient should receive an anatomical study. If renal function is normal, an intravenous urogram with nephrotomography delineates calyceal detail, cortical scarring, and nephrocalcinosis. Computed tomography may serve the same function. (See Chapters 3).

Specialized laboratory testing is divided into tests necessary to document tubular defects, and tests helpful in elucidating the etiology of TID. These tests are delineated in Table 6.

Tubular defects such as impaired water conservation are best documented with formal water deprivation testing. Similarly, the ability of the kidney to handle acid should be quantitated with formal acid-loading testing. If proximal renal tubular acidosis is suspected, bicarbonate infusions with subsequent determination of the transport maximum for bicarbonate may be required. Fortunately, however, isolated proximal renal tubular acidosis in adults is rare. Adults with proximal tubular dysfunction exhibit the acquired Fanconi's syndrome, with phosphatoria, aminoaciduria, glucosuria, and bicarbonaturia (See Chapter 1 for specific tests).

Tests to elucidate the etiology of TID are also listed in Table 6. Of particular importance

Table 14-6 Specialized Tests in the Evaluation of TID

1. To Document Tubular Defects

   A. Formal Water Deprivation with Pitressin
   B. Formal Acid Loading
   C. Determination of Glucose, Amino Acid, Phosphorus Excretion

2. To Clarify Etiology of TID

   A. Suspected Toxic Injury
      Analgesic Metabolites
      Heavy Metal Screen
   B. Suspected Plasma Cell Dyscrasia
      Urine Protein Electrophoresis
      Serum Protein Electrophoresis

are screens for analgesic metabolites, and urine and serum protein electrophoreses, because an analgesic nephropathy and plasma cell dyscrasias are increasingly important causes of TID.

Indications for biopsy of the kidney in patients with TID remain uncertain. Some indication include diagnosis after non-invasive tests have been unrevealing. Alternatively, a biopsy may be used to guide prognostic counselling. The reasons indicated above apply mainly to chronic TID. Indications for biopsy in acute TID are limited, but biopsy may be crucial if the distinction between rapidly progressive glomerulonephritis, acute renal failure, and acute TID cannot be made on clinical grounds (See Chapter 2 under renal biopsy).

THERAPY OF TUBULOINTERSTITIAL DISEASE

The treatment of acute TID is primarily limited to removal of the offending drug. It is extremely important that the physician identify any drug responsible for inducing TID. While a salutory influence of corticosteroids has been noted on azotemia in retrospective series, no contolled data are available to support the routine use of corticosteroids where a drug can be identified as causing acute TID. However, the use of corticosteroids may be considered in individual patients, when the benefits of such therapy appear to outweigh risks.

Successful treatment of chronic TID is primarily aimed at preventing further progression of injury. Thus, the cause of hypercalcemia or hyperuricemia must be eliminated. The plasma cell dyscrasias can be successfully treated in many patients with antineoplastic agents, and sarcoidosis responds favorably to corticosteroids. No therapy will reverse the established fibrosis and scarring characteristics of these diseases. At present, attenuation of the decline in renal function is the only realistic goal of therapy.

SELECTED READINGS

Appel GB, Kunis CL. Acute Tubulo-interstitial Nephritis. In: Cotran RS, eds. Tubulo-interstitial Nephropathies. New York, Churchill-Livingston, 1983:151–185.

Cogan MG. Classification and Patterns of Renal Dysfunction. In: Cotran RS, ed. Tubulo-interstitial Nephropathies. New York, Churchill-Livingston, 1983:35–48.

Cotran RS Tubulointerstitial Nephropathies. Hospital Practice, Jan 1982; 79–92.

Ditlove, J, Weidmann P, Bernstein M, Massry SG. Methicillin Nephritis. Medicine 1977; 56:483–491.

Kleinknecht D, Vanhille P, Morel-Maroger L, et al. Acute Interstitial Nephritis Due to Drug Hypersensitivity. An Up-to-Date Review with a Report of 19 Cases. In: Hamburger J, Crosnier J, Grunfield J, eds. Advances in Nephrology, Vol. 12. Chicago: Year Book medical Publishers, 1983:277–308.

Murray T. Drug-induced Chronic Tubulo-interstitial Renal Disease. In: Cotran RS, ed. Tubulo-interstitial Nephropathies. New York: Churchill-Livingston, 1983:187–210.

Murray T, Goldberg M. Chronic Interstitial Nephritis: Etiologic Factors. Ann Intern Med 1975; 82:453–459.

Pirani CL, Silva FG, Appel GB. Tubulo-interstitial Disease in Multiple Myeloma and other Nonrenal Neoplasias. In: Cotran RS, ed. Tubulo-interstitial Nephropathies. New York: Churchill-Livingston, 1983:287–334.

Watson AJS, Dalbow MH, Stachura I, Fragola JA, et al. Immunologic Studies in Cimetidine-Induced Nephropathy and Polymyositis. N Eng J Med 1983; 308: 142–145.

Rishpal Singh
Harry G. Preuss

15

Renal Vascular Diseases

INTRODUCTION

The kidney is a highly vascular organ. Accordingly, conditions influencing blood vessels affect kidneys. The following section is restricted to conditions involving the main blood vessels, namely the renal artery and renal vein, and to the embolic phenomena; because many disorders involving renal blood vessels such as vasculidities, hypertension, and renal stenosis are discussed in Chapters 13 and Chapter 6 of Volume 2 in this series, Management of Common Problems in Kidney Disease.

KIDNEY DISEASE FROM MAJOR ARTERIAL LESIONS

The renal artery may contain lesions or be involved indirectly from aortic lesions. A number of well recognized arterial disorders affecting kidneys are generally lumped together and referred to as nephrosclerosis. Nephrosclerosis includes more than one disorder involving the renal vasculature—arteriosclerosis, arteriolar nephrosclerosis, and the malignant phase of hypertension. These entities are associated with hypertension, and it is often difficult to determine whether the renal lesions precede or follow the hypertension. Renal lesions derived from these different entities are often patchy and in the case of the milder forms show no abnormalities other than minimal proteinuria.

Aortic Lesions

Aortic aneurysms and atherosclerosis commonly influence the renal artery. Eighty percent of aortic aneurysms arise below the origin of the renal artery and are caused in 95% of cases by atherosclerosis. The aorta may be involved by atheromata which lead to stenosis or blockage of the renal artery at the inlet. In turn, this causes hypertension or accelerates existent hypertension. Surgical correction without interruption of the blood supply to the kidney is often possible. Even when the blood supply is interrupted, the kidneys handle ischemia rather well—a 20-minute ischemic period may lead to no permanent damage. However, it is important to remember that ischemia is much better tolerated in the saline expanded state.

Renal Artery Stenosis. See Hypertension (Chapter 6 in Volume 2 of the series).

Renal Artery Aneurysms. The incidence of renal artery aneurysms varies considerably between diagnostic and autopsy series. A good overall approximation is 1%. Aneurysmal lesions are subdivided into 4 categories: 1) sacular, 2) fusiform, 3) dissecting and 4) mixed.

Sacular Aneurysms. These are the most common variety and occur at the bifurcation of the main renal branches. A dull ache in the flank is a not infrequent presentation. The aneurysms may be calcified or non-calcified and are generally unilateral. Atheromatous changes often develop secondarily in the aneurysm, restricting the renal arterial lumen, producing hemodynamically significant lesions, and leading to hypertension. Hypertension can disappear if the lumen completely closes.

These types of aneurysms may eventually invade the renal vein, producing an arterio-venous fistula. The most serious complication is rupture of the vessel. Small lesions less than 1 inch in diameter and wholly calcified seldom do. Larger uncalcified or partially calcified aneurysms rupture more often and should be surgically repaired. Surgical resection is almost always feasible since the aneurysms are generally located in the main branches.

Fusiform Aneurysms. These are really post stenotic dilatations. The dilatation is often at least 3 cm long and 3 times wider than the original renal artery. Therefore, they may mask stenosis, necessitating a careful search for the inciting cause.

Dissecting Aneurysms. A break in the intima leading to blood leakage into the vessel wall is, or course, a feared complication. While the dissection may remain localized to 1 cm of the renal artery, a more common outcome is thrombosis with subsequent renal infarction.

Acute abdominal pain associated with a non-obstructed non-functioning kidney is the hallmark of this lesion. Renal infarction often leads to elevated blood pressure, probably due to ischemia of the area surrounding the infarction. It may occur within 80 days to 150 days following infarction, then subside gradually. However, accelerated hypertension often necessitates emergency drug therapy. Surgical resection of dissecting aneurysms is the rule; and sometimes, partial or complete nephrectomy is necessary.

Mixed Aneurysms. Not infrequently 2 or even 3 forms of aneurysms may be discovered in the same major renal vessels.

RENAL ARTERY EMBOLISM AND THROMBUS

Emboli and/or thrombi may occlude the major renal vessels. When atheromatous mate-rial is released from the aorta or renal artery, it lodges in the small arteries, arterioles, and glomeruli. The atherosclerotic embolic phenomenon has been associated with surgery and the use of catheters during imaging procedures. Emboli arising from the heart have been known to completely occlude the renal artery. Depending on the magnitude of the vascular blockage and subsequent renal damage, acute or chronic renal failure, with or without subsequent hypertension, may ensue.

Pain may be prominent in the flanks, hypertension may develop or be accelerated, and the urine sediment often shows red cells, white cells, and a variety of casts. Since the resulting ischemia usually causes localized atrophy and infarction, renal biopsy may miss the lesions and not be diagnostic. Arteriography is undertaken for definitive diagnosis.

RENAL VEIN THROMBOSIS

Renal vein thrombosis has been well documented in infancy where a sudden onset of abdominal pain, hematuria, and a large kidney which later shrivels, are diagnostic. In adults, ante-mortem diagnostic capabilities have been slow to develop; most diagnoses are made post mortem. With increasing awareness and a high index of suspicion, more cases in the living adult are being diagnosed today.

Etiology. Renal vein thrombosis is associated with a number of conditions. Compression of the renal vein by a tumor or other external mass, and tumor extension from hypernephroma into the venous lumen may precipiate thrombosis. Thrombosis in leg veins and/or the inferior vena cava may enlarge to involve the renal veins. Association with systemic lupus, nephrotic syndrome, and the post partum period is probably due to hypercoagulability known to occur in these conditions.

Patients with amyloidosis and multiple myeloma develop renal vein thrombosis which extends from the peripheral vessels toward the central vessels, while sickle cell anemia may results in sludging of venous radicals with resultant thrombosis. The question still remains whether thrombosis occurs in otherwise healthy adult kidneys purely from hemoconcentration.

Presently, no concusive data are available to implicate severe dehydration as a primary cause.

Pathology. Acute blockage of the renal vein leads to hemorrhagic infarction of the kidney, and irreversible changes can develop within minutes. However, even in clinical situations suggesting acute thrombosis, treatment is still indicated as the possibility of reversal always exists.

Signs of chronic slow blockage are often difficult to distinguish from those caused by the underlying disease, e.g., signs and symptoms noted in membranous glomerulonephritis, lipoid nephrosis, or diabetes may be due to the underlying disease, rather than venous thrombosis. Interstitial changes such as edema, fibrosis and tubular atrophy out of proportion to glomerular changes, are suggestive of renal vein thrombosis. Additionally, a kidney that is initially enlarged but later shrinks, is compatible with renal vein thrombosis. Not infrequently, recanalization may occur.

At autopsy, thrombus in the renal vein is diagnostic. With chronicity, large collateral venous channels between the capsule of the kidney and surrounding tissue are noted. Microscopically, glomeruli appear normal, and the tubules are unchanged in the acute situation except when there is marked proteinuria. With proteinuria, the tubular cells contain lipoid and eosin staining material. Tubular atrophy appears with chronicity.

Clinical Diagnosis. Clinical findings depend upon whether the thrombosis is acute or chronic. In acute cases, flank pain with hematuria is a common presentation. A large kidney and hypertension are present in approximately one half of the cases. Proteinuria, massive in amount, is the hallmark of chronic obstruction. While abdominal pain is rare, thromboembolism to other areas, particularly the lungs, is commonly present. Left sided renal vein occlusion may result in a hydrocoele or venous engorgement in the left testes.

The most important factor in diagnosis is a high index of suspicion, because certain clinical signs, symptoms and associations point toward renal venous occlusion:

1. flank or abdominal pain with or without hematuria in the post-partum period, and in patients with systemic lupus erythematosis, nephrotic syndrome, amyloidosis, multiple myeloma and sickle cell disease.
2. a pulmonary embolus in a patient with nephrotic syndrome
3. a sudden marked increase in proteinuria in a patient with nephrotic syndrome. It is uncertain which appears first—the nephrotic syndrome or renal vein thrombosis.
4. the appearance of edema and proteinuria in patients with deep vein thrombosis of the lower extremity.

Intravenous pyelography is a good screening test. Unequally sized kidneys suggest unilateral disease. The large kidney, with a stretched out calyceal system similar to polycystic kidney, is a common finding. Round impressions from the dilated collateral vessels on the upper part of the ureter are also suggestive.

A large kidney with diminished function is consistent with acute thrombosis. Although renal scan and flow studies are not very helpful in chronic cases, a large kidney with poor perfusion is highly suggestive of acute renal vein thrombosis. Renal arteriography may show a flush in the renal subcapsular area and an absent venous flow phase; however, the venous flow is often not clearly seen in normal cases. Selective renal vein catheterization will diagnose a central obstruction, but attempts to push dye under pressure into renal venous radicals have been abandoned due to ensuing complications.

Treatment. Anticoagulant therapy has met with some success, especially in acute cases, and should be initiated as soon as the diagnosis is suspected. In cases such as SLE, there may be an initial prolonged PTT due to depressed concentrations of factor IX. Factor IX is consumed during coagulation. This should not be a deterrent to treatment which is initiated with heparin, and continued with coumadin. Treatment may be required for 6 weeks to 6 months until the collaterals are well established, or until it is determined that the kidneys are irreparably damaged. In chronic cases, the role of anticoagulation is less certain. However, it could be worthwhile, especially in cases where proteinuria is massive.

Clot lysis therapy is a potential, future mode of therapy, but there is insufficient data at the present time to make an accurate evaluation of its usefulness. Obviously, treatment of underlying diseases, such as lupus or myeloma, is indicated.

SELECTED READINGS

1. Heymann W, Hackel DB, Harwood S, Wilson SGF and Hunter JLP. Production of nephrotic syndrome in rats by Freund's Adjuvants and Rat Kidney Suspensions. Proc Soc Exp Biol Med 100:660–664, 1959
2. Llach F, Arieff AI, Massry SG: Renal vein thrombosis and nephrotic syndrome. A prospective study of 36 adult patients. Ann Intern Med 83:8–14, 1975.
3. Llach F, Koffler A, Finck E, and Massry SG. On the incidence of renal vein thrombosis in the nephrotic syndrome. Arch Intern Med 137:333–336, 1977
4. Moyer JD, Rao CN, Warren CW, Olsson, CA. Conservative management of renal artery embolism. J Urol 109:138–143, 1973
5. Sherry S. Low dose heparin prophylaxis for postoperative venous thromboembolism. N Engl J Med 293:300–302, 1975
6. Trew PA, Biava CG, Jacobs RP and Hopper JR., J. Renal vein thrombosis in membranous glomerulonephropathy: Incidence and association. Medicine 57:69–82, 1978

James F. Winchester
Michael C. Gelfand

16

Clinical Management of End-Stage Renal Disease (ESRD)

The successful management of the patient with uremic end-stage renal disease (ESRD) provides a challenge. In Chapter 1, it was pointed out that uremic complications arise from retention of wastes, principally end products of nitrogen metabolism, from alterations in essential metabolites, and also from failure of renal tissue to carry out important endocrine functions. In addition to chemical derangements and their effects on every organ system in the body, adaptive mechanisms become insufficient to preserve water and solute homeostasis. Often, there are accompanying psychiatric and psychological disturbances related to uremia, its treatment, or both.

Enormous variations in the individual patient's tolerance to uremia exist, but in general, patients remain asymptomatic and have no laboratory abnormalities, until 80% of nephrons are destroyed (i.e., a glomerular filtration rate below 20 ml/min). Ultimately, nephron loss is so great that dialysis and transplantation are required to sustain life. This usually occurs, however, near a creatinine clearance of 5 ml/min. It must be stressed that individual variations are so great that many patients can tolerate uremia down to glomerular filtration rates of 2 ml/min with conservative management, while others require dialysis at higher glomerular filtration rates.

Presently, patients undergo dialysis well before severe uremic symptoms occur.

MANAGEMENT OF ESRD IN THREE STAGES

In practical terms, the management of ESRD can be divided into three main phases, depending upon the degree of reduction in glomerular filtration rate. Phase I (GFR > 20 ml/min) consists of conservative management, defined here as measures other than dialysis and transplantation. Phase II (GFR 20 ml $\rightarrow\rightarrow\rightarrow$ 5 ml/min) consists of conservative therapy with dietary management, and Phase III (GFR < 5 ml) consists of dialysis and transplantation. In Phase I and II conservative management may retard or halt progression of renal disease and provide symptomatic therapy. Every measure is taken to fully exclude any reversible elements of the renal diseases, and such reversible elements are assiduously sought. A brief outline of the management of end-stage renal disease is shown in Table 1.

It is generally considered that life is incompatible with a glomerular filtration rate below 5 ml/min, although before widespread dialysis, patients were managed down to glomerular fil-

Table 16-1   Management of ESRD

PHASE 1—>(GFR 20 ml/min)
   Correction of the following reversible factors:

   1. Treatable renal diseases (e.g. systemic lupus erythematosus, polyarteritis nodosa)
   2. Control of hypertension
   3. Sodium/water balance
   4. Electrolyte/Acid-base balance
   5. Cessation of analgesics and avoidance of nonsteroidal anti-inflammatory agents
   6. Systemic or renal infection
   7. Cardiac failure
   8. Rule out or relieve obstruction

PHASE II—(GFR 5–20 ml/min)

   a. Correction of reversible factors as in Phase I
   b. Introduction of dietary protein restriction ± essential aminoacids/alpha keto acids
   c. Introduction of Vitamin D analogues and phosphate binders

PHASE III—(GFR <5 ml/min)

   Dialysis and/or transplantation
   Continued control of hypertension
   Continuation of Vitamin D analogues and phosphate binders

tration rates of 1 ml/min to 3 ml/min by severe protein restriction.

MANAGEMENT OF PHASE I OF CHRONIC RENAL FAILURE

As discussed in Chapter 1, progression of renal disease can be estimated by the reciprocal of serum creatinine, i.e., $1/S_{cr}$ versus time plotted semilogarithmically. This approximates the rate of GFR fall for an individual patient. For most patients, the progression to ESRD is inexorable; but there are several treatable diseases amenable to therapy. Included in this spectrum are collagen vascular diseases, particularly systemic lupus erythematosus and polyarteritis nodosa, and also noncollagen diseases such as Goodpasture's syndrome, rapidly progressive glomerulonephritis (nonoliguric), membranous glomerulonephritis, analgesic nephropathy, possibly diabetes mellitus, and secondary amyloidosis. Therefore, it is imperative that the clinician search carefully for any potentially treatable renal disease and use specific therapeutic approaches discussed elsewhere in this book. Even progressive diseases may be amenable to treatment by correcting factors which adversely in-

fluence their course. The most important of these contributory factors is hypertension, which potentiates glomerular injury in glomerulonephritis and contributes to progression of diabetes mellitus. Hypertension is now more easily treated than previously.

In patients with primary or secondary hypertension, renal damage may progress to the point where dialysis is required. Even here, there are many reports of patients who recovered enough GFR after antihypertensive therapy to eventually stop dialysis. Fear of further reducing GFR with antihypertensive therapy should be considered only briefly, because the benefits of maintaining blood pressure within normal limits far outweigh any temporary reduction in GFR. Even in Phase II chronic renal failure, any GFR reduction is normally followed by subsequent improvement. Modern drugs such as minoxidil, diazoxide, captopril and enalapril either slow progression of renal disease or help to the point that nephrectomy is rarely necessary to control hypertension. It is important to consider a rational approach to hypertension therapy, particularly in the choice of drugs. Often more success is achieved if drugs with different modes of action are chosen. Irrational use of two drugs of the same class (e.g. beta blockers) only increases the frequency of side effects without much increase in the antihypertensive effect.

As pointed out above, adaptive mechanisms occur in failing kidneys which preserve natriuresis and sodium balance, even to GFR's as low as 2 ml/min. On the other hand, when the GFR is below 25 ml/min, an acute change in sodium intake may not result in homeostasis. Below a GFR of 25 ml/min, the patient is unable to excrete more than 150 mEq to 200 mEq of sodium per day. Accompanying this, there is a degree of extracellular fluid volume expansion. In contrast, an obligatory excretion of 25 mEq of sodium occurs in chronic renal disease, i.e., abrupt reduction of sodium intake is not reflected in reduced sodium excretion. Rather, sodium continues to be excreted two to three times over the intake. This is generally true for most renal diseases whether glomerular or tubular. Excessive sodium loss is called "salt losing nephropathy" and is commonly associated with chronic pyelonephritis, polycystic renal disease, and nephronophthisis. Obviously, it is inappropriate to routinely restrict dietary sodium intake in renal patients. In those with evidence of total body sodium excess (congestive heart failure, edema and hypertension), dietary sodium should be curtailed. Alternatively, if negative sodium balance precipitated by pyrexia, gastrointestinal bleeding, vomiting, diuretics or dietary sodium restriction occurs in the patient with obligatory sodium loss, such patients may easily become volume contracted, thereby decreasing renal perfusion and GFR. Such precipitating events may occur in previously stable ESRD patients and create the need for dialysis.

In terms of water balance, a picture similar to sodium is seen. As renal function declines, excretion of isosmotic urine, i.e., isosthenuria occurs. In isosthenuria, the osmolality of urine is equal to that of plasma. Isosthenuria is present regardless of the intake of water, because patients are unable to concentrate or dilute the urine maximally. Therefore, the patient may become seriously volume contracted on fluid restriction, but rapidly fluid overloaded with excessive fluid intake. Because the rate of urine formation during chronic renal failure is relatively constant day and night, nocturia is an early feature of chronic renal disease. At very low filtration rates, fluid intake should be monitored and maintained around two liters per day.

Potassium, like sodium, is excreted at a greater rate per nephron due to decreased fractional reabsorption; however, potassium is also added to the urine via distal tubular secretion. Consequently, potassium balance is better maintained in chronic renal failure than sodium balance. In addition, the colon secretes potassium and shows an adaptive increase in fecal potassium secretion during ESRD. It follows that potassium intake should not be restricted until late stages of ESRD unless other circumstances exist, e.g. intercurrent illnesses or metabolic acidosis. Volume contracted patients and patients with oliguria are prone to develop urinary retention or acute reduction in GFR. In ESRD patients, constipation should be avoided since the contribution of the colon to potassium secretion is impaired. Finally, potassium sparing diuretics can upset the adaptive balance and should be avoided.

As renal failure progresses, the kidneys are unable to excrete an acid load, leading to metabolic acidosis. The immediate factor responsible is decreased ammonium excretion due to reduction in functioning nephrons. Clinically, the metabolic acidosis is associated with an excessive anion gap. The retained acid moieties are largely buffered in bone, eventually contributing to renal osteodystrophy. Treatment of the acidosis is weighed against the risk of sodium overload from sodium bicarbonate. In view of this, it is recommended that serum bicarbonate concentrations be maintained around 20 mEq/L. In addition, specific tubular disorders may produce hyperchloremic acidosis, and excessive use of phosphate binding gels (aluminum hydroxide) may restrict the availability of urinary phosphate. Thus, titratable acidity is limited for net acid excretion.

Systemic infections, i.e., viral, and bacterial infections (respiratory, gastrointestinal tract, and septicemia) or local renal infections may contribute to the marked acidosis. Also, volume contraction from vomiting or diarrhea may further reduce GFR. Accordingly, rapid treatment of such conditions is imperative.

Analgesic nephropathy caused by phenacetin was singled out for causing or for hastening ESRD, but other analgesics such as aspirin and other nonsteroidal anti-inflammatory agents have also been shown to reduce GFR as interstitial nephritis and/or papillary necrosis develop. In addition, the nonsteroidal anti-inflammatory agents reduce renal prostaglandin production, limit renal blood flow, and may result in further reduction of GFR in the renal impaired patient. A careful drug history is mandatory in patients in whom the etiology of the renal disease is not clear, since drug cessation can stabilize or improve renal function. Similar remarks apply to iodine containing radiology dyes and anticancer drugs such as cis-platinum. Drug induced renal disease is discussed more fully in Chapter 14.

Cardiac failure from relative volume expansion and anemia is common in ESRD patients. Not infrequently, cardiac failure is of the high output type, but may also be due to impaired left ventricular function (observed in over 1/3 renal disease patients). Pericardial effusion is frequent.

Any possible obstruction of the renal tract should be ruled out so that the obstruction might be relieved early. It is important that the classification of a patient's disease as "end-stage" should be made only after obstruction has been ruled out.

Management of Phase II of Chronic Renal Failure

The three major methods to manage Phase II chronic renal failure are outlined in Table 1. Obviously, correction of reversible factors is also important here, and each potentially reversible component should be addressed.

DIETS

Dietary protein restriction is useful to ameliorate symptomatology from chronic renal failure. Recent evidence strongly suggests that dietary nitrogen restriction with high biological value proteins providing 0.5–0.6 g protein/kg body weight/day may retard renal deterioration and delay dialytic therapy. Dietary phosphate restriction and calcium supplementation can also slow the progress of renal failure. In addition to these studies, phosphate itself may be a direct renal toxin, while other studies show that a low protein diet improves the blood pH, producing a rise in plasma bicarbonate which lasts for many years if the diet is maintained. Whatever mechanism, these dietary manipulatory observations have opened up new possibilities for managing ESRD.

Dietary protein restriction, however, has been tested and tried for at least 30 years in the management of chronic renal failure. Dietary protein restriction was introduced initially to manage patients before hemodialysis was widely available. The first (Giordano-Giovanetti) diet used 18 g protein largely composed of pasta and eggs. The diet eventually needed supplementation with 0.5 g of methionine in order to reverse negative nitrogen balance. Since this low nitrogen diet was abundant in essential amino acids, depletion of tissue amino acids and proteins was prevented, and nitrogen was conserved. The diet reduced serum creatinine, SUN, uric acid, and inorganic phosphate levels. Hemoglobin and hematocrit stabilized or rose and anorexia, nausea, vomiting, hiccuping, itching and drowsiness became less frequent. Many subsequent studies of restricted protein diets demonstrated that the quality rather than the duration of life was mostly improved. Many patients become euphoric, and terminally most patients developed acidosis, hyperkalemia, agitation, and died suddenly without overt symptoms of uremia. While most of these studies were encouraging, many other investigators found that negative nitrogen balance ensued with time; and consequently, it was determined that approximately 0.6 g of biological high value protein/kg/day was required to achieve neutral or positive nitrogen balance. Accordingly, the standard "renal diet" now consists of 40 g–60 g high biological value proteins (assimilable, and producing high quantities of essential amino acids with little residue), 60 mEq of sodium, 60 mEq of potassium, along with 1,000 to 1500 ml of fluid derived from foods ingested or drunk. At this point, it is worthwhile remembering that an average 24 hour urine sample contains 1500 ml of fluid, 20 g urea, (approximately 15 g urea nitrogen), 1.5 g creatinine, 0.75 g uric acid, 140 mEq of sodium and 60 mEq of potassium.

Recent attention has been devoted to the use of semi-synthetic diets containing very low quantities of protein but supplemented with essential amino acids or alpha ketoacids (the latter generate essential amino acids). By using appropriate combinations of the 8 classical amino acids (approximately 20 g) along with 20 g of primarily high quality protein, nitrogen balance will be neutral or positive, compared to isonitrogenous diets containing protein as the sole source of nitrogen. It is felt that the alpha-ketoacids and alpha-hydroxyacid analogues of essential amino acids, provide pure amino acids without increasing the nitrogen load. Several investigators have shown that adding ketoacid analogues of phenylalanine, valine and tryptophan allow a faster adaptation to the low nitrogen intake than with the nonketoacid diet. Moreover, renal function can be stabilized or increased using this regimen, although it is unclear whether it is due to the ketoacids or the low serum phosphate levels and/or the low calcium-phosphorus product.

Although compliance with restricted protein diets is variable, careful counselling will achieve a high rate of success. In highly compliant patients substantial delays in the introduction of substitution therapy may be achieved. Standard dietary interviews, supplemented by dietary diaries, are of some use in assessing outpatients, but the inaccuracy of the technique is well documented. Two better methods are available: serum urea nitrogen/serum creatinine and the urea nitrogen appearance (UNA). The SUN/serum creatinine correlates directly with the dietary protein intake in nondialyzed chronic uremic patients, if they are in a steady state without catabolic stress and have a urine volume greater than 1500 ml/day. In women, children and muscle wasted men, the reduced muscle mass causes less creatinine production and the SUN/creatinine is higher for any given protein intake. Urea nitrogen appearance (UNA) is the most accurate method that can be used in dialyzed and in nondialyzed patients. It is measured by the following formula: UNA (g/day) = urinary urea nitrogen + dialysate urea nitrogen + change in body urea nitrogen. The change in body urea nitrogen is derived from a more complex formula relating the changes in serum urea nitrogen to whole body water following introduction of a nitrogen restricted diet.

When substitution therapy becomes necessary, dietary protein restriction is relaxed somewhat with the standard diet containing 80 g protein, 60 mEq sodium and 60 mEq potassium. Protein restriction applies to patients who are not nephrotic or receiving peritoneal dialysis. In both of these conditions renal or peritoneal protein losses must be supplemented by additional dietary protein. For patients on continuous ambulatory peritoneal dialysis, discussed below, the average peritoneal protein loss is 8 g/day and patients' diets should contain 1.2 to 1.3 g protein/kg/day to obtain neutral or positive nitrogen balance. In addition to proteins, it is rec-

ommended that renal diets contain at least 2000 calories/day to prevent nitrogen catabolism.

One cautionary note should be sounded here. Most diets produce a rise in cholesterol and triglycerides which compound the propensity of the ESRD patients towards hyperlipidemia. In the dialyzed uremic patient there may be acceleration of atherosclerosis. For this reason, it is recommended that only one-third of the daily caloric intake be fat.

Phosphate Binders and Vitamin D Analogues

Renal osteodystrophy is a broad term that covers all osseous manifestations of uremia. Skeletal pathology includes osteitis fibrosa cystica (and other features of hyperparathyroidism), osteomalacia, osteoporosis and osteosclerosis. Unchecked, renal bone disease creates skeletal abnormalities: deformation, resorption, fractures, and retardation of growth. The etiology of renal osteodystrophy is multifactorial, but the basic common defects are varying combinations of Vitamin D resistance, Vitamin D deficiency (osteomalacia), and secondary hyperparathyroidism. Vitamin D_3 (cholecalciferol) from animal sources, and Vitamin D_2 (ergocalciferol) from plants, are the two major Vitamin D parent compounds. Vitamin D_3 is converted in the kidney to the biologically active 1,25 dihydroxy Vitamin D_3 ($1,25(OH)_2D_3$). It is apparent that the failing kidney exhibits impaired 1,25 hydroxy Vitamin D_3 production. Under normal physiological circumstances, the conversion of Vitamin D_3 to 1,25 dihydroxy D_3 (calcitriol) occurs in the proximal tubular cells. Hypocalcemia, calcium deficiency and hypophosphatemia normally augment 1,25 (dihydroxy D_3 formation. Calcitriol, transported by its carrier protein, enhances gastrointestinal absorption of calcium and phosphorus, acts on bone in the presence of parathyroid hormone to mobilize calcium, and stimulates mineralization of osteoid tissue. The latter occurs either through elevation of plasma calcium and phosphate or through its action on collagen metabolism, or both. Its activity on the parathyroids, pancreas, kidneys and salivary glands is uncertain. Calcitriol also has activity in skeletal muscle, possibly facilitating protein synthesis that allows calcium entry. Clinical features of Vitamin D deficiency are proximal myopathy and impaired mineralization of osteoid. In addition, there is low intestinal absorption of calcium and phosphate in the absence of Vitamin D. In turn, this leads to hypocalcemia and produces hyperparathyroidism, a renal phosphate leak, and subsequent hypophosphatemia. 24,25 dihydroxy Vitamin D_3 $(24,25(OH)_2D_3)$ is another sterol produced in the kidney which is absent in anephric animals and in man. Its exact biological role is controversial although it appears to lower plasma calcium, stimulate bone mineralization, and suppress parathyroid hormone secretion.

Parathyroid hormone (PTH) production is stimulated by lowered blood calcium, and even small changes in plasma calcium in the range of 7.5 mg/dl to 10.5 mg/dl can influence PTH secretion. Epinephrine and norepinephrine can augment PTH secretion, while hypermagnesemia suppresses it. PTH (9,500 daltons) secreted into the blood undergoes biotransformation in the liver and kidney with release of carboxy-terminal C-terminal fragments (7,000 daltons). The latter are biologically inactive. The active amino terminal (N-terminal) fragment (3500 to 4000 daltons) has a rapid half-life of 4–5 minutes. C-terminal fragments are removed by the kidneys, while the N-terminal fragments are metabolized in the skeleton. Consequently, C-terminal fragments achieve high levels in renal insufficiency. PTH acts in the kidney and bone through adenylase cyclic systems to inhibit renal reabsorption of phosphate, and stimulate renal conversion of 25 $(OH)D_3$ to 1,25 $(OH)_2D_3$. Most importantly, however, PTH allows the conversion of mesenchymal cells to osteoclasts, which increase bone resorption, as well as activating osteoblasts. The overall effect of PTH in bone is to increase bone resorption and formation, and increase bone turnover.

It is clear that renal bone disease begins early as renal function declines. Since even transient hyperphosphatemia may lower plasma calcium and stimulate PTH secretion, it is the therapeutic goal in Phase II chronic renal failure to reduce plasma phosphate and elevate serum calcium. Since hyperphosphatemia usually occurs when the GFR falls below 25 ml/min, modest dietary phosphate restriction combined with aluminum hydroxide gels to adsorb excessive dietary phosphate should be introduced. In addition, low plasma levels of 1,25 $(OH)_2D_3$ are almost invariable as renal failure advances. This

may or may not produce predominant osteomalacic bone disease.

To differentiate the predominant lesion in renal osteodystrophy, bone biopsies are performed and stained specifically for detection of the degree of bone mineralization. More recently, attention has turned to the involvement of toxic metals, particularly aluminum in renal bone disease. Some geographic areas have high tap water aluminum. The excess may deposit in bone and cause defects in mineralization. A specific stain for aluminum is available. Bone biopsy may reveal predominant osteitis fibrosa cystica, which would confirm the effects of high levels of parathyroid hormone. Another feature of renal bone disease is a mixed skeletal lesion which combines the effects of secondary hyperparathyroidism and osteomalacia. The many factors implicated in the pathogenesis of uremic bone disease are outlined in Table 2. Most of the pathogenetic factors are active in advanced renal failure (Phase III). The clinical features of renal osteodystrophy are shown in Table 3. Renal bone disease causes bone pain, particularly around the knees, ankles and tibia; advanced renal bone disease may produce spontaneous fractures of ribs and vertebrae. In Vitamin D deficient patients, a proximal myopathy may complicate osteomalacia. Pruritis, common in advanced renal failure, may be due to high ionized plasma calcium, and is associated with hyperparathyroidism. In children, the growth retardation and delayed epiphyseal ossification results from Vitamin D resistance and other as yet unidentified factors. In advance bone disease, fractures of the axial skeleton including ribs, vertebrae, hips and long bones are common. Patients may develop loss of height from vertebral body collapse and scoliosis. Aluminum may prevent osteoid mineralization in Vitamin D resistant adults. Occasionally, periarthritis occurs. Synovial fluid aspiration does not reveal uric acid or pyrophosphate crystals characteristic of gout and pseudogout respectively. The syndrome is due to hyperparathyroidism and responds to parathyroidectomy. On rare occasions, calcium deposits around joints of elbows, hands and shoulders particularly (x-ray diffraction reveals hydroxy apatite crystals). These cases respond to antiinflammatory agents, as well as parathyroidectomy. A feature of advanced hyperparathyroidism is the dissolution of the terminal phalanges through bone resorption with the for-

Table 16-2 Factors in the Pathogenesis
of Uremic Bone Disease

Altered Conversion of Vitamin D to Active
  Metabolites
Hyperparathyroidism
Calcium Deficiency
Prolonged Acidosis with Bone Buffering of H^+
Aluminum Deposition from Oral Phosphate Binders
Other Factors Decreasing Collagen Synthesis of
  Bone Formation
Fluoride Toxicity
Heparin
Trace Metal Derangements; zinc; strontium

Table 16-3 Clinical Features
of Renal Bone Disease

Bone Pain
Fractures
Pseudo Gout
Calcification in Extraosseous tissue
  (joints, eye, skin)
Proximal Myopathy
Pseudo Clubbing and Other Skeletal
  Deformities
Pruritus
Aluminum Deposition
Associated With Dialysis Dementia,
  Abnormal EEG

mation of "pseudo clubbing." In very severe hyperparathyroidism, "calciphylaxis" occurs due to advanced vascular calcification with gangrene of the terminal phalanges. Calciphylaxis is treated aggressively with subtotal parathyroidectomy.

In view of the above, the recommended measures for prevention of renal bone disease are as follows: dietary calcium should approximate 1 g/day and the calcium-phosphorus product should be maintained around 40–50. Since a higher calcium-phosphorus product is associated with vascular calcification and pruritis, the aim is to keep the product well below 50. Serum calcium is maintained around 9 mg/dl–10 mg/dl, although many physicians try to achieve a higher serum calcium, around 11 mg/dl. Serum phosphate within tight limits is achieved with aluminum hydroxide gels. Oral intake during any meal will adsorb phosphate from mixed foods. The dose of aluminum hydroxide is titrated against the serum phosphate. Magnesium hydroxide gels are used less frequently in order to avoid magnesium accumulation. Hypermagnesemia with increased skeletal magnesium is associated with abnormal bone mineralization. Although the exact role of magnesium in renal bone disease is unclear, persistent hypermagnesemia is undesirable. It is as yet unclear whether 1,25 dihydroxy Vitamin D_3 is the optimal agent for mineralization of bone, since Vitamin D_3 and 1, alphahydroxy D_3 may also promote calcium absorption and mineralization of bone. There are distinct differences between these sterol compounds. 1,25 dihydroxy D_3 and 1 alpha dihydroxy D_3 causes hypercalcemia, as does Vitamin D_3 itself. However, in the former the

hypercalcemia falls rapidly on cessation of the drugs, whereas in the latter the prolonged half life of D_3 produces prolonged hypercalcemia. Parathyroidectomy for secondary hyperparathyroidism or persistent hypercalcemia developing in the face of secondary hyperparathyroidism (formerly termed "tertiary hyperparathyroidism") may be necessary in patients who do not respond to the Vitamin D sterols, or in whom Vitamin D sterols produce complications. Because total removal of parathyroid glands may contribute to osteomalacia, subtotal parathyroidectomy with preservation of the parathyroid tissue in liquid nitrogen (for subsequent implantation should this be necessary) is recommended. Following parathyroidectomy, it is often necessary to infuse enormous quantities of calcium as excessive bone resorption along with improved mineralization, may result in the "hungry bone syndrome." Parathyroidectomy is most often required in Phase III treatment of chronic uremia.

Angioaccess

During the observation of a patient with slowly declining renal function, a time is reached when vascular access for subsequent hemodialysis should be created. The Cimino-Brescia fistula introduced in the 1960's has been the preferred method of angioaccess for hemodialysis. Since it requires 4–6 weeks of "maturity" for arterialization of the venous portion of the forearm fistula, the experienced nephrologist will anticipate this well in advance of the institution of hemodialysis. When presented with

ESRD where the GFR is less than 5 ml/min, other rapid but temporary access methods are available, i.e., the Scribner shunt, subclavian venous lines, and femoral venous lines. Arteriovenous fistula formation, although often attempted, may be unsuccessful in the diabetic patient with chronic renal disease, the elderly, female or failed vascular access patient. In this case, placement of a synthetic graft in the form of dacron, Goretex, polytetrafluroethylene vessels between artery and vein in the subcutaneous tissue of the forearm or upper arm may be preferrable.

Management of Phase III of Chronic Renal Failure

At this stage it is equally important to exclude reversible renal factors, introduce dietary protein restriction and control phosphate. Vitamin D analogues are also continued through Phase III chronic renal failure. The principal therapeutic intervention is substitution therapy in the form of dialysis and transplantation. The major diseases leading to ESRD requiring dialysis and transplantation varies throughout the world. In the western world, the major causes are glomerulonephritis, hypertension, diabetes mellitus, polycystic kidneys, chronic pyelonephritis, interstitial renal disease etc. By the late 1980's in the United States, however, it is expected that almost 1/4 of all patients receiving dialysis will have Type I diabetes mellitus. This trend in demographics has not yet been seen in the United Kingdom or in Europe, although the portion of diabetic patients being hemodialyzed or transplanted has increased remarkably in the last ten years. The number of patients on dialysis world-wide is approximately 200,000;

70,000 patients receive dialysis in the United States, 40,000 patients with functioning transplants are also being maintained in the United States.

The options for ESRD patients requiring substitution therapy are depicted in Figure 1. This algorithm shows that a life plan should be developed, and that all options be left open depending on the patient's medical status. While transplantation is generally restricted to patients under 55 years old, there is no age limitation to dialysis.

DIALYTIC THERAPIES

The term "dialysis" was coined by Thomas Graham in the 1950's to signify transfer of a solute across the semipermeable membrane. Graham predicted that dialysis would be utilized in the treatment of disease. Graham, however, was unable to predict the magnitude of, or the impact of his observations. The history of dialysis consists of a series of small technological advances to reach its present stage. At present, hemodialysis entails the passage of anticoagulated (heparin or citrate) blood, obtained via vascular access, through synthetic membranes in the form of flat plates, hollow fibers, or coil dialyzers. On the side of the membrane opposite the blood is dialysate (rinsing fluid) containing sodium, magnesium, calcium, glucose, chloride, acetate, and/or bicarbonate. The latter two compounds serve to buffer any hydrogen ion excess.

The major uremic toxins are not included in the dialysate, so that a concentration gradient for their removal is achieved. The major uremic toxins are shown in Table 4. The clinically important uremic toxins are urea, creatinine, uric acid, phosphate, hydrogen ion as well as so-

Options for the ESRD Patient*

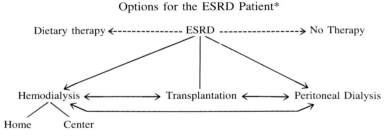

*At any point patient or family may wish to discontinue therapy.

Fig. 16-1.   Options for the ESRD Patient

Table 16-4   Major Uremic Toxins

Urea	Indican (Indoles)	Myoinositol
Cyanate, Ammonium,	Hippuric Acid	Oxalic Acid
Carbonate	Phenols (And Conjugates)	Water
'Organic Base'	Organic Acid	Acid/Base
Creatinine	Aliphatic Amines	Phosphate
Creatine	Dimethylamine	Hormones
Guanidinosuccinic Acid	Trimethylamine	Growth Hormone
Guanidinoacetic Acid	Pseudouridine	Renin
Methylguanidine	Acetoin	Glucagon
Guanidinopropionic Acid	2:3 Butylene Glycol	Natriuretic
Glycocyamine	Sulfates	Parathormone
Guanidinobutyric Acid	β-Hydroxybutyrate	Minerals
Taurocyamine	4 Amino 5 Imidazole	Ca
N-Acetylarginine	Carboxamide	Mg
Uric Acid	N-Methyl 2 Pyridoxine 5	As
Amino Acids	Carboxamide	
Polypeptides	3 a Hydroxy Androst	
Middle Molecules	5-EN-17 one	
Polyamines	Glucuronic Acid	

Winchester JF: Hemoperfusion in Uremia in SORBENTS AND THEIR CLINICAL APPLICATION. Ed Giordano C, New York: Academic Press, 1980, pp 387–397.

dium, potassium and water. Since volume expansion exists because of sodium retention in ESRD, as well as reduction by loss of urine volume, water and sodium removal is a necessary part of dialytic management.

The semipermeable membranes for hemodialysis originally were made of semisynthetic cellophone, then cuprophane and regenerated cellulose acetate and lately membranes composed of polyacrylonitrile and polysulfone. Each of these membranes exhibit different degrees of biocompatibility. During a single 5-hr dialysis, usually performed three times a week on alternate days in the outpatient setting or at home, serum urea nitrogen, creatinine and phosphate will be reduced by approximately 40–50 percent. Ultrafiltration through the membranes, achieved by negative or positive pressure on the blood compartment, removes between two and four liters of water per session. It can be appreciated that fluctuation in serum chemistries is experienced with intermittent hemodialysis. Accordingly, patients may experience shifts in osmolality, serum sodium, and fluid balance. Such shifts may produce hypotension and other symptomatic features, i.e., unphysiological responses to dialysate.

Unphysiological responses to dialysis are more common in the elderly by virtue of their impaired cardiovascular reflexes, in the diabetic and in other severely debilitated patients. However, most patients with experienced personnel or aides at home or in the outpatient setting undergo smooth dialysis. Many precautions are taken to insure the safety of standard hemodialysis. Monitors maintain safety standards for the following: temperature, dialysate conductivity (measure of dialysate sodium), air embolism, venous pressure and dialysate pressure.

Long dwell peritoneal dialysis (continuous ambulatory peritoneal dialysis (CAPD), and continuous cycling peritoneal dialysis (CCPD), utilize the natural peritoneal membrane for solute transfer. Intermittent peritoneal dialysis uses hourly cycling of peritoneal dialysate into and out of the peritoneal cavity. CAPD consists of 4 exchanges daily of 2–3 L of peritoneal dialysate, in adults (less in children). A "dwell" time in the peritoneal cavity of approximately 6 hrs during the day and longer overnight is used. CCPD is a mirror image of CAPD, utilizing a long dwell time during the daytime hours, and machine controlled instillation and removal of peritoneal dialysate every 2.5 hrs during sleep.

Both techniques are employed daily, in contrast to intermittent peritoneal dialysis where a total treatment of 40 hrs/wk is divided into two or three sessions. CAPD has grown rapidly since its introduction in the late 1970's and at the time of writing, 17,000 patients are receiving long dwell peritoneal dialysis throughout the world. Approximately half of these patients reside in the United States. By virtue of the peritoneal membrane characteristics, solute transfer is less efficient than with hemodialysis. However, the total quantity of solute removed often exceeds that with hemodialysis for certain molecules because of longer dwell time, with larger molecules termed "middle molecules" being more efficiently removed with CAPD than intermittent hemodialysis. Table 5 shows the weekly clearance rates for the various forms of dialysis.

An advantage of long dwell peritoneal dialysis is achievement of relatively stable serum chemistries and abolition of the large fluid and electrolyte shifts occurring with hemodialysis. In addition, systemic hypertension is more easily controlled in these patients, compared to hemodialysis because of constant fluid removal. Other advantages include improved nutrition and a rise in hematocrit. On the other hand, there are serious disadvantages of peritoneal dialysis. The major complication is peritonitis which develops in more than one-half of patients within the first year. Peritonitis accounts for approximately 27% of all "dropouts" from CAPD programs and is responsible for frequent hospitalizations. While efficiency for solute removal through the peritoneal membrane does not appear to diminish with time, there are isolated reports of membrane failure due to thickening of its mesothelial surface. Obstructive sclerosing peritonitis has been reported now in 15 patients worldwide. The etiology of peritoneal membrane thickening is uncertain. It does not seem to relate to frequency of peritonitis, and current evidence favors either the type of dialysate involved, possibly plastic particles contained within the dialysate, or perhaps the drugs employed e.g., beta blockers.

Two therapies used infrequently in the United States for Stage III ESRD patients are hemofiltration and sorbent hemoperfusion. Hemofiltration uses an artificial membrane which allows equal transfer of solutes up to a molecular weight cut off of 40,000 to 50,000 daltons. To remove all molecules equally, large quantities of dilute plasma are filtered through the membrane, and the filtrate substituted with sterile intravenous fluid. Large volumes of sterile fluid are required for replacement, the technique is more expensive than hemodialysis, more cumbersome than hemodialysis, and has not seen widespread clinical use in the United States. By virtue of lesser sodium flux than hemodialysis, hemofiltration is associated with less hypotension and cramps and may also be associated with less systemic hypertension during long term therapy. Sorbent hemoperfusion uses the adsorptive capacity of activated charcoal for removing uremic toxins, in some respects, more efficiently than with hemodialysis. Interestingly, urea, water, electrolytes, sulfates and phosphates are not efficiently removed. Accordingly, hemoperfusion needs to be combined with dialysis for their removal. Again, the expense mitigates against the widespread use of hemoperfusion. Sorbent hemoperfusion combined with hemodialysis, however, has reduced dialysis time, stabilized the patient, and perhaps is associated with reduced frequency of severe peripheral neuropathy, pericarditis, and feelings of being ill.

Both hemoperfusion and hemofiltration with various modifications may find widespread use in the future. Sorbents in the form of activated charcoal along with urease zirconium phosphate and hydrated zirconium oxide in a cannister are

Table 16-5

	Weekly Solute Clearance Rates		(L/wk)		
	HD (15 hrs/wk)	CAPD (196 hrs/wk)	CCPD (196 hrs/wk)	IPD (40 hrs/wk)	Normal Kidneys (196 hrs/wk)
Urea	135	76	67	60	604
Creatinine	90	58	58	28	1008
Vitamin B_{12}	30	50	45	16	1008

used widely for the regeneration of dialysate to reduce the total volume of dialysate in a single hemodialysis session. Urea is split by urease into ammonium which is absorbed on activated charcoal. Zirconium phosphate exchanges ammonium, calcium, magnesium and potassium for hydrogen and sodium ions. Hydrated zirconium oxide also exchanges phosphate for acetate. Activated carbon will adsorb creatinine, uric acid, phosphate and other organic compounds. Regeneration of dialysis fluid is a convenient form of reducing dialysate volume; thus, it increases the portability of such dialysis equipment and reduces the need for expensive plumbing in the home dialysis setting.

Alternatives to all forms of dialysis include oral sorbents (activated charcoal, oxidized starch, and oxidized cellulose), locust bean gum, and liquid membrane capsules, all of which have been used clinically or experimentally to treat uremia. The results of these treatments are far below acceptable standards for maintenance of ESRD patients, and have not yet found widespread clinical use. Diarrhea therapy was another alternative to dialysis, initially tried in Taipei, (Taiwan). It is employed thrice weekly for three hours per session. The uremic patient swallows 7 L of solution at the rate of 200 ml every five minutes to be followed by diarrhea. These solutions contain various electrolytes along with mannitol and produce substantial creatinine and urea clearances. This low cost diarrheal treatment was initially used in patients who had modest residual renal function. The trials in 17 patients lasted approximately seven months. The major problem was achievement of stable fluid blance; and at the time of writing, only one patient is currently receiving such treatment. Diarrhea therapy may find some use in countries with limited financial resources for managing a large ESRD population.

SURVIVAL WITH DIALYSIS

As might be expected, age and other medical conditions complicating renal failure significantly influence survival in patients undergoing substitution therapy. In Europe and in the United States many patients are still alive after 10 years of hemodialysis. All studies show that a greater survival occurs in the home hemodialysis patient. In contrast to the center dialysis patients, home patients are selected because of improved medical status, compliance,

etc. The majority of deaths in ESRD are due to cardiovascular complications—myocardial infarction and cerebrovascular accidents. The second commonest cause is sepsis, most likely introduced via arteriovenous needles. Another factor contributing to the frequency of sepsis, is that ESRD patients are immunocompromised. Mortality rates do not appear to differ significantly between hemodialysis and CAPD when age corrections are made, but "dropout" from the CAPD is a significant problem. This is predominantly related to peritonitis.

COMPLICATIONS ASSOCIATED WITH UREMIA AND ESRD THERAPIES

At best, dialytic techniques achieve a state of mild chronic uremia; and the complications of uremia progress. In addition, complications do arise from dialytic techniques and contribute to both morbidity and mortality. The complications of uremia and its therapy are outlined in Table 6.

QUALITY OF LIFE AND REHABILITATION

The therapy of ESRD is a palliative one and does not entirely substitute for all natural renal functions. However, dialysis has resulted in a substantial savings of life, a substantial increase in return to work, and even full rehabilitation. Unfortunately, rehabilitation does not reach its full potential in most patients, because of many factors, including continued illness, blindness (particularly in the diabetic), psychiatric problems, social factors, compliance, etc.

SELECTION OF PATIENTS FOR ESRD SUBSTITUTION THERAPIES

The number of patients treated in any one country is related to the gross national product. By choice, third world countries do not have large numbers of dialysis facilities, since they are faced with even greater social problems—malnutrition, infectious disease, etc. Accordingly, ESRD therapy in some countries is limited, and selection criteria are employed to choose patients for

Table 16-6 Complications of Uremia and Its Therapy*

System involved	Complications of uremia persisting with dialysis therapy	Complications of dialysis therapy
Cardiovascular	Refractory hypertension; pericarditis; accelerated atherosclerosis	Accelerated atherosclerosis
Dermatological	Pruritis; pigmentation	
Endocrine	Lipid abnormalities; carbohydrate disturbances; protein malnutrition; renal osteodystrophy; thyroid functional abnormalities; infertility; sexual dysfunction	Psychosexual disturbances
Gastrointestinal	Peptic ulceration	Refractory ascites
Hematological	Anemia; platelet dysfunction; leucocyte dysfunction; sepsis; derangements of iron metabolism	Spontaneous hemorrhage; hypersplenism; dialysis-associated blood loss
Immunological	Depressed immune response	? Increased incidence of neoplasia; autoantibody formation; hepatitis; sepsis
Neurological	Peripheral neuropathy	Dialysis encephalopathy syndrome; psychosocial problems, disequilibrium syndrome
Pharmacological	Derangements of drug metabolism	
Other		Deficiencies of vitamins, amino acids, metals; metal intoxication; lung dysfunction; osmolality changes

*From Winchester, J.F., "Hemoperfusion In Uremia" in Giordano, C., *Sorbents and Their Clinical Applications*. New York: Academic Press, 1980, p. 387.

dialysis or transplantation, criteria include: age, systemic disease, cardiovascular complications, etc. In the United States only patients with severe psychiatric problems, advanced cerebrovascular disease or metastatic carcinoma are excluded. In the United States more often the physician is faced with the moral/ethical decision of discontinuing dialysis, rather than selecting patients for dialysis.

It cannot be overstressed that a program which integrates all forms of therapy for the ESRD patient is the ideal. Patients may choose to begin with home dialysis, but later (if a partner is indisposed or dies) be more suitably dialyzed in an outpatient center or offered transplantation. Such a comprehensive program allows patients to move between all the therapeutic modalities, providing they are medically and psychologically suitable for each therapy. Such

movement encourages and significantly improves patient morale and outlook.

GUIDELINES FOR DRUG USAGE IN RENAL FAILURE

In renal failure, the use of many pharmacological agents becomes a sometimes difficult and delicate task because of impaired renal clearance of the drug. This impairment in renal clearance usually results from decreased urinary excretion; however, in some instances, most notably the clearance of insulin, the kidney actually participates in the metabolism of the drug. In most cases, specific information regarding alterations in drug dosage in renal failure is contained in the manufacturer's product information inserts; however, the following will provide

Table 16-7   Some Important Drugs Requiring Significant Alterations in Renal
Failure

Drug	Removal by Hemodialysis	Removal by Peritoneal Dialysis
Aminoglycosides	yes	yes
Cephalosporins		
General	yes	yes
Cefazolin	yes	no
Digoxin	yes (minimal)	yes (minimal)
Ethambutol	yes	yes
Lincomycin	no	no
Penicillins*		
Ampicillin	yes	no
Amoxicillin	yes	no
Carbenicillin	yes	no
Ticarcillin	yes	yes
Sulfamethoxazole-		
Trimethoprim	yes	yes (?)
Sulfisoxazole	yes	yes
Tetracyclines**	no	no
Vancomycin	no	no

*No alteration for penicillin G, oxacillin or nafcillin.
**No alteration for doxycycline, minocycline and chlortetracycline.

some principles and guidelines for the use and adjustment of drugs in renal failure.

Table 7 provides a partial listing of important drugs which are dependent on renal excretion for clearance, thereby frequently requiring adjustment in patients with renal failure. The range of the adjustment depends on the level of renal failure (i.e., endogenous creatinine clearance) and the frequency of dialysis being given the patient as well as the degree of renal metabolism, toxicity and dialyzability of the drug. In addition, other medications may affect the effective half-life of the drug. It is important, therefore, in evaluating any particular situation that all variables be considered. Nevertheless, the following principles may be helpful in guiding the clinician in the proper use of drugs in renal failure.

Principle I: Monitor blood levels when possible.

Measurement of peak and/or trough blood levels of a particular drug if possible remains the single most effective way to monitor drug administration in renal failure. In general, the therapeutic blood level for a drug in a patient with renal failure is the same as that for a patient without renal failure.

Principle II: The initial ("loading") dose of drug need not be adjusted.

In most cases the initial or "loading" dose of a particular drug is about the same as that which might be given to a patient without renal failure. For example, in using the aminoglycoside Tobramycin, an initial dose of 1 mg/kg can be given in most cases without complications. Subsequent doses, however, depend on many factors such as dialysis schedule, severity of infection, route of administration.

Principal III: Subsequent doses should be altered to reflect prolonged drug half-life.

Although techniques vary, a good guiding principle is that subsequent doses after the initial loading dose are usually the same in patients with renal failure as in patients without renal failure—*except* that the *interval* between doses is appropriately adjusted. This adjustment is the essence of the use of drugs in renal failure, because the appropriate interval requires knowledge of the biological half-life of the drug, the effect of renal failure on the biological half-life, the effect of dialysis on the biological half-life and any other factors affecting the half-life such as protein binding, change in volume of distribution, drug interactions, etc. Thus, drugs whose major route of excretion is via the urinary tract tend to require adjustment in dose interval and the dose interval tends to become greater the more impaired the renal function.

Table 7 lists some drugs requiring significant prolongation of dose interval. Dose interval changes may be as little as a 2-fold increase for drugs such as cephalexin and ampicillin to the administration of vancomycin once every 10 to 14 days.

Principle IV: Drugs excreted by the kidneys tend to be removed by dialysis and require replacement post dialysis.

Drugs which are predominantly excreted in the urinary tract tend to be drugs which are removed by dialysis. Thus, as a guideline, dialysis results in considerable lowering of blood levels, and it is frequently necessary to repeat the loading dose post dialysis to maintain adequate blood levels. Conversely, drugs which tend to be more highly protein bound tend to be less reliant upon urinary excretion. These drugs tend to be less significantly or not affected by dialysis.

Principle V: Do not guess.

When in doubt, check an appropriate source for the proper use of drugs in renal failure.

SELECTED READINGS

Anderson, RJ Drug Prescribing for Patients in Renal Failure. Hosp Prac 18(2)145–160, 1983.

Avram, MM (Ed) Prevention of kidney disease and long-term survival. Plenum Publishing Corp, 1982

Kurtzman, NA Chronic renal failure: metabolism and clinical consequences. Hosp Prac 17(8):107–122, 1982

Lazarus, JM Dialytic Therapy: principles and clinical guidelines. Hosp Prac 17(10):111–133, 1982

Maher, JF Dialysis, hemofiltration and hemoperfusion, in: Contemporary Nephrology, Vol 2 (Eds Klahr, S, Massry, SG) Plenum Publishing Corp. 1983, pp 649–698, 1983

Walser, M Nutritional support in renal failure: Lancet 1: 340–342, 1983

Michael C. Gelfand, MD
James F. Winchester, MD
Antonia C. Novello, MD

17

Renal Transplantation and Rejection

Renal transplantation is the surgical replacement of functioning renal tissue from a human cadaver or living related donor into a recipient. The transplanted kidney is the *renal allograft,* or in short, the *graft*. Since the graft is a foreign body, the immune system may fail to accept the transplant. This is *rejection,* and attempts to clinically reduce the rejection process are called *immunosuppression*. A graft may be obtained from a living donor (in the case of duplicated organs such as the kidney) or from a recently deceased individual (mandatory for essential organs such as the heart, lungs, pancreas, or liver). Grafts from the former are called *living donor grafts;* and from the latter, *cadaveric donor grafts*.

Four types of grafts are identified according to the relationship of donor to recipient. An *autograft* is a graft taken from and transplanted into the same individual, e.g., skin transplanted from the thigh to the chest in a patient with severe burns. This is of no clinical importance in renal transplantation. Autografts are not rejected, since they derive from the recipient. A graft from an identical twin is called an *isograft*. This type of graft is also not rejected, since it is antigenically identical to the recipient. The vast majority of grafts are *allografts,* an exchange between individuals of the same species having different tissue antigens. With the exception of the identical twin transplant, all human-to-human organ grafts are allogeneic grafts. The *xenograft* is not used often in clinical organ

transplantation. In this case, different species are involved, e.g., a baboon liver transplanted into a human with liver failure. Xenografts are generally rejected rapidly.

RENAL TRANSPLANTATION IN ADULTS

Cell surface proteins that give organs their recognizable antigenicity and evoke rejection are referred to as histocompatibility antigens. In various species, similar antigens have been identified on the nucleated cell surfaces of transplanted tissue. These glycoprotein molecules induce rejection and appear to be inherited in a systematic fashion, bearing a relationship to parental antigens.

Histocompatibility Complex

The strip or chromosomes that codes histocompatibility antigens in man is known as the histocompatibility or HLA complex. Mice and rats have analogous systems, H-2 and AGB respectively, which have provided much of our understanding of the human HLA complex. In these systems, genes code for production of cell surface antigens, recognized by recipients as self or foreign. On each of two chromosomes there are at least four known loci, containing a series of codominant allelic forms. In man, more than 51 antigens have been recognized in the HLA system; there are Type I or antigens of the HLA-A, B and C loci and Type II or antigens of the DR locus. Individuals inherit one chromosome from each parent, e.g., one allele for four loci from the mother and father. While a parent shares exactly half of his/her antigens with an offspring, siblings may share all, some, or none of these antigens, depending on the inherited genetic makeup. Importantly, gene product antigens of the various loci stimulate recognition by different limbs of the immune response. Type I or the A, B and C loci antigens stimulate recognition by the humoral immune system, whereas the D/DR locus appears to stimulate recognition by thymus-derived (T-) lymphocytes participating in a mixed lymphocyte reaction. Accordingly, sensitization against antigens of the A, B or C loci induces circulating antibodies against specific antigens of these loci. Indeed, this is the basis of the technique by which individuals are screened for renal transplant acceptance. If the recipient has antibodies against the antigens of the donor kidney *before* the transplant, it will usually be rejected. This is referred to as a positive pre-transplant cross match.

Renal Transplantation

The successful renal transplant provides the most effective rehabilitative therapy for patients with end-stage renal disease; for it provides not only excretory function but a number of metabolic functions, such as vitamin D metabolism and erythropoietin production. Hemodialysis or peritoneal dialysis is a satisfactory substitute for excretory function, but metabolic functions are not adequately replaced. A dramatic example of this is transplantation of a normal kidney into a patient with Fabry's disease. In Fabry's disease, renal failure results from renal deposition of a glycolipid due to absence of a galactosidase. After renal transplantation, enzyme levels rise as high as 10 percent or more, suggesting that transplantation has caused partial reversal of the underlying enzyme deficiency.

Over 85,000 renal transplants have been performed, providing the majority of current clinical experience in organ transplantation. This experience emphasizes the importance of careful management of the transplant recipient with avoidance of excessive immunosuppressive therapy.

Relatively recent developments have resulted in a dramatic improvement in renal allograft survival: 1) improved matching of tissue antigens of the recipient with those of the donor, especially in the Type II (D/DR) series of antigens; 2) liberalized use of blood transfusions in renal transplant recipients; and 3) development of a new, highly potent immunosuppressive drug, cyclosporine. At most centers, the renal transplant current success rate at two years is about 75 percent for living related donor transplants and 70 percent for cadaveric donor transplants. Living related donor transplantation is generally associated with fewer and more easily reversible complications, allowing for a smoother post-transplantation course. Transplant centers, therefore, frequently prefer to perform living related donor transplantation. Patient survival rates as distinct from graft survival rates, have progressively improved, suggesting improved medical management of the transplant recipient.

Proper attention to good surgical and medical care of the renal transplant recipient is of prime importance in renal post-transplantation follow-up. Two types of complications may occur. First, technical or surgical problems, such as leakage of urine from the implanted ureter, stenosis of the anastomosed renal artery, or the collection of lymph around the kidney, may be evident in a small number of patients. These technical problems can cause graft loss; although prompt surgical intervention is usually corrective.

The second complication is graft loss secondary to return of the original disease. This was first noted in identical twins. Although rejection should have occurred in this situation, a large proportion of recipients of twin renal grafts lost function. Analysis revealed that loss of renal function resulted from return of glomerulonephritis, the original disease. More recently, the list of diseases that recur after renal transplantation has grown to include anti-glomerular basement membrane disease, focal glomerular sclerosis, diabetes and oxalosis (Table 1).

The closer the match between donor and recipient, the more likely the success. This is clearly apparent when graft survival in identical twin donor-recipient pairs is compared to unrelated pairs. Indeed, bone marrow transplantation invariably met with failure until methods

Table 17-1 Diseases Found to Recur After Renal Transplantation

Glomerulonephritis

1. Focal sclerosing glomerulonephritis
2. Membranoproliferative glomerulonephritis
3. Rapidly progressive glomerulonephritis (Anti-GBM-type)
4. Berger's IgANephropathy

Henoch-Schönlein purpura

Polyarteritis Nodosa

Oxalosis, cystinosis, Fabry's disease

Diabetes

Systemic Lupus erythematosus
Hypertensive renal disease

Table 17-2 Some Factors Affecting Organ Transplantation Between Individual Donor-Recipient Pairs

Recipient

1. Immunologic integrity
2. Previous sensitization
3. Presence of other diseases affecting immune response (e.g., uremia)
4. Presence of disease that might affect metabolism of immunosuppressive drug (e.g., liver disease)
5. Presence of systemic condition that might be exacerbated (e.g., diabetes or hypertension)
6. Need for other medication (e.g., allopurinol)
7. Nutritional status
8. Patient compliance

Donor

1. Type of organ being transplanted
2. Degree of match with recipient
3. Pre-treatment of donor
4. If cadaver donor, cause of death

for typing and matching donor bone marrow were developed. General principles of donor-recipient matching are illustrated in Table 2.

Transplantation will not succeed where there is ABO group incompatibility. It can, however, be performed in the presence of incompatibilities of minor blood groups, including, Rh. A positive cross-match, i.e., when the recipient demonstrates circulating antibodies against donor tissue antigens, is also a contraindication. Circulating cytotoxic antibodies are routinely assessed by incubating donor lymphoid cells in recipient serum in the presence of a complement source. After incubation, a marker of cell death (such as trypan blue) is added to the cell suspension, and the proportion of dead cells is counted. A significant number of dead cells indicates a positive cross-match. The first two principles are considered inviolable, whereas the others are relative.

The lack of histocompatibility between recipient and donor is not an absolute contraindication to transplantation; however, every effort is made to obtain the closest possible antigenic match through tissue typing, i.e., identifying antigens of loci A, B, and C and DR of the recipient. This is accomplished by using monospecific antisera obtained from sensitized individuals to perform a series of individual cross-match tests with the recipient's lymphoid cells.

The same is done with cells from potential donors and in the absence of other critical factors, the donor with the closest match is selected. Critical factors elminating a potential donor include ABO incompatibility, recipient antibodies against the donor's cells, medical disability of the donor, and unwillingness to donate an organ.

Living related donors may also be matched to recipients by evaluating D locus compatibility. Compatibility is assessed by mixed lymphocyte culture reactivity (MLC), i.e., the degree to which recipient lymphocytes undergo blast transformation on exposure to donor lymphocytes. To date, the mixed lymphocyte response is evaluated only prospectively in the living donor transplantation situation. The MLC test requires days to perform, which is too much time to determine the recipient's response to cells from a cadaver. In retrospective studies, low response of recipient lymphocytes to cadaveric donor cells relates to better allograft survival. Such laboratory evaluation tests the D-related (DR) locus part of the D/DR locus. This latter antigen can be identified and matched serologically. Such matching has resulted in significant improvement in the success of renal transplantation.

PATHOPHYSIOLOGY OF REJECTION

Rejection is the process by which the host immune system recognizes, becomes sensitized against, and attempts to eliminate the antigenic differences of the donor organ. With the exception of autografts and isografts, some rejection occurs with every transplant. At present, the role of immuno-suppression is to control the host's natural response in order to prevent graft rejection.

The prototype of immunobiological rejection is *primary (first-set) rejection.* In this form of rejection, the host encounters, for the first time, the histocompatibility antigens on the surface of the transplanted cells. In some as yet poorly understood manner, macrophages process antigenic material, locally or within regional lymph nodes, and present it to B- and T-lymphocytes for sensitization. Sensitized lymphocytes then enter the peripheral circulation directly or proceed via lymphatics to the thoracic duct prior to entering the peripheral circulation. After encountering the specific antigens of the graft, sensitized lymphoid cells initiate immune injury. Immune injury may be mediated by either the humoral or cellular limb of the immune response in a variety of ways: (1) directly, by cytotoxic T-cells (K-cells); (2) indirectly, by soluble T-cell mediators of immune injury (lymphokines); (3) by B cell-mediated (humoral) antibody; or (4) by antibody-dependent cellular cytotoxicity (ADCC) attack on the target organ. Primary rejection can become clinically evident one week post transplantation.

Another type of rejection is *hyperacute rejection,* where the recipient has been sensitized to the histocompatibility antigens of the graft by previous transfusions, pregnancy, or transplantation. Circulating cytotoxic antibodies to the HLA antigens of the graft may be found in the serum of recipients. After vascular anastomosis, prompt deposition of antibody occurs along vascular endothelium with activation of the complement and coagulation systems, resulting in fibrin deposition, polymorphonuclear leukocyte infiltration, platelet thrombosis, and prompt coagulative necrosis. Invariably, loss of graft follows.

Acute rejection is associated with abrupt signs and symptoms of rejection. The graft is tender, and heavily infiltrated with mononuclear and inflammatory cells. Nevertheless, this type of rejection may resolve following immuno-suppression therapy.

Chronic rejection, which occurs after an extended period, is characterized by gradual loss of graft function. On histopathological examination, the chronically rejected organ is infiltrated with large numbers of mononuclear cells, predominantly T-cells, although B-cells may also be involved. This type of rejection is indolent and often unresponsive to immunosuppresive therapy.

DIFFERENTIAL DIAGNOSIS OF RENAL FAILURE

The differential diagnosis of renal transplant failure is shown in a temporal fashion in Table 3.

Acute tubular necrosis (ATN). The graft may be impaired due to ATN resulting from any of the multiple etiologies (See Chapter 5), including hypotension, sepsis, drug reaction, etc. In addition to the usual causes of ATN, the graft may develop ATN after sustained and prolonged periods of non-perfusion during handling of the kidney prior to transplantation. To avoid ATN, every effort is made to minimize the warm ischemia time (the time needed to remove the kidney from the deceased cadaver) and the cold ischemia time (the time required to perform the transplant after removal).

Rejection. (see above)

Infection. Frequently, it is difficult to distinguish renal infection from rejection in the presence of impaired function. The diagnosis is established by careful urinalysis and culture of urine. Distinction may also be made on the basis of cell types found in the urine. Rejection is associated with predominant T lymphocyturia, infection with B lymphocyturia.

Surgical complications. A wide variety of surgical complications can occur postoperatively. These include, among others, obstruction usually by stenosis or kinking of renal artery or vein, ureteral obstruction, disruption of the ureteral anastomosis, and appearance of lymphoceles.

Table 17-3 Differential Diagnosis
of Renal Transplant Failure

1–5 Days Post-Transplantation

1. Technical Problem
2. Hyperacute or Accelerated Rejection
3. Acute Tubular Necrosis

5 Days to Weeks Post Transplantation

1. Acute/Chronic Rejection
2. Infection
3. Vascular Occlusion
4. Urinary Leak

Weeks to Years Post Transplantation

1. Chronic Rejection
2. Return of Original Renal Disease
3. De Novo Renal Disease

Table 17-4 Symptoms and Signs
of Rejection

Symptoms

Fever
Malaise
Graft tenderness

Signs

General

Hypertension	OKT4/OKT8 ratios
Leukocytosis	Spontaneous
	blastogenesis
Hypocomplementemia	B-2
	microglobulinemia
Elevated	C reactive protein
sedimentation rate	

Renal Specific Signs

Rising BUN	Thromboxanuria
Rising creatinine	Immunoglobulinuria
Lymphocyturia	Cytotoxic antibody
Hematuria	
Proteinuria	
Oliguria	

De novo renal disease. The renal transplant is not totally invulnerable to *de novo* renal diseases, such as post streptococcal GN, diabetes mellitus, hypertensive nephrosclerosis, and urolithiasis.

Return of original renal disease. The transplant may develop the original disease such focal sclerosing GN, Berger's IGA-nephropathy, Goodpasture's anti-GBM disease, or diabetes, and metabolic disorders, such as oxalosis, cystinosis, and Fabry's disease (Table 1).

Renal artery and renal vein thrombosis. These complications are catastrophic in the transplant situation, since the patient has only one kidney.

DIAGNOSIS OF REJECTION

The clinical diagnosis and treatment of allograft rejection are extremely challenging for immunologists, since there is neither a precise method to diagnose nor any universally accepted "correct" treatment. This, no doubt, relates to the fact that no recipient, donor, or recipient-donor pair are identical, except for identical twins. For example, the health of one recipient or the type of organ being transplanted may differ.

Nevertheless, a number of clinically helpful symptoms and signs of rejection have been identified (see Table 4). Fever, myalgias, and localized graft tenderness are frequently observed symptoms; hypertension, leukocytosis, and hypocomplementemia are useful biochemical signs to diagnose graft rejection. It has also been suggested that transplant rejection may be determined by the relative proportion of helper/inducer, (OKT4+) T cells in the blood relative to the proportion of suppressor (OKT8+) lymphocytes. Generally, but not invariably, rejection is associated with increased levels of OKT4+ T cells.

TREATMENT OF REJECTION

The treatment of rejection varies considerably depending on the type of transplant and the institution; however, there are a number of generally applicable principles of immunosuppression as shown in Table 5. The goal of immunosuppression is to prevent or minimize sensitization, because once sensitization occurs, suppression of the immune response becomes

Table 17-5 Principles of
Immunosuppression

1. Use highest dose of treatment during early post-transplantation period to prevent sensitization

2. Combination drug regimens are often more effective than a single-drug regimen

3. Taper immunosuppression when possible

4. If effective, low-dose or alternate-day regimens are associated with reduced side-effects

5. Treat rejection promptly and aggressively

6. In severe infection or leukopenia, immunosuppression may have to be greatly reduced or stopped to prevent patient death

7. Do not overtreat

considerably more difficult. For this purpose, the recipient receives the largest dose of immunosuppression just prior to or during the first week after transplantation, the period during which primary sensitization occurs. When the recipient has been presensitized, prompt graft rejection (hyperacute or accelerated) will ensue, usually defying the most strenuous attempts at immunosuppression. If no early rejection occurs, drugs used for immunosuppression are gradually reduced over succeeding days and weeks until a stable maintenance dose is achieved.

In the event of an acute rejection, the dose of immunosuppressive agents may be increased or different drugs may be added to the regimen until the rejection is brought under control, or the graft is lost.

Drug Therapy

The drugs used for immunosuppression fall into three general categories: anti-inflammatory agents, antimetabolites, and cytotoxic agents. Table 6 lists the commonly used immunosuppressive agents and their mechanisms of action.

ANTI-INFLAMMATORY AGENTS

The major anti-inflammatory and perhaps the major agents used for immunosuppression are adrenocortical steroids, e.g., prednisone, prednisolone, and methylprednisolone. These agents provide broad, nonspecific, anti-inflammatory action by stabilizing lysosome membranes. In addition, steroids have a variety of

Table 17-6 Immunosuppressive Agents Used in Organ Transplantation

I. Anti-inflammatory
   Adrenocortical steroids: Prednisone,
   prednisolone, methylprednisolone
	Stabilizes lysozomes, impairs antigen
	   recognition and processing
	Lymphocytolysis, impairs antibody
	   synthesis

II. Antimetabolites
   Azathioprine, 6-mercaptopurine
	Impairs nuceic acid synthesis in pyrimidine
	   ribonucleotides

III. Cytotoxic
   Alkylating agents
   Cyclophosphamide, chlorambucil
	Causes inter- and intrastrand DNA cross-
	   linkage with alteration of DNA helix

X-irradiation	Karyorrexis, destruction of DNA helix
Antilymphocyte globulin	Immune cytolysis

IV. Cyclosporine	Not clearly defined; may stimulate
	   suppressor T cell activity or reduce
	   helper cell activity

V. Other—Thoracic Duct Drainage Plasmaleukapheresis	Sensitized T cell removal Immunoglobulin removal Immune-Complex removal

other functions that suppress the immune response, including prevention of antigen recognition and suppression of the effector limb of lymphocyte function.

ANTIMETABOLITES

A number of agents with antimetabolic properties have been used in immunosuppression. The purine antagonist, azathioprine, and its active metabolite, 6-mercaptopurine, competitively inhibit effective purine nucleotide synthesis, thereby causing faulty RNA synthesis. The alkylating agents, cyclophosphamide and chlorambucil, also have antimetabolic effects, since these agents induce breaks in the cross-linkage of the DNA helix with faulty relinkage and subsequent cell death.

CYTOTOXIC AGENTS

This large category includes a variety of agents. X-irradiation, whether total-body, local to the graft, or delivered extracorporeally to cells of the bloodstream, has cytolytic properties especially on rapidly reproducing cellular elements, such as lymphoid cells undergoing sensitization. In addition, X-irradiation has antilymphocyte properties especially on rapidly reproducing cellular elements, such as lymphoid cells undergoing sensitization. Antilymphocyte serum (ALS) or globulin (ALG), antibodies produced in animals (usually the horse) against human lymphocytes, are helpful in suppressing the immune response by destroying or inactivating circulating lymphocytes. Steroids, azathioprine, the alkylating agents, and certain antibiotics such as actinomycin-D also possess cytotoxic capabilities. The steroids are predominantly effective in ablating recirculating lymphocytes. The alkylating agent cyclophosphamide is effective against both T- and B-lymphocytes. Azathioprine predominantly affects T-lymphocytes, and actinomycin-D is cytotoxic for a variety of dividing cells.

CYCLOSPORINE

A relatively new agent which has just been approved for release by the U.S. FDA, is cyclosporine. This agent appears to be one of the most powerful immunodepressive drugs yet discovered. Its mechanism of action is not definitively proven, but cyclosporine may either inhibit helper T cells or potentiate suppressor T cells. Unfortunately, the development of lym-

phomas and toxic renal failure have been described in renal transplant recipients treated with cyclosporine.

Thoracic Duct Drainage (TDD) and Plasmaleukopheresis

These techniques remove circulating sensitized T cells and may thus be helpful in controlling the immune reaction to a particular graft. TDD achieves this goal by directly draining the thoracic duct, while plasmaleukapheresis uses extracorporeal removal of immunoglobulins and lymphocytes from the peripheral blood.

Immunosuppressive Treatment Regimens

Most treatment regimens include a combination of immunosuppressive agents that provide a multifocal attack on the immune response. For example, many regimens include a corticosteroid to prevent sensitization, ablate lymphocytes, impair antibody synthesis, and suppress inflammation plus an antimetabolite to inhibit the transmission of the message of antigen sensitization and to provide additional lymphocytolysis. An alkylating agent, cyclophosphamide, may be added for its additional cytotoxic properties, especially against B-lymphocytes. X-irradiation or antilymphocyte serum may be included to enhance cytotoxicity. During rejection, boluses of intravenous corticosteroids are frequently added to the standard regimen, with tapering upon successful reversal of rejection. An alternative to bolus steroids is antithymocyte globulin (ATG). Steroid resistant rejection may respond to ATG or plasmaleukopheresis.

Consequences of Immune Response Suppression

Immunosuppressive therapy provides one of the rare opportunities in clinical medicine of being too successful. Since most immunosuppressive regimens are non-specific assaults on immune responsiveness, successful efforts to prevent normal graft rejection are invariably accompanied by depression of host immune defenses. Fortunately, in most instances, alterations in immunocompetence do not result in major complications. For example, delayed hypersensitivity to an intradermal antigen such as PPD may disappear during immunosuppressive therapy. While this is a rather trivial consequence, the reactivation or acquisition of tuberculosis during therapy is a more significant complication.

The three major complications of immunosuppression include: (1) increased susceptibility to infection; (2) development of neoplasms; and (3) graft-versus-host disease (Table 7). Infection represents the most important category and occurs secondary to common and uncommon agents. When approaching the diagnosis of infection in the immunosuppressed host, it is appropriate to consider the more common organisms first. Pneumonia is still more likely to be caused by pneumococcus, and urinary tract infection by Escherichia coli. Nevertheless, the immunosuppressed individual has a considerably increased risk of developing pneumonia from Pneumonocystis carinii or cytomegalovirus and of having a urinary tract infection caused by Candida.

In most instances, infections in the transplant recipient can be successfully treated routinely. In the event of overwhelming infection or infection caused by an uncommon organism for which treatment may be ineffective (such as

Table 17-7 Consequences
of Immunosuppression

1. Infections
       Common organisms
         Pneumococcus
         Escherichia coli
       Uncommon organisms
         Pneumocystis carinii
         Cytomegalovirus
         Candida

2. Neoplasms
       Lymphomas
       Reticulum cell sarcoma
       Skin and lip carcinomas

3. Graft-versus-host disease
       Dermatitis
       Diarrhea
       Fever
       Failure to thrive
       Death (if severe)

disseminated herpes), it is of utmost importance to restrict or even stop immunosuppressive treatment. This would allow recruitment of host/immune defenses. In addition, one might try antiviral chemotherapy, e.g., ARA-a. In some cases, infections will cause graft loss; however, the ultimate survival of the host must be the primary objective. Frequently, the goals of host survival and graft survival are not easily separated. In renal transplantation, the host may return to hemodialysis in the event of graft failure; however, in cardiac transplantation, it is virtually impossible to save the patient who loses his graft.

The second major complication of immunosuppression is neoplastic transformation. Since the normal immune response provides surveillance against the development of neoplasms, the immunosuppressed host is obviously at higher risk for developing neoplasms. The risk of lymphoma developing in the immunosuppressed transplant recipient is increased 35-fold, with reticulum cell sarcoma occurring at 300 times the expected frequency. During early trials of cyclosporine, there was striking high incidence of lymphomas, thought to be related to excess dosage. Of less serious clinical consequence, but also occurring with considerably increased frequency, are cancers of the skin and lip.

Major side effects attributable to corticosteroids include infection, induction of diabetes mellitus, obesity, cataracts and osteopenia. With regard to the latter, aseptic femoral head necrosis may necessitate operative intervention.

Perhaps the clearest example of excessive host immunosuppression is the development of graft-versus-hosts (GVH) disease. This entity lies at the far end of the spectrum of host-graft symbiosis. It results when the host is so totally immunosuppressed that the donor lymphoid cells transplanted along with the graft are able to become sensitized and mount an unchallenged immune response against the host. The parental cells recognize and mount an immune response against the F_1 host cells, but the neonatal host cells fail to recognize the parental cells as foreign. In experimental transplantation, recipient mice develop a clinical syndrome characterized by failure to thrive, runting, diarrhea, dermatitis, and eventually death. Accordingly, the host is "rejected" by the uninhibited immune assault of donor lymphoid cells in GVH disease. GVH occurs infrequently (or only subclinically) in most instances; however, because the recipient is spontaneously or intentionally severely depleted of immunocompetent cells in bone marrow transplantation, GVH disease is not an uncommon complication.

THE DONOR AND RECIPIENT WORK-UP

Prior to transplantation, the donor and the recipient must undergo evaluation to confirm their medical acceptability to give or receive a renal transplant.

Donor Work-Up

Since the donor is voluntarily agreeing to undergo a major operative procedure resulting in the removal of one half of his/her renal mass, it is imperative that all precautions be taken to assure that no medical or psychological contraindications exist.

The basic donor work-up is outlined in Table 8. As a matter of course, the donor should be interviewed prior to beginning the work-up by both the nephrologist (internist) and the surgeon. Donors who are obviously coerced and are afraid or unwilling should be eliminated during these interviews. A careful history and physical examination should be performed with special emphasis on discovering any significant illnesses that might contraindicate organ donation such as hypertension, renal disease, hematogenously spread tumors, or active infectious diseases. If the donor has been cleared to this

point, the examinations listed in Table 8 may be pursued. These exams are approached from least invasive to the more invasive (the most invasive being the renal arteriogram). If a donor cannot be cleared at one level, he/she should not be tested at the next level, unless such an exam is indicated for the health of the donor.

Recipient Work-Up

The recipient evaluation also begins with an interview with the nephrologist and the transplant surgeon and a frank discussion about renal transplantation. This discussion should cover the pros and cons fairly, recognizing that a physician must develop certain value judgments which he/she is obligated to discuss with an inquiring patient. If the patient desires to proceed, blood groups and tissue typing are performed, and a decision is made with possible living related donors as to the source of the transplant. The recipient receives a work-up designated to assure a functioning lower urinary tract and bladder and the absence of active infections. A routine screening for neoplasm is accomplished depending on age. After the studies listed in Table 9 are completed, the recipient may be activated on the cadaver recipient list or scheduled for a living related donor transplant when the donor has been evaluated.

In some centers, a number of immunological studies are performed on the recipient to develop an immune response "profile." These studies include skin reactivity to DNCB and other skin allergens, immunoglobulin levels, lymphocyte, T and B cell levels, T cell subsets and their

Table 17-8 Donor Evaluations

Level I: Interview to explain renal donation and to determine if donor understands the risk and is willingly volunteering, blood group and tissue typing.

Level II: History and the physical exam to rule out significant illness, excluding illnesses such as active bacterial, viral diseases, hypertension, renal disease, etc.

Level III: Routine laboratory, chest x-ray, EKG, urinanalysis, culture and sensitivity of urine, creatinine clearance X3.

Level IV: IVP

Level V: Bilateral Renal Arteriogram

*The donor has to pass each level before proceeding to the next level.

Table 17-9   Recipient Evaluations

1. Interview with surgeon and nephrologist for a candid discussion of the pros and cons of transplantation.

2. History and physical examination to rule out contraindicatory condition such as infection, diseases or neoplasms, etc.

3. Chest x-ray, voiding cystourethrogram (or cystoscopy).

4. Dental exam, eye exam.

5. Proctosigmoidoscopy if over 45 years of age.

6. Additional test based on history, such as coronary angiography, gall bladder series, etc.

ratios, mitogen responsiveness, mixed lymphocyte reactivity, and other tests. These studies are neither universally performed nor universally accepted as indicative of the potential outcome of the transplant.

RENAL TRANSPLANTATION IN CHILDREN

The annual incidence of end stage renal disease (ESRD) in children is 1.5 per million total population. In the pediatric population transplantation is the preferred goal for the correction of chronic renal failure; because over a long period of time, a successful renal transplantation provides the best opportunity to maximize return of renal functions.

Important Considerations when Performing Renal Transplants in Children

AGE

In pediatrics, psychosocial and developmental age are of great importance when considering transplantation. Chronologically, the age range for considering transplantation is from 6 months onward.

RECURRING RENAL DISEASE

Three main categories of diseases may cause native kidney failure and may potentially recur in the graft: 1) Primary glomerulonephritis, 2) generalized systemic diseases, 3) inherited metabolic diseases. Despite a relatively high incidence of histological recurrence of the glomerular lesion, the frequency of graft loss attributable to recurrence is low ($\pm$)10%.

Primary Glomerulonephritis

The most common specific primary glomerular disease creating ESRD is focal glomerulosclerosis (FGS). The incidence of recurrence varies from center to center, depending on documentation criteria. A factor known to influence recurrence is the degree of histocompatibility between donor and recepient. Thus, a higher recurrence rate has been noted in recipients of live-related donors when compared to cadaver donors (65% vs. 35%), and a 52% recurrence rate occurs in HLA identical sibling grafts. The recurrence of FGS in subsequent grafts implies that a circulating factor, the identity of which is unknown, may be responsible for the primary disease. To date, it is impossible to predict which patients will manifest recurrence, and so patients with FGS should not be excluded from transplantation. If recurrence develops, in the initial graft, however, caution in retransplantation is advised. Another histological recurrent disease in children is membranoproliferative glomerulonephritis (MPGN) type II and, less frequently, type I.

Generalized Systemic Diseases

Of the systemic glomerular diseases, systemic lupus erythematosus (SLE) and hemolytic uremic syndrome (HUS) are the most significant. With SLE the graft has rarely been affected despite the systemic nature of the primary disease. With respect to HUS, it has been suggested that transplantation be deferred for at least six months after purpura has abated.

Inherited Metabolic Diseases

The two mosts common metabolic diseases resulting in recurrence are cystinosis and oxalosis. In cystinosis, despite adequate graft function, the cystine content of white blood cells and cultured skin fibroblasts remains elevated after transplantation. Cystine accumulates in the interstitium and occasionally in the mesangium, but not in the tubular or glomerular epithelial cells, which is the case in the cystinotic kidney. The extra renal manifestations of cystinosis generally persist following transplantation. In oxalosis, the disease recurs in the graft. It was for this reason that patients with oxalosis were previously excluded as transplant candidates. Recently, prolonged survival has been reported.

Technical Considerations

The technical aspects for renal transplantation in children are similar to those for adults, except for the obviously small child, where the question of extraperitoneal vs. transabdominal placement is important. The latter is utilized when the organ is adult size and the child weighs less than 20 kg.

One of the most critical moments in pediatric transplantation comes when an adult organ is placed in a small child. Intraoperative fluid management and careful monitoring of central venous and arterial pressure are necessary to maintain adequate vascular volume. Likewise, physicians recommend vasodilators to perfuse the graft, and central to peripheral temperature measurements as an indication of perfusion. In children, the ureter is usually reimplanted by means of a ureteroneocystostomy or an ileal conduit, the latter only if the bladder is inadequate.

Immunosuppression

In children, corticosteroids and azathioprine are the primary drugs of choice. An initial dose of corticosteroids (20–30 mg daily) has been used without compromising allograft functions. Once the allograft function is stabilized (6–12 months post transplant), alternate day corticosteroids can be introduced. In children, this is of utmost importance since it has been associated with improvement in growth velocity and no adverse effect on allograft function. Recently, as with adult patients, cyclosporine has been used following renal transplantation. The initial reports are encouraging, although few pediatric recipients have received the drug.

Post Operative Medical Complications

INFECTION

Pediatric patients are exposed to the same host of infections, when they are immunocompromised, as are adults. Thus, the same precautions are warranted. Of special note is varicella,

where azathioprine should be discontinued with the onset of symptoms and not reinstituted until 24 to 48 hours after new crops of vesicles cease.

GROWTH AND PUBERTAL DEVELOPMENT

One of the most important parameters to follow in pediatric allograft transplant recipients is their growth potential. The lack of uniformity in linear height following transplantation depends on many factors, among them chronological age versus growth potential at the time of transplantation, allograft function and corticosteroid dosage. Children with a bone age greater than 12 years at transplantation normally grow minimally, if at all, after transplant. Recent reports, however, have shown that substantial growth post transplant can occasionally be achieved despite a bone age greater than 12. The reasons for this are not apparent. At present, precise mechanisms that adversely affect growth are unknown. However, linear growth can be maximized following transplantation by maintaining optimal allograft function, by using alternate day steroids and by performing transplantation early in children who develop chronic renal failure. Puberty proceeds normally in amenorrheic females after transplantation, with menses returning within 6 to 12 months following successful transplant. Again, this exists mainly in children whose bone age has been less than 12 years. In males, genital maturation has been significantly delayed both in bone and chronological age. The pituitary-testicular axis has been normal in those recipients with good renal function.

With children, some additional factors should be considered when performing a transplant evaluation. The transplantation team needs to be sensitive to the problems of children who have behavioral and/or psychiatric problems. There is no unequivocal contraindication for transplantation of ESRD patients with mental retardation. The primary difficulty with this group of patients is noncompliance with the therapeutic regime. Furthermore, the decision to use a parental or sibling donor allograft is a parental one. Dispassionate counseling is needed to assist in making this decision. Once the transplant has been performed, the patient should be helped to cope with the undesirable side effects of steroids, namely, obesity, growth failure, acne, hirsuitism and Cushinoid facies. Otherwise, there may be emotional and social problems for chil-

Table 17-10   Long-Term Outcome

Author	# Patients	Actuarial Graft Survival (%)			
		Live-Related		Cadaver	
		5 years	10 years	5 years	10 years
DeShazo, et al (1974)	100		74		44
Fine, et al (1978)	69	73*		39*	
Chantler, et al (1980)	75	55		43**	
Arbus, et al (1980)	78				59
Potter, et al (1980)	145		55		31

*Actual
**3 Years

dren beyond infancy. Finally, despite all occasional problems, the rehabilitation potential of those with a functioning allograft is excellent.

Long-Term Outcome

As shown in the table, the allograft survival for 5 and 10 years in pediatric recipients depicted in Table 10 does not guarantee continued allograft function. Despite adequate function at 5 years, attrition ensues secondary to chronic rejection or death. Since an indolent immunological attack may occur in any recipient, pediatric patients can anticipate undergoing three to four transplants in their lives in order to achieve longevity.

SELECTED READINGS

Cameron, J.S. Effect of the recipient's disease on the results of transplantation, (other than diabetes mellitus). Kidney Int., 23(suppl. 14), S24–S33, 1983.

Gelfand, M.C. Transplantation in Immunology. J. Bellanti, ed., Saunders, 1978.

Novello, A.C. and Fine, R.N. Renal transplantation in Children. Int. J. Ped. Neph. 3:87–98, 1982.

Gradus, D. Ettenger, R.B. Renal transplantation in Children. Pediatric Clinics of North America. 29. 1013–1038, 1982.

Schreiner, G.E. Past, present and future of Renal Transplantation. Kidney Int., 23(suppl. 14), S4–S9, 1983.

Starzl, T.E., Rosenthal, J.T., Hakala, T.R., Iwatsuki, S., Shaw, B.W., Klintmalin, G.B.G. Steps in Immunosuppression for renal transplantation. Kidney Int., 23 (suppl. 14), S60–S65, 1983.

Vinod K. Bansal
Leonard L. Vertuno

18

Total Parenteral Nutrition in Renal Failure

Parenteral nutrition is the supply of nutrients via the intravascular route. Parenteral nutrition may be total when it is the patient's only source of energy; or partial when it is used to supplement an inadequate oral intake.

Intravenous nutritional supplementation has been available for many years, but the concept of total parenteral nutrition (TPN) as a therapeutic modality dates from 1968. Initially, TPN was used to correct nutritional deficiencies; its role has now expanded to include specific management of enterocutaneous fistula, inflammatory bowel disease, burns, chemotherapy of malignant disease, acute renal failure and during the post operative management of all types of renal failure. It is the role of TPN in the treatment of renal failure that forms the basis of this chapter.

TPN attempts to provide sufficient protein and calories to meet the patient's metabolic needs and produce a state of positive nitrogen balance. In a typical postoperative patient, 3000 to 4000 calories may be required and, if not supplied, a catabolic state develops in a short period of time. In renal failure the situation is more complex because of the disruption of the normal excretory function of the kidneys and the accumulation of nitrogenous waste products which may be partly responsible for uremic symptoms. Therefore, until very recently, protein has been severely restricted in renal failure and energy requirements supplied as fat and carbohydrates.

Calories were given to prevent endogenous protein breakdown. With this approach, almost all patients were in negative nitrogen balance; and mortality in acute renal failure (ARF) remained distressingly high, especially in post surgical patients. The use of TPN in renal failure is an attempt to prevent or reverse the negative nitrogen balance and promote faster recovery from surgical stress.

Our understanding of the role of specific amino acids in improving nitrogen balance is derived from the work of Rose. He established the concept of essential amino acids (EAA) and non-essential amino acids (NEAA). EAA (isoleucine, leucine, lysine, methionine, phenylanine, threonine, tryptophan and valine) cannot be synthesized in the body. Histidine may be another essential amino acid in the uremic state. NEAA can be synthesized in the body provided that EAA are supplied in sufficient quantity. The caloric requirement when amino acids are the only source of nitrogen (N) is 35 to 40 Kcal/Kg/day. Rose also demonstrated that urea could be utilized as a source of non-protein nitrogen for synthesis of NEAA if: (1) adequate calories are provided; (2) EAA are used exclusively as the nitrogen source; and (3) the gut functions normally. Under these circumstances, urea is hydrolyzed by bacterial urease to ammonia and carbon dioxide in the intestine. Ammonia then enters the enterohepatic circulation and is transaminated to form NEAA. This concept was confirmed by feeding groups of normal and uremic patients a diet with a high EAA content and observing a decrease in SUN. Next, a diet with a very high EAA content containing only 1.5 g N and 2000 to 3000 Kcal/day was devised. Then the concept of TPN utilizing protein hydrolysates as the N source was introduced. The initial solutions contained 6 g N/L (equivalent to 36 grams of protein) in 50% glucose. This supplied 2000 Kcal/L as carbohydrate and yielded a N:non-N caloric ratio of 1:333. Crystalline amino acids are now available as the N source.

In 1973, the efficiency of TPN utilizing a mixture of eight EAA (1.46 g N) in 70% dextrose to hypertonic glucose alone was compared in a group of patients with acute renal failure. An increased patient survival and shorter recovery time in the patients receiving TPN was demonstrated. Although these early landmark results have been difficult to duplicate, the study provided strong impetus to provide adequate parenteral nutrition to all acute renal failure patients and post-surgical or septic chronic renal failure patients who cannot be supported adequately by oral or enteral routes.

CLINICAL APPLICATION

Technique

TPN utilizes fluids of high osmolality, so administration via a large caliber vein with a high blood flow rate is necessary to prevent sclerosis. The technique most commonly employed is the percutaneous insertion of a catheter into the subclavian vein by the infraclavicular approach. Other large central veins can be used, but subclavian vein catheterization offers the most practical route and does not inhibit the patient's mobility. Catheter insertion and maintenance must be performed by a team skilled in catheter care to minimize traumatic and infectious complications. The complication rate of catheter insertion is 1–2% and includes: pneumothorax, hemothorax, hydrothorax, subcutaneous emphysema, subclavian artery injury and air embolism. A post-insertional chest radiograph is done to check whether catheter placement is appropriate and whether complications have occurred. The role of the internist or nephrologist is to determine nutritional and fluid require-

Table 18-1   General Principles for Use of TPN in Renal Failure

Guidelines	Parameter
Protein Requirement	0.5–1.0 g/Kg B.W. Rarely possible to exceed 1.2–1.5 g/Kg B.W.
Nitrogen Component	16% of calculated protein requirement
Calories	300 calories/g N
Glucose	Total calories ÷ 4 = g glucose required. Glucose concentration varies with fluid allowance.
Fluid Requirement	Varies with urine flow and total output. In anuric patients, 750 ml a day.
Electrolytes	Potassium: Varies with clinical states Phosphorus: Due to hyperphosphatemia, early replacement not required, subsequent replacement necessary Magnesium: In general, replacement rarely required
Trace Elements	Zinc Chromium
Emulsified Fat	Administered weekly to prevent essential fatty acid deficiency

ments, determine the type and amount of solution to be administered, and prescribe required additives. This is especially important in the patient with ARF in whom careful assessment must be made daily.

TPN PRESCRIPTION

The major determinants of the TPN prescription are: (1) protein requirement and, thus, type and amount of amino acids to be given, (2) caloric requirements, (3) volume, and (4) required additives to the basic solution.

Protein Requirement and Types of Amino Acid Solutions

The goal of TPN is to achieve positive N balance. In a nondialyzed patient, the recommended protein intake is 0.5 g/Kg/BW daily. In a dialyzed patient, the intake will need to be increased to 1.0 to 1.5 g/Kg BW. Further increments in nitrogen intake do not increase utilization but may exacerbate azotemia.

Solutions of EAA or a mixture of EAA + NEAA are available. Early studies of TPN in renal failure emphasized the particular suitability of EAA because of the lesser rise of SUN. It was hoped that dialysis might be delayed or obviated. It has since become clear that dialytic requirements or the duration of ARF are not altered by TPN. Since nitrogen balance may be more favorably affected by a combination of EAA + NEAA, we utilize a mixture of EAA − NEAA for the dialyzed renal failure patients. The greater increment in SUN with these solutions is an insignificant factor in the well dialyzed patient. In the rare circumstance where dialysis is neither feasible nor available, the use of EAA as Nephramine® or Aminosyn-RF® will slow the rate of progression of azotemia and should be utilized.

Caloric Intake

The caloric requirements in ARF have yet to be determined with precision. To maintain a 70 Kg man in a basal non-catabolic state, 1500 cal/day are required. This would appear to be a minimum in ARF. In the stressful postsurgical state, 3000–4000 calories might be required. In severe catabolic stress such as the badly burned patient, up to 8000 Kcals/day has been the estimated requirement. Sufficient non-protein calories must be administered to promote N utilization. In patients with normal renal function, a ratio of 100 Kcal/gN is sufficient. The ratio required in renal failure is not established with certainty, but appears to be three or four times greater. It is our practice to administer 300 calories as glucose for every g N required. We calculate:

a.) g amino acids required = BW × 1.0
b.) g N = 16% × g amino acids

Table 18-2 Composition of Amino Acid Solutions for Use in Parenteral Nutrition

A.A. Solution		Vol. (ml)	A.A. Content		N Content		NPC:N Ratio When Mixed c̄ 500 ml	
			g/100 ml	gm/T.V.	g/100 ml	gm/T.V.	D50W	D70W
Aminosyn-RF	5.2%	300	5.2	15.6	0.78	2.34	427:1	598:1
Aminosyn	10 %	500	10	50	1.57	7.85	108:1	152:1
Nephramine	5.4%	250	5.4	13.4	0.6	1.5	—	745:1
FreAmin II	8.5%	500	8.5	42.5	1.25	6.25	135:1	189:1
RenAmin	6.5%	250	6.5	16.2	1.0	2.5	—	476.1
	6.5%	500	6.5	32.5	1.0	5.0	200:1	280:1
Travasol	5.5%	500	5.5	27.5	0.92	4.6	217:1	313:1
	8.5%	500	8.5	42.5	1.42	7.1	140:1	202:1

Information compiled from Manufacturers' product brochure. 1 g of glucose taken to provide 4 calories per gram.

c.) non N calories required $= 300 \times$ g N

d.) g glucose required $=$ non N calories $\div 4$

Glucose Concentration and Volume

Glucose is administered in concentrations from 25% to 70%. One L of 70% glucose will provide 2800 Kcal (700 g $\times$ 4). Thus, in a situation where high caloric intake with a reduced volume is desired, a higher glucose concentration can be used to advantage. Volume of infusate that is tolerated is determined by urine output plus other measurable and insensible losses. In the anuric patient, 250 ml of EAA plus 500 ml of 70% glucose will give 12.5 g of amino acids and 1400 non-N calories. These stringent restrictions may be liberalized considerably by frequent dialysis when appropriate.

Additives

Many other substances must be added to the basic amino acid-glucose solution. Because the needs of patients with renal failure are so disparate, additives should be individualized from patient to patient. A solution without electrolytes is preferable provided daily assessment of electrolyte needs is made. Electrolyte free solutions allow one to add various constituents as required.

Since hyperkalemia and hyperphosphatemia are features of renal failure, initiation of TPN with potassium and phosphate free solutions is appropriate. As anabolism occurs, the intracellular transport of potassium and phosphate may result in hypokalemia and hypophosphatemia. Phosphate may be replaced as double phosphate (10 mEq/ml), potassium phosphate (3 mEq/ml) or sodium phosphate (3 mEq/ml). Acetate ions (sodium acetate) provide a base equivalent. Bicarbonate cannot be administered in TPN fluids. Vitamins, trace metals (zinc, copper and chromium) are routinely supplied. Some weekly or bi-weekly infusions of emulsified fat to provide supplemental calories and prevent essential fatty acid deficiency should be given.

TPN is administered as a continuous infusion; the rate is determined by the total volume

Table 18-3 Available Electrolyte Additives

Ions	Salts	Conc/ml	Usual Daily Requirement
Sodium	Sodium Chloride Conc.	4 mEq/sml	60–150 mEq
	Sodium Acetate	2 mEq/ml	
	Sodium Phosphate	4 mEqNa/ml	
Potassium	Potassium Chloride	2 mEq/ml	Varies. If hyperkalemia is present none required. Usually,
	Potassium Acetate	2 mEq/ml	
	Potassium Phosphate	4.4 mEqK/ml	40–150 mEq
Calcium	Calcium gluconate 10%	4.5 mEq/10 ml	3–30 mEq
	Calcium Chloride 10%	13 mEq/10 ml	
Magnesium	Magnesium Sulfate	4 mEq/ml	10–45 mEq
Phosphate	Potassium Phosphate	3 mMP/ml	5–10 mM
	Sodium Phosphate	3 mMP/ml	If hyperphosphatemia is present, none required. Requirement necessary when anabolism occurs
Trace Elements	Zinc		2.5–4.0 mg/day
	Copper		0.5–1.5 mg/day
	Chromium		10–15 μg/day

requirement of the patient. It is started slowly with low glucose concentrations to prevent the precipitation of a hyperosmolar syndrome. In the renal failure patient, 2000 ml/day or slightly higher volumes is the practical limit.

SYSTEMIC COMPLICATIONS

Apart from problems associated with catheter insertion, systemic complications can be grouped into three categories:

a.) thrombosis of the great veins
b.) sepsis
c.) metabolic complications

Thrombosis of the great veins is uncommon. Long term catheter use, hyperosmolality of the TPN fluid, and coagulopathy associated with the patient's illness are contributing factors. The silastic catheter has replaced the polyethylene catheter and has reduced the incidence of thrombosis. The diagnosis is suspected when edema of the face or arm develops or embolic events occur. Diagnosis is confirmed by angiography. Treatment is catheter removal, anticoagulation and reinsertion of the catheter elsewhere.

Patients receiving TPN have complex medical and surgical illnesses, and sepsis remains the most frequent and serious complication, occurring in 4–6% of cases. Roughly half the instances of sepsis are fungemias: *Candida albicans, Candida parapsilosis,* and *Torulopsis glabrata* are the most common. Staphylococcus aureus and staphylococcus epidermitis are the most frequent cause of bacterial sepsis. Clinical signs include chills, fever, and leukocytosis. Since other sources of infection are common, all possible sites should be evaluated by history, physical examination and other indicated studies. If blood culture is positive, the catheter must be removed and the catheter tip cultured as well. In septic shock, the catheter should be removed unless the cause of sepsis is obvious. When infection is controlled, a new catheter may be replaced at a distant site.

Metabolic complications include:

a.) abnormalities of glucose metabolism: hyperglycemia, hyperosmolar nonketotic coma, and hypoglycemia
b.) hyperchloremic acidosis
c.) hypophosphatemia
d.) hypokalemia
e.) hyponatremia
f.) magnesium deficiency
g.) trace element deficiency
h.) essential fatty acid deficiency

The large glucose loads utilized frequently produce hyperglycemia. Blood glucose must be monitored frequently and if it exceeds 250 mg/dl, insulin must be provided. This may be done by adding insulin to the TPN solution, 15 units/L initially. This can be increased to 100–200 units/L if necessary. Early reports that adding insulin directly to the TPN solution results in a significant loss of activity have not been substantiated. It appears that inactivity is minimal, probably less than 2% of administered dose.

Hyperchloremic acidosis was a common occurrence with early TPN solutions. This is less of a problem now and is easily corrected by the administration of a base equivalent, lactate or acetate.

Most renal failure patients are hyperphosphatemic so it is appropriate to start TPN without added phosphate. As TPN promotes anabolism, profound hypophosphatemia and hypokalemia may occur precipitously. Very low levels of serum phosphate are associated with red cell dysfunction, central nervous system dysfunction, rhabdomyolysis, as well as cardiac and pulmonary abnormalities. Careful monitoring is required to prevent this and provide adequate supplementation.

Trace metals and fatty acids can be administered on a regular basis to avoid deficiencies.

To date, few studies of TPN in renal disease have been able to show positive nitrogen balance or alter the course of the basic disease process. It has proven very useful in the management of these critically ill patients who cannot be otherwise adequately nourished.

SELECTED READINGS

1. Abel, RM, Beck, CH, Abbott, WM, Ryan, JA Jr., Barnett, GO and Fischer, JE Improved survival from acute renal failure after treatment with intravenous essential L-amino acids and glucose. N. Eng J Med. 288: 695–699, 1973.
2. Feinstein, EI, Blumenkrantz, MJ, Healy, M, Koffler, A, Silberman, H, Massry, SG, and Kopple, JD Clinical and metabolic response to parenteral nutrition in acute renal failure. Medicine 60: 124–137, 1981.

3. Miatallo, JM, Schneider, PJ, Majko, K, Rubey, RL and Fabri, PJ Comparison of essential and general amino acid infusions with the nutritional support of patients with compromised renal function. JPEN 6: 109–113, 1982.

4. Rose, WC The amino acid requirements of adult man. Nutr. Abst. Rev. 27: 631, 1957.

5. Wilmore, DW and Dudrick, SJ Treatment of acute renal failure with intravenous essential L-amino acids. Arch. Surg. 99: 669–673, 1969.

James Winchester
Lester Haddad

19

Poisoning

The nephrologist aids the management of poisoned patients in several ways: through his knowledge of forced diuresis and dialytic techniques, and more recently through expertise in sorbent hemoperfusion. Prior to outlining the special use of the latter techniques, it is worthwhile to review the history of poisoning, to update the epidemiology of modern poisoning, and to briefly describe the general approach to the emergency management of poisoning.

Poisoning, defined in Webster's dictionary (1981), as "to injure or kill with poison; a substance through which its chemical action usually kills, injures or impairs an organism," is not a new phenomenon. The history of poisoning dates back to antiquity, originally in the province of ancient magicians and priests. The first documented recognition of poisons came from Egypt, in the form of the Smith Papyrus (1600 B.C.) citing the use of charms against snake poisoning. Subsequently, the Hearst Medical Papyrus and the Ebers Papyrus referred to poisons and therapeutic agents (1500 B.C.). Paracelsus related the toxin dosage to the severity of poisoning and coined the phrase "dosage alone determines poisoning." However, it was not until the 19th century that Orfila established toxicology as a discipline. Since that time, toxicology has become an established discipline in clinical medicine.

Figures from the National Center for Health Statistics for 1978 underline the importance of poisoning mortality—12,171 cases attributable to poisoning were reported. Of this number, 2,452 were due to carbon monoxide, a situation almost identical to that in the United Kingdom. Most deaths are in adults since the figures for children over the last 20 years show a consecutive decline in accidental poison deaths. Only 100 deaths were reported for 1980. The declining pediatric mortality may be due to the safety closures on drug containers, improved medical training, consumer awareness, and voluntary industrial efforts limiting the toxicity content of commercial products.

DIAGNOSIS

The diagnosis of poisoning may or may not be straightforward, and it is the physician's duty to ascertain from all sources any possibility of toxic ingestion, particularly in psychiatric patients, trauma victims, comatose patients, patients rescued from fires, or patients with an unexplained metabolic acidosis. If poisoning is suspected, simple chromatographic urinary drug screening methods are widely available and take less than three hours to make a tentative diagnosis. Following diagnosis, the approach to the poisoned patient can be divided into seven phases (Table 1).

In emergency stabilization of patients, the physician should direct his attention to cardiac and respiratory care, resuscitation, and fluid balance before any attempt at diagnosis is made.

Table 19-1   General Approach to the
Management of Poisoning

1. Emergency stabilization of the patient

2. Clinical evaluation

3. Elimination of poison from the gastrointestinal
   tract, skin or eyes

4. Administration of an antidote (if available)

5. Elimination of the absorbed substance

6. Supportive therapy and observation

7. Disposition

An IV should be set up with normal saline, and comatose patients may be given naloxone hydrochloride followed by 50 g of glucose as an IV bolus after blood and urine samples have been obtained for toxicological screening. In the comatose patient, particular attention should be paid to respiration, and the respiratory system, pupils, the body surfaces, the breath, heart and abdomen, since all may give clues to the etiology of poisoning. For example, in the comatose patient, pinpoint pupils suggest organophospate insecticides, opiates, brain stem hemorrhage, or phenothiazines; whereas dilated pupils suggest tricyclic antidepressants, anticholinergic drugs, and sedatives such as glutethimide. Metabolic acidosis can be caused by several poisons. The following specifically contribute to the acidosis; salicylates, methanol, ethylene glycol and paraldehyde.

Elimination of the poison from the gastrointestinal tract, skin, and eyes, is a major therapeutic goal in clinical toxicology. Most attention is directed towards the gastrointestinal tract. For organophosphates, it is imperative that the skin, eyes, and other body surfaces are thoroughly cleansed of organophosphate. Soap and water is used initially, followed by alcohol rinses on exposed surfaces. Absorption of poisons from the gastrointestinal tract can be reduced by dilution with milk or water, gastric emptying (lavage or emesis), administration of activated charcoal, and administration of neutralizers or cathartics.

Syrup of ipecac and gastric lavage are the two most common techniques employed in gas-

tric emptying, the former being particularly useful in children. Ipecac syrup is formulated from the dried root of cephaelis ipecacuanha or acuminata which grows primarily in Central Brazil and Central America, and gives the principle alkaloids emetine and cephaeline. The recommended dosage of syrup of ipecac is 15 ml for children up to age 12 and 30 ml for teenagers and adults. It is even effective when antiemetics (phenothiazines) have been ingested. Ipecac is contraindicated in comatose patients or patients with epileptiform seizures, following caustic ingestion, and in petroleum distillate ingestion, unless the latter is a carrier for substances such as organophosphate insecticides. Gastric lavage using a #36 French Catheter or Ewald tube is common practice in adults. Gastric lavage is clearly indicated for the comatose child and adult and when ipecac fails to produce emesis. Contraindications to gastric lavage include the comatose patient prior to endotracheal intubation, kerosene ingestion, and lye ingestion. Drugs which can produce concretions in the stomach include meprobamate, barbiturates, aspirin, carbromal, glutethimide and carbamazepine. In this circumstance, warm saline lavage with abdominal massage, endoscopy, and endoscopic gastric removal of drug masses have been recommended.

"Activated" charcoal is the residue from destructive distillation of wood pulp, bone, coconut shells, peat, starch, lactose, and sucrose. Charcoal is rendered "activated" by chemical or physical creation of numerous surface pores; the small pores (micropores) determine the surface area and binding efficiency. Charcoal is administered by mouth in the form of a water based slurry. Despite the fact that activated charcoal was used by Hippocrates in the 5th century B.C. for gastrointestinal disorders and despite some dramatic human demonstrations in the early 19th century, it was not until 1964 that it was demonstrated that the morbidity and mortality of barbiturate and salicylate poisoning in children could be dramatically reduced by the simple expedient of frequent administration of oral activated charcoal. The adult dose of activated charcoal is 50 to 100 g in 8 ounces of water and the pediatric dose is 30 to 50 g in 4 ounces of water. Activated charcoal will adsorb most drugs and alcohols and other toxic compounds. There are very few contraindications to charcoal; however, it must be remembered that charcoal will absorb ipecac and n-acetyl-cysteine, the antidote for acetaminophen poisoning. Activated charcoal may also have a role in the management of poisoning from drugs that enter the enterohepatic circulation, such as barbiturates, digoxin, tricyclic antidepressants and glutethimide.

In certain situations such as mercury poisoning, iron, iodine ingestion, strychnine, nicotine, and quinine, there are specific neutralizing agents which can be used instead of activated charcoal. Although cathartics are usually used in poisoning, there is no direct evidence of benefit, except for intestinal lavage with an osmotic agent in paraquat poisoning.

Very few antidotes are available for the treatment of general drug poisoning. The following is a partial listing, the drug being followed in parentheses by its antidote: acetaminophen (n-acetyl-cysteine); cyanide (amylnitrite, sodium nitrite); methanol and ethlene glycol (ethanol); iron, lead, mercury, gold, arsenic (chelating agents such as deferoxamine, calcium disodium versenate, and British antilewisite); opiates, propoxyphene and Lomotil (naloxone); organophosphates (atropine, pralidoxime); and atropine (physostigmine).

Elimination of the absorbed substance from blood will be dealt with in more detail below. Supportive therapy is the prime tested and proven therapeutic intervention for poisoning. This requires intensive care and a multidisciplinary approach in the management of respiration, circulation, and other vital functions. Only when intensive supportive care fails and the patient is deteriorating should recourse be made to considering other techniques such as dialysis or hemoperfusion. It must be remembered that certain poisons such as iron, acetaminophen, paraquat amanita phalloides, carbon tetrachloride, mercury, and tricyclic antidepressants produce delayed effects. Accordingly, prolonged periods of observation may be necessary. Finally, attention should be paid to medical and psychiatric followup, where appropriate, in the recovered drug-intoxicated patient.

Forced Diuresis

Most drugs are weak acids or bases that exist in the nonionized or ionized form; the nonionized molecules are lipid soluble and diffuse across the cell membrane by nonionic diffusion. In contrast, the ionized form is unable to penetrate lipid membranes. In the kidney, drug excretion involves three main processes (*glomerular filtration,* whereby weakly protein bound substances are ultrafiltered; *tubular secretion* at the proximal convoluted tubule with transport systems for acidic or basic drugs, and finally *passive tubular reabsorption*). The latter process involves bidirectional movements of drugs across tubular epithelium, and a concentration gradient is created for absorption of the soluble drug back into the blood. Reabsorption requires little energy and is limited to lipid soluble drugs in the nonionized form. Increasing the pH of the tubular fluid increases the degree of ionization of weak acids and reduced tubular reabsorption. The reverse applies to weak bases. The dissociation of a weak acid or base is determined by both its dissociation constant (pK_a) and pH gradient across the tubular membrane. Elimination of weak acids by the kidney is increased in alkaline urine if the pK_a of the drug lies between 3.0 and 7.5. For the weak bases elimination is increased if the pK_a of the drug is 7.5 to 10.5. Drugs amenable to forced diuresis must be predominantly eliminated in the unchanged form via the kidney, be weak electrolytes with a pK_a in the appropriate acidic or basic pK_a range and be distributed with minimal protein binding mainly in the extracellular fluid compartment. Forced diuresis is also called "ion trapping." Since forced diuresis involves the administration of fluid in large quantities, alkaline and acidic agents, close vigilance must be paid to urine pH (hourly) and plasma pH and electrolytes (every one to two hours). Changes in blood pH induce shifts of potassium into and out of cells. Therefore, it is essential to monitor and replace potassium during the use of this treatment method. Since urine flow rates should be accurately accessed, a Foley catheter is placed in the bladder; and when appropriate, a Swan-Ganz line should be used to assess fluid balance.

Alkaline diuresis is attained by using one liter of 5% dextrose containing 25 mEq of bicarbonate and 75 mEq of sodium. Appropriate levels of potassium are given along with mannitol or furosemide every one to two hours until a urine flow of 300 to 500 ml/hr is reached. Alkaline diuresis is suitable for phenobarbital poisoning when the plasma levels exceeds 10 mg/dl, barbital poisoning when the plasma level exceeds 10 mg/dl, salicylate poisoning when the plasma levels exceed 50 mg/dl and also 2,4-

dichlorophenoxyacetic acid (2,4 D). On the other hand, acid diuresis is attained by using 5% dextrose with added arginine, lysine, or ammonium chloride, 4 g every two hours given by mouth or intravenously. The dose should be adjusted to maintain a urinary pH near 6.5. Plasma potassium should be measured frequently. Forced diuresis increases excretion of amphetamines, fenfluramine, phencyclidine and also quinine. Ascorbic acid, one g every six hours, can also be given orally to acidify the urine. A water and chloride diuresis increases the excretion of bromides, whereas lithium excretion is not enhanced further with alkaline or acid diuresis.

Dialytic Techniques for Removing Poisons

Dialysis, the term coined in 1854 by Thomas Graham, describes the transfer of solute across a semipermeable membrane. Although introduced in 1913 in an experimental form for the removal of diffusable toxins, it was not used successfully in man until 1955 in a patient poisoned with aspirin. Since then, many substances have been reported to be removed by hemodialysis and peritoneal dialysis. Exhaustive reviews concerning individual poisons are available.

Factors governing drug removal are solute (or drug) size, lipid-water partition coefficient (or lipid solubility) protein binding, the apparent volume of distribution, and the maintenance of a concentration gradient. Physical factors governing drug removal by the dialyzer itself are blood flow rate, dialysate flow rate, surface area, and characteristics of the dialysis membrane. The ideal drug for efficient removal by dialysis should be low molecular weight, fully distributed in whole body water, not lipid soluble and have no plasma protein binding; lithium fulfills these criteria and is highly dialyzable. On the other hand tricyclic antidepressants possess large molecular weights, are to some degree lipid soluble, and are highly protein bound with a large volume of distribution; consequently, tricyclic antidepressants are poorly dialyzable.

The term "dialysance" or "clearance" of drugs is identical to that of other uremic solutes described in the chapter on Management of Chronic Renal Failure (Chapter 16). Briefly, clearance of drugs equals blood flow rate through the dialyzer multiplied by A-V/A, where A is arterial (or inlet) concentration, V is venous (or outlet) concentration of drug. The A-V/A is equivalent to the extraction ratio across the dialyzer.

Drug removal rates are frequently calculated from bench-type experiments, which for the most part use aqueous drug containing solutions. This usually overestimates the drug removal rates since plasma protein binding is missing. It is more correct to use whole blood flow rates and whole blood drug measurements in the calculation of drug clearances. Certain drugs such as salicylates, although saturating plasma protein binding sites at high drug concentrations, are weakly bound and highly ultrafilterable. Thus, salicylates are ideal dialyzable drugs. Lipid solubility of drugs also governs their removal by dialysis. Lipid dialysis using soybean oil emulsion with dialysis fluid was used for partitioning. In modern times, however, large surface area dialyzers have replaced lipid dialysis and consequently the technique has fallen into disfavor. In addition, lipid soluble drugs can be removed with charcoal or resin hemoperfusion.

The peritoneal route is the least effective dialytic method for removing drugs, in view of the maximal achievable drug removal rates of between 5 and 10 ml/min with intermittent (short dwell time) peritoneal dialysis. Peritoneal dialysis is used for treating dialyzable poisons only if other methods are unavailable. Peritoneal dialysis, however, can be used to increase the central ("core") temperature in patients severely hypothermic from drug intoxication.

The dialyzable poisons are shown in Table 2.

Sorbent Hemoperfusion

Hemodialysis and hemoperfusion require passage of anticoagulated blood through dialyzer lines. Blood pumps should maintain blood flow rates, depending on the patients blood pressure, as high as possible (up to 300 ml/min). Since dialysis and hemoperfusion can remove pressor substances such as dopamine or dobutamine, these drugs should be placed distal to the dialyzer or hemoperfusion column when required.

Hemoperfusion is the passage of anticoagulated blood through a column containing sorbent particles—basically activated charcoal and the resin XAD4, an amberlite nonionic polysty-

Table 19-2   Drugs Removed with Various Dialytic Techniques

ALOCHOLS*
ethanol
ethylene glycol
isopropanol
methanol

ANALGESICS*
acetaminophen/paracetamol
acetophenetidin
acetylsalicylic acid
methylsalicylate
propoxyphene
salicylic acid

ANTIDEPRESSANTS*
(amitriptyline)
amphetamine
(imipramine)
isocarboxazid
methamphetamine
(nortriptyline)
(pargyline)
(phenelzine)
tranylcypromine

ANTIMICROBIALS/
   ANTICANCER AGENTS
amikacin
ampicillin
azathioprine
azlocillin
bacitracin
carbenicillin
cefamandole
cephaloridine
cephalothin
chloramphenicol
chloroquine
colchicine
colistin
(cyclophosphamide)
(cycloserine)
(ethambutol)
5-fluorouracil
flucytosine
fosfomycin
gentamicin
(hexachlorophene)
(isoniazid)
kanamycin
(methotrexate)

nafcillin
neomycin
nitrofurantoin
penicillin
polymyxin
quinine
streptomycin
sulfonamides
tetracycline
tobramycin
vancomycin

BARBITURATES*
amobarbital
aprobarbital
barbital
butabarbital
butalbital
cyclobarbital
pentobarbital
quinalbital
(secobarbital)

METALS/INORGANICS
(aluminum)*
ammonia
arsenic*
borates
boric acid
bromide
carbromal
chloride
(chromates)
(chromic acid)
copper
fluoride*
iodide
(iron)
lead
lithium
(magnesium)*
(mercury)
nitrite
phosphate*
potassium*
sodium*
strontium
thallium
(tin)
(zinc)

NONBARBITURATE
   HYPNOTICS,
   SEDATIVES, AND
   TRANQUILIZERS
carbamazepine
carbromal
chloral hydrate
(chlordiazepoxide)
(chlorpromazine)
(diazepam)
diethyl pentenamide
(diphenhydramine)
(diphenylhydantoin)
ethchlorvynol
(ethinamate)
gallamine triethiodide
glutethimide
(heroin)
meprobamate
(methaqualone)
(methsuximide)
methyprylon
paraldehyde
primidone
PLANT/ANIMAL TOXINS,
   HERBICIDES, AND
   INSECTICIDES
alkyl phosphate
Amanita phalloides
amanitin
(atropine)
demeton-S-methylsulfoxide
dimethoate*
dinitrophenol
diquat
(ergotamine)
methyl mercury complex
(organophosphates)
paraquat
snake bite
sodium and potassium chlorate

SOLVENTS/GASES
acetone
camphor
carbon monoxide
(carbon tetrachloride)
(dichloroethane)
(dinitro-*o*-cresol)
(eucalyptus oil)
thiols

169

Table 19-2 Drugs Removed with Various Dialytic Techniques

SOLVENTS/GASES (cont.)	methyldopa	(chlorpropamide)
(toluene)	ouabain	cimetidine
(trichloroethylene)	practolol	mannitol*
	procainamide	methyl mercury complex
CARDIOVASCULAR	propranolol	methylprednisolone
AGENTS	(quinidine)	nitrates
N-acetylprocainamide	(quinine)	(orphenadrine)
atenolol	sotalol	oxalate
(chloroquine)		oxalic acid
(diazoxide)	MISCELLANEOUS	sodium citrate
(digitoxin)	(acetohexamide)	(theophylline)
(digoxin)	aniline	thiocyanate*

*Extensively studied in vivo.
Drugs in parentheses indicate dialysis is ineffective or data are insufficient. Reprinted from Haddad LM, Winchester JF Eds. Clinical Management of Poisoning and Drug Overdose, WB Saunders Co., Philadelphia, 1983.

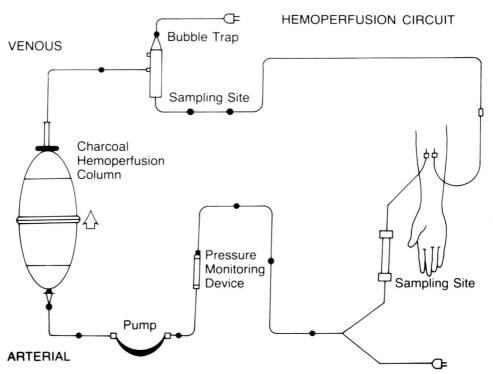

Fig. 19-1. Clinical hemoperfusion circuit. With permission. Haddad LM, Winchester, JF eds., Clinical Management of Poisoning and Drug Overdose. WB Saunders Co., Philadelphia, 1983

rene resin which specifically removes lipid soluble drugs. Description of the devices is beyond the scope of this text. The reader is referred to reviews on hemoperfusion.

Hemoperfusion relies on drug adsorption for its efficacy; and in many instances, drug clearance rates are higher than with hemodialysis, peritoneal dialysis, or forced diuresis. Activated charcoal binds drugs so tightly that they may be unextractable from the perfusion devices. The resin preparations bind the drug tightly but not irreversibly within the bead matrix, such that the drug can be eluted with organic solvents. A typical hemoperfusion circuit for treatment of drug intoxication is shown in Figure 1. In general, hemoperfusion is instituted within a column which contains between 100 and 300 g of activated charcoal (mostly 300 g), or 650 g (wet weight) of polystyrene resin. Devices come sterilized. Blood is passed through the devices using arterio-venous shunt or veno-venous shunt as for hemodialysis. Blood flow rates are determined by the clinical condition of the patient. The most efficient drug removal is achieved with blood flow rates of approximately 300 ml/min. Table 3 shows the plasma drug extraction ratios for many drugs with hemodialysis, charcoal hemoperfusion and XAD4 resin hemoperfusion. As can be seen, the efficiency for drug removal is highest for XAD4 resin, except for paraquat and acetylsalicylic acid. A representative list of drugs that can be removed with hemoperfusion are shown in Table 4.

CRITERIA FOR CONSIDERATION OF HEMODIALYSIS OR HEMOPERFUSION IN POISONING

Basically the decision whether or not the patient undergoes active drug removal with dialysis or hemoperfusion is a clinical one; the prime consideration being whether the patient's condition is progressively deteriorating despite intensive supportive management. Criteria have been developed for instituting hemoperfusion based on the clinical picture and plasma drug concentrations. These are shown in Table 5.

It is not easy to choose between hemodialysis and hemoperfusion. Hemodialysis should be reserved for molecules which have a low molecular weight and low protein binding such as lithium, bromide and ethanol and also drugs which produce metabolic acidosis or generate toxic metabolites. The latter are methanol, ethylene glycol, and salicylates. Hemoperfusion should be reserved for lipid soluble drugs, particularly barbiturates, nonbarbituric hypnotics, sedatives, and tranquilizers. In addition, hemoperfusion is useful treatment for poisoning by digitalis glycosides. Although recommended, there is little evidence to support the use of hemodialysis or hemoperfusion in antidepressant (tricyclic) drug overdose.

Complications arising from hemodialysis or hemoperfusion are usually managed easily. Hemodialysis may cause electrolyte abnormalities if the dialysis solution is not properly prepared

Table 19-3   Plasma Drug Extraction Ratios with Different Drug Removing Devices*

Drug	Hemodialysis	Charcoal Hemoperfusion	XAD-4 Resin Hemoperfusion
Acetylsalicylic acid	0.5	0.5	—
Amobarbital	0.3	0.3	0.9
Digoxin	0.2	0.3–0.6	0.4
Ethchlorvynol	0.2	0.7	1.0
Glutethimide	0.2	0.65	0.8
Methaqualone	0.1	0.4–1.0	1.0
Paraquat	0.5	0.6	—
Pentobarbital	—	0.5	0.85
Phenobarbital	0.3	0.5	0.85
Theophylline	0.5	0.7	0.75

*Calculated for blood flow rate of 200 ml/min at the midpoint of the procedure. Reprinted with permission from Haddad LM, Winchester JF Eds. Clinical Management of Poisoning and Drug Overdose, WB Saunders Co., Philadelphia, 1983.

Table 19-4 Drugs Removed with Hemoperfusion

ALCOHOLS
(ethanol)
(methanol)

ANALGESICS
(acetaminopen/paracetamol)*
acetylsalicylic acid*
methyl salicylate*
phenylbutazone
propoxyphene

ANTIDEPRESSANTS
(amitriptyline)
amphetamine
(clomipramine)
(desipramine)
imipramine
(nortriptyline)

ANTIMICROBIALS/
ANTICANCER AGENTS
ampicillin
chloramphenicol
clindamycin
doxorubicin*
erythromycin
gentamicin
isoniazid
(methotrexate)*

BARBITURATES*
amobarbital
barbital
butabarbital
hexabarbital
pentobarbital
phenobarbital
qulnalbital
secobarbital
thiopental
vinalbital

CARDIOVASCULAR
AGENTS
N-acetylprocainamide
(digitoxin)
(digoxin)*
diisopyramide
methylproscillarin
procainamide
quinidine
quinine

METALS/INORGANICS
(calcium)
(phosphate)
(thallium)

NONBARBITURATE
HYPNOTICS,
SEDATIVES, AND
TRANQUILIZERS
(acetamides)
carbromal
chloral hydrate
chlorpromazine
(diazepam)
diethyl pentenamide
diphenhydramine
ethchlorvynol*
gluiathimide*
meprobamate
methaqualone*
methsuximide
methyprylon*
N-desmethsuximide
pentenamide
promazine
promethazine

PLANT/ANIMAL
TOXINS, HERBICIDES/
INSECTICIDES
Amanita phalloides
amanitin
camphor
chlordane
chlorinated insecticides
demeton-S-methyl sulfoxide*
dimethoate*
nitrostigmine
paraquat*
parathion
phalloidin
polychlorinated biphenyls

SOLVENTS/GASES
carbon tetrachloride
ethylene oxide
trichloroethanol

MISCELLANEOS
aminophylline
angiotensin
camphor
dopamine
epinephrine
(fluoroacetamide)
heparin
norepinephrine
oxalic acid
(phencyclidine)
phenols
(podophyllin)
theophylline

*Extensively studied in vivo.
Drugs in parentheses indicate hemoperfusion is ineffective or data insufficient.
Reprinted with permission from Haddad LM, Winchester Eds.
Clinical Management of Poisoning and Drug Overdose, WB Saunders Co., Philadelphia, 1983.

Table 19-5 Clinical and Blood Level Criteria for Consideration of
Hemodialysis or Hemoperfusion

Drug	Plasma Concentration (mg/dl)	Method of Choice
Phenobarbital	10	HP > H
Other barbiturates	5	HP
Glutethimide	4	HP
Methaqualone	4	HP
Salicylates	80	H > HP†
Ethchlorvynol	15	HP
Meprobamate	10	HP
Trichloroethanol	5	HP
Paraquat	0.1	HP > H
Theophylline	5	HP
Methanol	50	H†
Ethylene glycol	unknown	H†

1. Progressive deterioration despite intensive supportive therapy.
2. Severe intoxication with depression of midbrain function leading to hypoventilation, hypothermia, and hypotension.
3. Development of complications of coma, such as pneumonia or septicemia, and underlying conditions predisposing to such complications (e.g., obstructive airways disease).
4. Impairment of normal drug excretory function in the presence of hepatic, cardiac, or renal insufficiency.
5. Intoxication with agents with metabolic and/or delayed effects, e.g., methanol, ethylene glycol, and paraquat.
6. Intoxication with an extractable drug or poison, which can be removed at a rate exceeding endogenous elimination by liver or kidney.

*In "mixed" poisonings, hemodialysis or hemoperfusion may be considered at lower plasma drug concentrations. Hemodialysis also corrects metabolic complications. H = hemodialysis, HP = hemoperfusion
Reprinted with permission Haddad LM, Winchester JF Eds.
Clinical Management of Poisoning and Drug Overdose, WB Saunders Co., Philadelphia, 1983.

and hypothermia if the temperature is not maintained. Additionally, hemoperfusion is associated with loss of platelets (generally a 30% fall in platelet count with activated charcoal and approximately 50% fall in platelet count with the resin). Blood exposed outside the body in the extracorporeal circuit may reduce body temperature one to 2° F. Therefore, body temperatures should be measured in deeply comatosed patients. Hypotension may arise from the volume of blood (approximately 0.5 L) in the extracorporeal circuit. This can be corrected with fluid administration and/or pressor agents. Calcium and glucose should also be monitored since these may be affected. Observed falls in platelet counts are generally transient since hemoperfusion only requires a single use. Because observed falls in platelet counts are small, bleeding with central nervous system effects are uncommon.

While most hemoperfusions last between 4 and 6 hours, repetitive hemoperfusion may be required in paraquat poisoning, and for highly lipid soluble drugs such as glutethimide. Plasma paraquat levels must be maintained below a critical concentration of 0.1 μg/ml to prevent induction of pulmonary fibrosis; and with glutethimide redistribution of drug from the deep tissue compartment to the plasma compartment may cause relapse into coma unless repetitive hemoperfusion is instituted. Any active treatment method should be proven to have a greater efficiency in removing drugs than naturally occurring endogenous organ biotransformation or excretion. Hemodialysis and hemoperfusion enhance drug elimination rates for acetaminophen, amobarbital, ethchlorvynol, adriamycin, digoxin and digitoxin. It cannot be overemphasized that hemoperfusion or any dialytic technique may be followed by "rebound" in drug concentration, since drug redistribution from tissues into the plasma occurs following their removal from the plasma compartment. As pointed out above, this may return coma. Glutethimide poisoning commonly causes such happenings.

EXCHANGE BLOOD TRANSFUSION AND PLASMA EXCHANGE

Both techniques have been used in a small number of patients with poisonings. Plasma exchange (plasmapheresis) removes the patients plasma by centrifugal or filtration devices with subsequent replacement with fresh plasma or colloid. Exchange blood transfusions involve the removal of blood and its replacement with fresh whole blood. Plasma exchange involves 3–4 L exchange of plasma over approximately 4 hours. Therefore, the total maximal quantity of drug removed will be its plasma concentration multiplied by the volume of plasma removed. The technique is most applicable to highly protein bound drugs that are not well removed with hemodialysis (for example chromic acid and chromate). Exchange blood transfusion, especially in children, has been utilized particularly when hemolysis and methemoglobinemia complicate the poisoning, for example with sodium chlorate. Few reports of the effectiveness of plasmapheresis in various poisonings have been published.

IMMUNOPHARMACOLOGIC REVERSAL OF DRUG TOXICITY

Antibodies consist of two Fab fragments and one Fac fragment. The Fab fragments containing binding sites for antibodies and have a molecular weight around 50,000 daltons. By binding drugs to hapten, antibody responses can be mounted. The antibody fractions are subjected to splitting (papain) to obtain Fab fragments which injected combine with specific drug antigens with a high degree of specificity. This neutralizes drug toxicity. Potentially fatal cases of digoxin poisoning have been treated by this means with a high degree of successs. It is likely that in the future, drugs with a high toxicity ratio and poor removal with hemodialysis or hemoperfusion (tricyclic antidepressants) or drugs with delayed effects (paraquat) may be treated with immunopharmacological methods.

CLINICAL APPLICATIONS OF ACTIVE TREATMENT METHODS

As with any branch of clinical medicine, the over-riding tenet in treatment of poisoning should be "primum non nocere." Active treatment methods should only be used after due consideration of severity. Inappropriate use of analeptic agents (for example nikethimide) was shown in the early 60's to be associated with a higher mortality. Intensive supportive therapy alone, without the use of such central nervous system stimulation, was associated with a reduction in mortality in barbiturate poisoning. Similarly, hemodialysis and hemoperfusion should be considered only if the severity of poisoning merits such intervention. Consideration might also be paid to cost reductions brought about by hemoperfusion since rapid awakening from coma with barbiturates or nonbarbiturate hypnotics is likely to reduce hospitalization.

SELECTED READINGS

1. Colburn, WA. Specific antibodies and Fab fragments to alter the pharmacokinetics and reverse the pharmacologic/toxicologic effects of drugs. Drug Metab Rev 11:223–262, 1980
2. Haddad, LM, Winchester, JF eds, Clinical Management of Poisoning and Drug Overdose, WB Saunders Co., Philadelphia, 1983
3. Seyffart A, Poison Index. Fresenius Foundation, Bad Hamburg, West Germany, 1971
4. Vale JA, Meredith TJ, eds, Poisoning Diagnosis and Treatment, Update Books, London, 1981
5. Winchester, JF, Gelfand, MC, Knepshield, JH, Schreiner, GE, Dialysis and Hemoperfusion of Poisons and Drugs—Update Trans Am Soc Artif Intern Organs, 23:762–842, 1977.

INDEX

Page numbers in *italics* indicate a figure, "t" following a page number indicates a table.

Abdominal mass, in newborn, 83
Acid challenge, 13, 13t
Acid load procedure, short, 13, 13t
Acid-base regulation, in pregnancy, 71
Acidification of urine, assessment of, 13
Acute nephrotic syndrome. *See* Nephrotic syndrome, acute
Allografts, 147
Amino acid excretion, urinary, assessment of, 17
Amino acid solutions, in total parenteral nutrition prescription, 161, 161t
Ammonia, blood, assessment of, 17
Amyloidosis, 117
Analgesic nephropathy, 123, *124*
Anemia, in chronic renal failure, 49
Aneurysms, dissecting, 130
    fusiform, 130
    mixed, 130
    renal artery, 129
    sacular, 129–130
Angiography, renal, 29
    in renal cell carcinoma, 60, *60*
Anticoagulant therapy, in renal vein thrombosis, 131
Anti-glomerular basement membrane disease, 36
Anti-inflammatory agents, for immunosuppression, 152–153
Antimetabolites, for immunosuppression, 153
Anti-platelet therapy, in hemolytic uremic syndrome, 115
    in thrombotic thrombocytopenic purpura, 114
Anuria, in newborn, 78–83, 78t, 79t
Aorta, lesions of, kidney disease from, 129–130
Arteriography, renal, 29
Arteriosclerosis, hyaline, in diabetes mellitus, 116
Artery(ies), major, lesions of, kidney disease from, 129–130

renal, embolism and thrombus of, 130
Arthralgias, in Henoch-Schönlein nephritis, 110
Arthritis, in Henoch-Schönlein nephritis, 110
Artificial membranes, in acute renal failure, 45
Atherosclerosis, accelerated, in nephrotic syndrome, 56
Autograft, 147
Azotemia, in diabetes mellitus, 115–116
    "post-renal," 42–43
    "pre-renal," 42

Bacteriuria, detection of, 7–9
    in pregnancy, 71
Bedwetting. *See* Enuresis
Bence Jones proteins, test for, 4t
Bicarbonate titration, 13
Biopsy, renal, closed, 21, *21*
    complications of, 21
    contraindications to, 20–21
    indications for, 20
    in localization of kidney, 21–22
    in nephrotic syndrome, 57
    open, 21
    in pregnancy, 71
    in primary glomerulopathies, 98t
    specimens, handling of, 22
    techniques for, 21
    in tubulointerstitial disease, 127
Bladder exercises, in enuresis, 84
Bleeding tendencies, in chronic renal failure, 49
Blood, in urine, 4
Blood flow, renal, development of, 76
    measurement of, 11–12
Blood pressure, distribution, in newborn, *82*
Blood transfusion(s), in chronic renal failure, 49
    exchange, in poisoning, 174

Blood urea nitrogen, in acute renal failure, 43
  in pregnancy, 69, 70
Boiling test, 4t
Bone disease, uremic. See Osteodystrophy, renal

Calcium, excretion, urinary, test of, 16
  metabolism, in chronic renal failure, 50
Caloric intake, in total parenteral nutrition prescription,
    161–162
Carbohydrate intolerance, in chronic renal failure, 50
Carcinoma(s), of prostate, 62–63, 63
  renal cell, diagnosis of, 59–60, 60
    pathology of, 60
    symptoms of, 59
    treatment of, 60
  of renal pelvis, 62, 62
Cardiac failure, in end-stage renal disease, 136
Cardiac problems, in chronic renal failure, 49
Charcoal, "activated," in poisoning, 166–167
Child(ren), renal transplantation in, 156–158
    complications of, 157–158
    long-term outcome in, 158, 158t
Clot lysis therapy, in renal vein thrombosis, 131–132
Collagen vascular disease, 36
Complement assessments, in acute nephritic syndrome,
    37
Computed tomography, 28–29, 29
  in renal cell carcinoma, 60, 60
Computer-assisted functional data analysis, 30
Concentrating ability test, 14, 15t
Contrast medium, reactions to, 28t, 29
Cope needle, 21, 21
Corticosteroids, in Henoch-Schönlein nephritis, 111
  in lupus nephritis, 105
  in nephrotic syndrome, 57–58
  side effects of, 154
  in systemic vasculitis, 107–108
  in thrombotic thrombocytopenic purpura, 114
  in Wegener's granulomatosis, 109
Creatinine, serum, in pregnancy, 69, 70
Creatinine clearance tests(s), 10–11, 11t, 12
  in acute nephritic syndrome, 37
Cryoglobulinemia, 18, 118
Cyclophosphamide, in lupus nephritis, 106
  in systemic vasculitis, 108
  in Wegener's granulomatosis, 109
Cyclosporine, for immunosuppression, 153
Cystic disease of kidney, 63–66
  in newborn, 83
Cystic kidney, multiocular, 65–66
Cystinosis, in children, 156
Cysts, simple, 65
Cytotoxic agents, for immunosuppression, 153

DDAVP, in enuresis, 85
Dehydration and pitressin-stimulation procedure, 14, 15t
Desmopressin, in enuresis, 85
Diabetes mellitus, azotemic phase of, 116–117

glomerulosclerosis in, 115, 116
  pregnancy in, 72
  proteinuria in, 115
  renal pathology in, 116
  renal syndromes in, 115–116
  risk factors for, 116
  treatment of, 116–117
Dialysis, in acute renal failure, 44
  in chronic renal failure, 140–143
  complications associated with, 143, 144t
  peritoneal, long dwell, in end-stage renal disease, 141,
    142
  in poisoning, 168, 169–170t
  in renal failure, drug replacement following, 146
  responses to, in elderly, 141
  survival with, 143
  weekly clearance rates for forms of, 142
  in Wegener's granulomatosis, 109
Diarrhea therapy, in end-stage renal disease, 143
Diazoxide, in hypertension in pregnancy, 74
Diet(s), in chronic renal failure, 136–137
Dipstick examination, of urine, 3
Ditropan, in enuresis, 85
Diuresis, forced, in poisoning, 167–168
Diuretics, in acute renal failure, 44
  in nephrotic syndrome, 57
  in pregnancy, 74
  in renal perturbations in newborn, 81
Dopamine, in acute renal failure, 44
Drug(s), adjustments, in renal failure, 145, 145t
  antidotes, in poisoning, 167
  causing acute tubulointerstitial disease, 122–123, 122,
    122t
  causing chronic tubulointerstitial disease, 123–124
  levels, monitoring of, in renal failure, 145
  poisoning, immunopharmacologic reversal of, 174
  removal by dialysis, in poisoning, 168, 169–170t
  replacement of, 146
  usage, in renal failure, guidelines for, 144–146

Eclampsia, survival following, 72, 73
Edema, in newborn, 81
  in pregnancy, 71
  refractory, in nephrotic syndrome, 56
Electrolyte additives, in total parenteral nutrition
    prescription, 162–163, 162t
Electromicroscopy, of renal biopsy specimens, 22
Electrophoresis, hemoglobin, in nephrotic syndrome,
    56–57
Embolism, renal artery, 130
Encephalopathy, in chronic renal failure, 48
Endocrine alterations, in chronic renal failure, 50–51
End-stage renal disease, angioaccess in, 139–140
  chronic renal failure in, phase I, management of,
    134–135
    phase II, management of, 136–137
    phase III, management of, 140–143
  clinical management of, 133–146

management of, options for, *140*
  in three stages, 133–134, 134t
  rehabilitation following, 143
  substitution therapies in, selection of patients for,
    143–144
  treatment of, complications associated with, 143, 144t
    quality of life following, 143
Enuresis, assessment and evaluation in, 84
  associated findings in, 84
  etiology of, 84
  prevalence of, 83–84
  treatment of, 84
Enuresis alarms, 84–85
Enzyme studies, 17
Exercises, bladder, in enuresis, 84

Fabry's disease, 148
Fluid restriction, in acute renal failure, 44
Furosemide, in acute renal failure, 44
  in renal perturbations in newborn, 81

Gastric emptying, in poisoning, 166
Gastrointestinal tract, problems of, in chronic renal
    failure, 49
Geriatric nephrology, anatomy and, 86
  background of, 86
  clinical studies in, 88–89, 88t, 89t
  pathophysiology of, 88
  physiology of, 86–88, 87t
Glomerular diseases, primary, features of, 90
  morphologic classification of, 90–100
Glomerular filtration rate, development aspects of, 76
  effect of age on, 77t
  in end-stage renal disease, 135
  measurement of, 10–11, 11t, *12*
  in pregnancy, 69
Glomerulonephritis, acute, acute renal failure in, 42
  in pregnancy, 71
  chronic, 100
    management of, 100
    pregnancy in, 71–72
  crescentic, 35–36
  post-infectious, 38
  post-streptococcal, in nephritic syndrome, 35
  primary, in children, 156
  rapidly progressive, 35–36, 99
Glomerulopathy(ies), in malignancies, 118
  post-infectious, 119
  primary, 90
    classification of, 97t
    clinical diagnosis of, 92–96
    clinical syndromes associated with, 96–100
    morphologic classification of, 90–100 *92–93,
      94–95*
    renal biopsy in, 98t
    therapy of, 98t
  systemic, 102–120

Glomerulosclerosis, in diabetes mellitus, 115, 116
  focal, in children, 156
Glomerulus(i), endocapillary proliferative changes in, 91
  extracapillary proliferative changes in, 91
  membranoproliferative changes in, 91
  membranous changes in, 91
  minimal changes in, 90–91
  primary sclerosing changes in, 91
Glucose, in total parenteral nutrition prescription, 162
  in urine, 3
Glycosuria, in pregnancy, 69–70, *70*
Goodpasture's syndrome, 36
Graft(s), cadaveric donor, 147
  living donor, 147
Graft-versus-host disease, following immunosuppression,
    154–155
Granulomatosis, Wegener's. *See* Wegener's
    granulomatosis
Growth, in chronic renal failure, 50
Growth and development, post-transplant, in children,
    157–158

Heart failure, in end-stage renal disease, 136
Heart problems, in chronic renal failure, 49
Heavy metal screen, in nephrotic syndrome, 56
Hematuria, isolated, 96
  in newborn, 83
  and proteinuria, in Henoch-Schönlein nephritis, 110
Hemodialysis, in acute renal failure, 44–45
  angioaccess for, in end-stage renal disease, 139–140
  in diabetes mellitus, 117
  in poisoning, 168–171, 171t
    criteria for consideration of, 171–173
  semipermeable membranes for, in end-stage renal
    disease, 141
Hemofiltration, in end-stage renal disease, 142
Hemoglobin electrophoresis, in nephrotic syndrome,
    56–57
Hemolytic uremic syndrome. *See* Uremic syndrome,
    hemolytic
Hemoperfusion, sorbent, drugs removed with, 172t
  in end-stage renal disease, 142–143
  in poisoning, 168–171, 171t
    criteria for consideration of, 171–173
Hemoperfusion circuit, *170,* 171
Henoch-Schönlein nephritis, diagnosis of, 109
  pathology of, 111
  renal syndromes in, 110
  treatment of, 111
Histocompatibility complex, renal transplantation and,
    147–148
History taking, in chronic renal failure, 46
Hodgkin's disease, renal involvement in 118
Hydronephrosis, 66
  in newborn, 83
Hyperchloremic acidosis, in total parenteral nutrition, 163
Hyperfiltration, in diabetes mellitus, 115
Hyperglycemia, in total parenteral nutrition, 163

Hyperkalemia, in elderly, 88
Hypertension, chronic, with superimposed preeclampsia, 73
    in chronic renal failure, 48–49
    in end-stage renal disease, 143–145
    in nephrotic syndrome, 57
    in newborn, 81–83
    in pregnancy, 72–73, *72*
        treatment of, 74
    in scleroderma, treatment of, 112
    in systemic vasculitis, 107
    transient, in pregnancy, 73
Hypothermia, in chronic renal failure, 51
Hypovolemia, in nephrotic syndrome, 56

Imaging, in acute renal failure, 44
    techniques, in evaluation of kidneys, 23–33, *32*
Imipramine, in enuresis, 85
Immunofluorescence, of renal biopsy specimens, 22
Immunoglobulin deposits, in diabetes mellitus, 116
Immunological complications, in chronic renal failure, 50
Immunosuppression, 147
    complications of, 153–155, 154t
    drugs used for, 152–153, 152t
    post-transplant, in children, 157
    principles of, 151–152, 152t
    regimens, 153
    therapy, consequences of, 153–155, 154t
Immunosuppressive agents, in nephrotic syndrome, 58
Infants, *See* Newborns
Infection(s), causing acute tubulointerstitial disease, 123
    in end-stage renal disease, 135
    following immunosuppression, 154
    glomerulopathies following, 119
    in nephrotic syndrome, 56, 57
    post-transplant, in children, 157
    renal transplant failure in, 150
    in total parenteral nutrition, 163
Infectious complications, in chronic renal failure, 50
Interstitial nephritis, chronic, pregnancy in, 72
Isograft, 147

Ketone bodies, in urine, 3–4
Kidney(s), decreased size of, common causes of, 26t
    disease(s) of. *See* Renal disease(s)
    enlargement of, common causes of, 26t
    function of. *See* Renal function

Laboratory evaluation(s), in acute nephritic syndrome, 37, 37t
    in chronic renal failure, 46–47
    of renal patients, 1–19
    in tubulointerstitial diseases, 127
Lead inclusion bodies, in tubulointerstitial disease, 123, *124*
Light microscopy, of renal biopsy specimens, 22
Lupus erythematosus, systemic, 36, 38
    in children, 156

classification criteria for, 103t
diagnosis of, 102
immunological disturbances in, 102
pregnancy in, 72
renal pathology in, 103–104
renal syndromes in, 102–103
treatment of, indications for, 104–105, 105t
    options in, 105–106, 105t
Lupus nephritis. *See* Nephritis, lupus

Macroglobulinemia, 118
Magnesium excretion, urinary, test of, 16–17
Magnetic resonance imaging, nuclear, 33
Malignancies, glomerular lesions in, 118–119
Mannitol, in acute renal failure, 44
Medullary cystic diseases, 64–65
Medullary sponge kidney, 65
Metabolic diseases, inherited, in children, 156–157
Methyldopa, in hypertension in pregnancy, 74
Methylprednisolone, in lupus nephritis, 105–106
β_2-Microglobulin screening test, 17–18
Multicystic kidney, congenital unilateral, 65, *66*
Multiocular kidney, 65–66
Multiple myeloma, 117

Neoplasm(s), following immunosuppression, 154
Neoplastic diseases, glomerular lesions in, 118–119
Nephritic syndrome, acute, 99–100
    background of, 34, 35t
    differential diagnosis of, 35t
    etiologies of, 34, 35t
    features of, 34–35, 35t
    in Henoch-Schönlein nephritis, 110
    laboratory values in, 37, 37t
    pathology of, 38
    treatment of, 38–39, 38t
Nephritis, Henoch-Schölein. *See* Henoch-Schönlein nephritis
    lupus, renal biopsy features in, 104, 104t
        treatment of, indications for, 104–105, 105t
            options in, 105–106, 105t
        WHO classification of, 103–104, 103t
Nephroblastoma, diagnosis of, 61
    incidence of, 60
    pathology of, 61
    symptoms of, 60–61
    treatment of, 61–62
Nephrological laboratory values for adults, 16t
Nephrology, geriatric. *See* Geriatric nephrology
    pediatric, 76–85
    pregnancy-related, 69–75
Nephropathy, analgesic, 123, *124*
Nephrosclerosis, 129
Nephrotic syndrome, 96–99
    complications of, 55–56, 55
    definition of, 52
    in diabetes mellitus, 115
    differential diagnosis of, 52

etiology of, 52–53, 53t
evaluation in, 56–57, 56t
idiopathic, causes of, 53t
clinical features of, 53t
treatment of, 57–58
management of, 57
pathophysiology of, 52, 52
pregnancy in, 72
secondary, causes of, 54–55t
Nephrotomography, 24–25, 25
abnormalities of renal parenchyma on, 24, 27t
Neuropathy, peripheral, in chronic renal failure, 48
Newborns, abdominal mass in, 83
acidifying capacity of, 78
acute renal failure in, 79–81, 80t
anuria or oliguria in, 78–83, 78t, 79t
blood pressure distribution in, 82
edema in, 81
glomerular filtration rate in, 77t
hematuria in, 83
hypertension in, 81–83
renal excretion of Na⁺ in, 76–77
renal perturbations in, 78–83
renal water metabolism in, 78
Nitroprusside, in hypertension in pregnancy, 74
Nocturia, in pregnancy, 70–71
Nuclear magnetic resonance imaging, 33
Nuclide renal imaging, 30–33, 31
Nutrition, in chronic renal failure, 50
total parenteral. See Total parenteral nutrition

Oliguria, in acute nephritic syndrome, 35
in newborn, 78–83, 78t, 79t
Osteodystrophy, renal, in chronic renal failure, 50
clinical features of, 138–139, 139t
etiology of, 137
pathogenesis of, 138, 139t
Oxalosis, in children, 157–158
Oxybutynin, in enuresis, 85

Paraproteinemias, 117
Parathyroid hormone, production, in end-stage renal
disease, 138
secretion, in chronic renal failure, 50
Pediatric nephrology, 76–85
Pericarditis, in chronic renal failure, 49
Peritoneal dialysis, in acute renal failure, 44
in diabetes mellitus, 117
pH, serum, in elderly, 88
of urine, 3
Phosphate binders, in end-stage renal failure, 137–139
Phosphate infusion test, 14
Phosphate levels, in total parenteral nutrition, 163
Phosphorus, excretion, urinary, test of, 16–17
metabolism, in chronic renal failure, 50
Physical examination, in chronic renal failure, 46
in renal perturbations in newborn, 78
Plain films, 24

Plasma exchanges, in poisoning, 174
in Wegener's granulomatosis, 109
Plasma flow, renal, in pregnancy, 69
Plasma therapy, in thrombotic thrombocytopenic purpura,
114
Plasmaleukopheresis, following renal transplantation, 153
Plasmapheresis, in Henoch-Schönlein nephritis, 111
Poisoning, 165–174
active treatment of, clinical applications of, 174
definition of, 165
diagnosis of, 165
dialysis in, 168, 169–170t
drug, immunopharmacologic reversal of, 174
exchange blood transfusion in, 174
forced diuresis in, 167–168
hemodialysis in, 168–173, 171t, 173t
history of, 165
management of, general approach to, 165–171
mortality, 165
plasma exchange in, 174
sorbent hemoperfusion in, 168–173, 171t, 172t, 173t
Polycystic kidney disease, 64, 64
pregnancy in, 72
Polyuria, in pregnancy, 70–71
Potassium, excretion, in end-stage renal disease, 135
urinary, test of, 15–16
Prednisone, in lupus nephritis, 105
in systemic vasculitis, 107–108
in Wegener's granulomatosis, 109
Preeclampsia, 72–73, 73
in chronic hypertension, 73
Pregnancy, acid-base regulation in, 71
anatomical changes of, 69
bacteriuria in, 71
following renal transplantation, 72
hypertension in, 72–73, 72
treatment of, 74
nocturia in, 70–71
physiological changes of, 69–70
polyuria in, 70–71
proteinuria in, 71
-related nephrology, 69–75
renal disease in, 71–74
weight gain and edema in, 71
Prostate, carcinoma of, 62–63, 63
Protein(s), Bence Jones, test for, 4t
requirement, in total parenteral nutrition prescription,
161
restriction, in acute renal failure, 44
in chronic renal failure, 136–137
in urine, 3, 4t, 5t
Proteinuria, in acute nephritic syndrome, 35
causes of, 53t
in diabetes mellitus, 115
hematuria and, in Henoch-Schönlein nephritis, 110
isolated, 96
in pregnancy, 71
Pyelography, antegrade, 27–28

intravenous, in renal cell carcinoma, 59, *60*
  retrograde, 26–27, *28*
Pyelonephritis, chronic. *See* Tubulointerstitial diseases

Quadruple therapy, in Henoch-Schönlein nephritis, 111

Radionuclide renal function analysis, 30–33, *31*
Refractive index, 2–3, *3*
Refractometer, 2
Rejection, following transplantation, 147
  acute, 150
  chronic, 150
  diagnosis of, 151, 151t
  hyperacute, 150
  pathophysiology of, 150
  primary, 150
  treatment of, 151–155, 151t
Renal biopsy. *See* Biopsy, renal
Renal agenesis, bilateral, in newborn, 78–79
Renal concentrating and diluting assessment, 14
Renal disease(s), chronic, acute renal failure in, 42
  cystic, 63–66
  following renal transplantation, 151
  from arterial lesions, 129–130
  in pregnancy, 71–74
  recurring, following transplantation in children, 156
  urologic-related, 59–68
Renal failure, acute, causes of, 41t
    diagnosis of, 42–43
    differential diagnosis of, 42–43
    established, treatment of, 44–45
    incidence of, 40
    mortality associated with, 40–41, 45
    in newborn, 79–81, 80t
    pathogenesis of, 41–42
    in pregnancy, 71
  in acute nephritic syndrome, 38–39
  chronic, cardiovascular manifestations of, 48–49
    clinical manifestations of, 48–51
    definition of, 46
    diagnostic evaluation in, 46–48, 48t
    etiologies of, 47t
    hematological manifestations in, 49–51
    neurological manifestations of, 48
    phase I of, management of, 134–136
    phase II of, management of, 136–137
    phase III of management of, 140–143
    reversible problems in, 47t
    stages of, 46
    treatment of, 51
  total parenteral nutrition in. *See* Total parenteral
    nutrition
Renal function, age-related changes in, 86–87, 87t
  development aspects of, 76–78
  tests of, 9–17
Renal insufficiency, in pregnancy, 71
Renal pelvis, carcinoma of, 62, *62*

Renal transplantation, advantages of, 148
  in adults, 147–149
  allograft survival in, 148
  in children, 156
    complications of, 157–158
    long-term outcome in, 158, 158t
  complications of, 148, 150
  definition of, 147
  diseases recurring after, 148, 149t
  donor work-up for, 155, 155t
  donor-recipient matching in, 149, 149t
  failure of, differential diagnosis of, 150–151, 151t
  histocompatibility complex and, 147–148
  pregnancy following, 72
  recipient work-up for, 155–156, 156t
  rejection following. *See* Rejection, following
    transplantation success of, factors influencing,
    148–149

Sarcoidosis, tubulointerstitial disease in, 125
Scleroderma, 112
Sclerosis, systemic, 112
Serological tests, 18–19
Skin, in chronic renal failure, 49–50
Sodium excretion, urinary, test of, 15
Sodium ions, renal excretion of, in infants, 76–77
Sodium sulfate infusion test, 14
Sorbent hemoperfusion. *See* Hemoperfusion, sorbent
Sorbents, oral, in end-stage renal disease, 143
Sponge kidney, medullary, 64–65
Steroids. *See* Corticosteroids
Sulfosalicyclic acid test, 4t
Supra vide, nephritic syndrome in, 36

Thoracic duct drainage, following renal transplantation,
  153
"Three-glass text," 1–2, 2t
Thromboembolism, in nephrotic syndrome, 55–56, 57
Thrombosis, renal artery, following transplantation, 151
    in newborn, 82
  renal vein, clinical diagnosis of, 131
    etiology of, 130–131
    following transplantation, 151
    in newborn, 83
    pathology of, 131
    treatment of, 131
  in total parenteral nutrition, 163
Thrombotic thrombocytopenic purpura, diagnosis of, 113
  hemolytic anemia in, 112
  renal pathology in, 114
  renal syndromes in, 113–114
  treatment of, 114
Thrombus, renal artery, 130
Tofranil, in enuresis, 85
Total parenteral nutrition, clinical application of,
    160–161
  goals of, 159
  history of, 159, 160

nitrogen balance in, 159–160
prescription, 161–163
in renal failure, 159–164
general principles for use of, 160t
systemic complications of, 163
Toxins, endogenous and exogenous, causing chronic
tubulointerstitial disease, 123
uremic, 140–141, 141t
Transfusions, blood, in chronic renal failure, 49
exchange, in poisoning, 174
Transplantation, renal. *See* Renal transplantation
Tubular excretory maxima, assessment of, 12–13
Tubular necrosis, acute, renal transplant failure in, 150
Tubulointerstitial diseases, acute, disorders presenting as,
122–123
biopsy in, 127
causes of, 121
chronic, disorders presenting as, 123–125, 123t
clinical syndromes of, 125, 125t
diagnosis of, 126–127
drug-induced, 122–123, *122,* 122t
evaluation in suspected, 126t
and glomerular disease, differential diagnosis of, 126
infection-induced, 123
laboratory testing in, 127
pathogenesis of, 121
recognition of, 121
treatment of, 127
tubular defects in, 125
urinary abnormalities in, 125
Tubulointerstitial nephritis, acute, acute renal failure in,
42
Tumors, renal, 59–63
classification of, 61t
diagnosis of, 61
pathology of, 61
treatment of, 61–62
of renal pelvis, 59–63

Ultrasonography, 23, *24*
in renal cell carcinoma, 59–60
Urea nitrogen, serum, in pregnancy, 69, *70*
in renal failure, 43
Uremia, and end-stage renal therapies, complications
associated with 143, 144t
Uremic syndrome, hemolytic, 36–37, 38
in children, 156
diagnosis of, 113
hemolytic anemia in, 112
in oral contraceptive use, 113
postpartum, 113
renal pathology in, 114
renal syndromes in, 114
treatment of, 114–115

Uric acid excretion, urinary, assessment of, 17
Urinalysis, in acute nephritic syndrome, 37
in acute renal failure, 43
in chronic renal failure, 46
collection and handling of sample in, 1–6
Urinary abnormalities, isolated, syndrome of, 96
(Urinary Arterial)pCO$_2$ test, 13–14
Urine, acidification of, assessment of, 13
blood in, 4
casts in, 6, *8–9*
color and transparency of, 2
concentration of, age-related decrease in, 87
dipstick examination of, 3
examination of, routine, 1–6
glucose in, 3
ketone bodies in, 3–4
microscopic examination of, 4–6, 6t, *6–7, 8–9*
pH of, 3
proteins in, 3, 4t, 5t
sediment, elements in, 6, *6–7*
specific gravity of, 2–3, *3*
volume of, 2
Urography, direct opacification, 26–28
excretory, 25–26
Urologic-related renal diseases, 59–68

Vascular diseases, renal, 129–132
Vasculitis, systemic, clinical course of, 107
diagnosis of, 106–107
diversity of symptoms in, 106
renal pathology in, 107
renal syndromes in, 107
treatment of, 107–108
indications for, 107
Veins, renal, thrombosis of. *See* Thrombosis, renal vein
Venography, renal, in nephrotic syndrome, 57
Vesicoureteral reflux, 66–67
classification of, 67t
grades of reflux in, *67*
Vim-Silverman needle, Franklin modification of, 21, *21*
Vitamin D, deficiency of, 137–138
Vitamin D analogues, in end-stage renal failure, 137–139

Water deprivation test, 14–15
Water metabolism, renal, in newborns, 78
Wegener's granulomatosis, clinical features of, 108
mortality in, 109
renal syndromes in, 108–109
treatment of, 109
indications for, 109
Wilms' tumor. *See* Nephroblastoma

Xenograft, 147
X-ray examination, renal, 24–28